Math for Meds
DOSAGE AND SOLUTIONS

Math for Meds

DOSAGES AND SOLUTIONS

8th edition

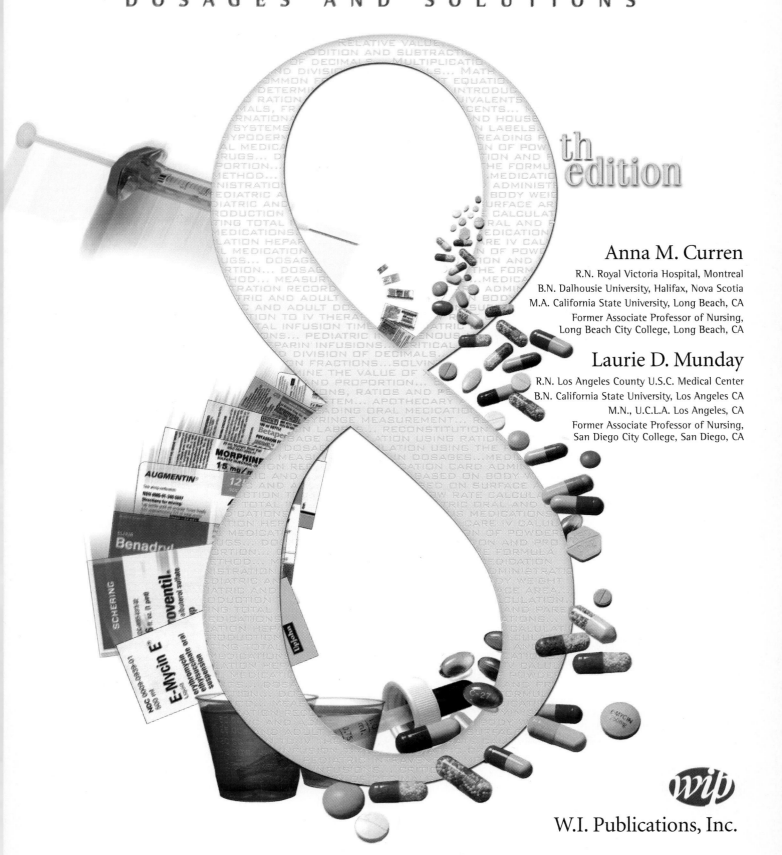

Anna M. Curren

R.N. Royal Victoria Hospital, Montreal
B.N. Dalhousie University, Halifax, Nova Scotia
M.A. California State University, Long Beach, CA
Former Associate Professor of Nursing,
Long Beach City College, Long Beach, CA

Laurie D. Munday

R.N. Los Angeles County U.S.C. Medical Center
B.N. California State University, Los Angeles CA
M.N., U.C.L.A. Los Angeles, CA
Former Associate Professor of Nursing,
San Diego City College, San Diego, CA

wip

W.I. Publications, Inc.

ACKNOWLEDGMENTS.

Our thanks once again to those pharmaceutical companies who were generous in their provision of drug labels for use in the text: Abbott, American Cyanamid, Ascot, Astra USA, Ayerst, Beecham, Berlex, Bristol/Apothecon, Bristol Meyers Squibb, Burroughs Wellcome, Cetus Oncology, Ciba-Geighy, Dupont, Eli Lilly/Dista, Elkins-Sinn, Geneva, Glaxo, Hoechst-Roussel, Invenex, Lederle, Lypho Med, Marion Merrill Dow, McNeil, Mead Johnson, Merck, Miles, Nova-Nordisk, Parke Davis/Warner-Lambert, Pharmacia, Pfizer/Roerig/Pratt, A.H. Robins, Roxane, Searle, Schering, SmithKline Beecham, E.R. Squibb/Squibb-Marsham, Travenol, Upjohn, Whitby, and Wyeth-Ayerst.

We thank the following companies and health centers for permission to reproduce product photos and medication administration records: Retractable Technologies, Inc.; Becton Dickinson and Company; Sherwood-Davis & Geck; B.Braun-MacGaw, Inc.; Ivac Corporation; Abbott Laboratories; Lionville Systems, Inc.; University Hospital, San Diego, CA.; The University Health Network, Toronto, ONT.; Scripps Memorial Hospital, La Jolla, CA; and Veterans Administration Hospital, Long Beach, CA.

Our special thanks to Rae Richard, RN, ANP-C, MSN, CRNI, of Scripps Hospital, La Jolla, CA., for her excellent review of and suggestions on IV therapy and IV medication content.

Our final thank you goes to the hundreds of educators continent wide who wrote and phoned with suggestions. As always, their input was indispensable.

BOOK AND COVER DESIGN
Peter T. Noble Associates, Encinitas, CA

PHOTOGRAPHY
Kim Brun Photography
Starkman Photography, San Diego, CA

COMPOSITION AND PAGE MAKEUP
Janice Thompson Graphics, San Diego, CA

ELECTRONIC PREPRESS, PRINTING AND BINDING
Banta Book Group

PUBLISHER'S NOTICE.

The authors have designed this text to assist allied health students to develop professional competence. The authors have taken every reasonable precaution to ensure that the instructional content contained in the text is current and accurate. However, the authors and publisher specifically make no implied or expressed warranties, representations or guarantees of any kind with respect to or responsibility for, any material included in the text. The authors and publisher shall not be liable for any special, consequential or exemplary damages resulting in whole or in part, from the readers use of, or reliance upon, this material.

All instructional information, including but not limited to examples, illustrations, and equations are offered here for the limited purposes of illustrating and explaining general techniques. Still, the facts and circumstances of every case inevitably require variations and unique medical knowledge.

The determination of amounts and proportions and the administration of prescription drugs is the rendering of medical services and no text can assume that responsibility. The responsibility ultimately rests with the individual medical practitioner.

Printed in the United States of America

10 9 8 7 6 5 4 3

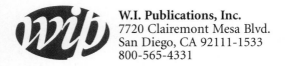

W.I. Publications, Inc.
7720 Clairemont Mesa Blvd.
San Diego, CA 92111-1533
800-565-4331

Preface

The updating of a text requires taking into account a number of factors: educator evaluations/requests, current clinical practice as observed by the authors on hospital visits, the input of experts in specific clinical areas, and, finally, author choice.

In making content decisions we begin by identifying student competency outcomes, and these become our guidelines for all changes. What exactly does the student need to know to meet identified objectives? How can this content be structured to make learning easy, enjoyable and lasting? At what point does "too much" instruction serve only to confuse? Given that different programs/instructors have different requirements, how do we structure content to please the majority? The last is an essential consideration if the text is to continue to be successful.

Philosophically we feel that content should be kept as simple as possible. We believe that our most important task is to give the student sound basics, and a sense of accomplishment to overcome the natural fear of such a major responsibility as clinical calculations. There is no point teaching to an "ideal" which is unrealistic, yet as educators we fall readily into the trap of trying to teach "everything".

On the subject of calculations we come immediately upon a point of contention: the use of calculators. Advanced clinical calculations are routinely done with calculators in the clinical setting. Indeed, it would be foolhardy not to use them, both from a time and accuracy standpoint. Yet students are barred from using calculators in licensing examinations. Should this policy not be reevaluated in the light of realistic clinical practice? As authors the calculator dichotomy has plagued us for years. So, we continue to teach the basic math required for simple calculations, most of which can be done mentally, and which we feel each practitioner should be competent to do. It is these skills which *Math For Meds* addresses first and forcefully in it's content. It is also the reason the use of ratio and proportion is not discussed until mid text, where more complicated calculations are introduced, and where it rightfully belongs.

All calculations in this text were checked with a calculator. If one is not used by students, or their calculator setting varies, an occasional discrepancy at the hundredth or tenth may be experienced, and should be considered correct. This is clearly explained in "Directions To The Student" on page vii, but may need to be reinforced as instruction progresses.

Once again we wish to express our thanks to the hundreds of educators who completed and returned an evaluation of the previous edition of *Math for Meds*. We are very pleased with our landmark 8th edition, and trust you will be too.

Anna M. Curren
Laurie D. Munday

San Diego, CA. November 1999

Directions to the Student

Welcome, to what we anticipate will be one of the most enjoyable texts you have ever used. *Math For Meds* is about to reassure you that math is nothing to be afraid of; that even the most difficult clinical calculations you encounter will present no problem for you; and that, on completion of your instruction, you will have the calculation skills you need to practice safely in your profession. You don't have to be a math expert to use this text. All that is required is average ability and a desire to learn. If you have not used your math skills for a number of years you will still have no difficulty, because the refresher math section will quickly bring you up to date. *Math For Meds* lets you move at your own pace through the content, which ranges from easy to thought provoking. Hundreds of examples and problems will keep your learning on track. You will enjoy learning from *Math For Meds*, and here are the tips you need to get started.

1. Gather a pencil or pen and plenty of scratch paper.

2. Record the answers to calculations in your text as well as on the scratch paper. It makes checking your answers against those we provide much easier.

3. As you work your way through the programs do exactly as you are instructed to do, and no more. Programmed learning proceeds in small steps, and jumping ahead may cause confusion. All chapters are designed to let you move at your own speed. If you already know some of the basics you will move through them more quickly than you can imagine.

4. The refresher math section must be completed without a calculator. **However, be aware that the multiple steps of ratio and proportion calculations will result in a variety of answers to some problems. Small differences should be considered negligible, and answers correct.** If your instructor allows the use of a calculator for advanced calculations set it, if possible, to round to hundredths. All calculations in the text were checked on a calculator at the hundredth setting. If you use a calculator that does not have optional settings, you may experience answers which vary at the hundredth, or tenth. This difference may be considered negligible, and your answers correct.

5. Once you have completed your instruction we suggest you keep *Math For Meds* in your personal library. As you move to different clinical areas during your career you will encounter different types of calculations. A quick refresher with *Math For Meds* will be invaluable when that occurs.

REFRESHER MATH PRE-TEST

If you can complete the following pre-test with 100% accuracy you may wish to bypass the Refresher Math section of this text, as all the pertinent math concepts are covered in the test items included. You should be aware, however, that this section offers many memory cues and short cuts for solving clinical calculations without a calculator.

Identify the decimal fraction with the highest value in each of the following.

1.   a) 4.4   b) 2.85   c) 5.3   _____
2.   a) 6.3   b) 5.73   c) 4.4   _____
3.   a) 0.18   b) 0.62   c) 0.35   _____
4.   a) 0.2   b) 0.125   c) 0.3   _____
5.   a) 0.15   b) 0.11   c) 0.14   _____
6.   a) 4.27   b) 4.31   c) 4.09   _____

Add the following decimals.

7. $0.2 + 2.23$ = _____
8. $1.5 + 0.07$ = _____
9. $6.45 + 12.1 + 9.54$ = _____
10. $0.35 + 8.37 + 5.15$ = _____

Subtract the following decimals.

11. $3.1 - 0.67 =$ _____
12. $12.41 - 2.11 =$ _____
13. $2.235 - 0.094 =$ _____
14. $4.65 - 0.7 =$ _____

15. If tablets with a strength of 0.2 mg are available and 0.6 mg is ordered you must give how many tablets? _____

16. If tablets are labeled 0.8 mg and 0.4 mg is ordered how many tablets must you give? _____

17. If the available tablets have a strength of 1.25 mg and 2.5 mg is ordered how many tablets must you give? _____

18. If 0.125 mg is ordered and the tablets available are labeled 0.25 mg how many must you give? _____

Express the following numbers to the nearest tenth.

19.   2.17 = _____
20.   0.15 = _____
21.   3.77 = _____
22.   4.62 = _____
23.   11.74 = _____
24.   5.26 = _____

Express the following to the nearest hundredth.

25.   1.357 = _____
26.   7.413 = _____
27.   10.105 = _____
28.   3.775 = _____
29.   0.176 = _____

30. Define "product."

_____

_____

Multiply the following decimals. Express answers to the nearest tenth.

31. $0.7 \times 1.2 =$ _____
32. $1.8 \times 2.6 =$ _____
33. $5.1 \times 0.25 \times 1.1 =$ _____
34. $3.3 \times 3.75 =$ _____

Divide the following fractions. Express answers to the nearest hundredth.

35. $16.3 \div 3.2 =$ _____
36. $15.1 \div 1.1 =$ _____
37. $2 \div 0.75 =$ _____
38. $4.17 \div 2.7 =$ _____

39. Define "numerator."

_____

_____

40. Define "denominator."

_____

_____

41. Define "highest common denominator."

_____

_____

Solve the following equations. Express answers to the nearest tenth.

42. $\frac{1}{4} \times \frac{2}{3} =$ _____

43. $\frac{240}{170} \times \frac{135}{300} =$ _____

44. $\frac{0.2}{1.75} \times \frac{1.5}{0.2} =$ _____

45. $\frac{2.1}{3.6} \times \frac{1.7}{1.3} =$ _____

46. $\frac{0.26}{0.2} \times \frac{3.3}{1.2} =$ _____

47. $\frac{750}{1} \times \frac{300}{50} \times \frac{7}{2} =$ _____

48. $\frac{50}{1} \times \frac{60}{240} \times \frac{1}{900} \times \frac{400}{1} =$ _____

49. $\frac{35,000}{750} \times \frac{35}{1} =$ _____

50. $\frac{50}{2} \times \frac{450}{40} \times \frac{1}{900} \times \frac{114}{1} =$ _____

ANSWERS: 1. c 2. a 3. b 4. c 5. a 6. b 7. 2.43 8. 1.57 9. 28.09 10. 13.87 11. 2.43 12. 10.3 13. 2.141 14. 3.95 15. 3 tab 16. 1/2 tab 17. 2 tab 18. 1/2 tab 19. 2.2 20. 0.2 21. 3.8 22. 4.6 23. 11.7 24. 5.3 25. 1.36 26. 7.41 27. 10.11 28. 3.78 29. 0.18 30. the answer obtained from the multiplication of two or more numbers 31. 0.8 32. 4.7 33. 1.4 34. 12.4 35. 5.09 36. 13.73 37. 2.67 38. 1.54 39. the top number in a common fraction 40. the bottom number in a common fraction 41. the highest number which can be divided into two numbers to reduce them to their lowest terms (values) 42. 0.2 43. 0.6 44. 0.9 45. 0.8 46. 3.6 47. 15,750 48. 5.6 49. 1633.3 50. 35.6

Contents

SECTION ONE

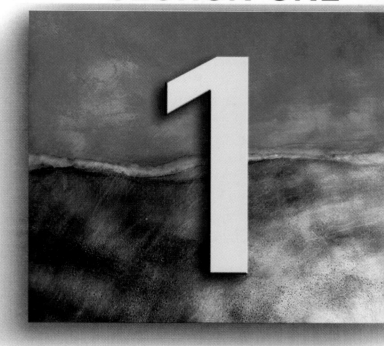

Refresher Math

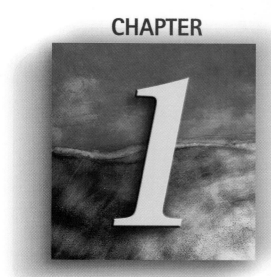

Relative Value, Addition and Subtraction of Decimals

1 n the course of administering medications you will be calculating drug dosages which contain decimals, for example 2.5 mg. The first two chapters of this text will provide a complete and easy refresher of everything that you must know about decimals. Let's begin with a review of the relative value of decimals, so that you will be able to recognize which of two or more numbers has the highest (and lowest) value.

OBJECTIVES
The student will
1. identify the relative value of decimals
2. add decimals
3. subtract decimals

PREREQUISITE
Recognize the abbreviation mg, for milligram, as a drug measure.

Relative Value of Decimals

The easiest way to begin a review of decimal numbers is to visualize them on a scale which has a decimal point at its center. Look for a moment at Figure 1.

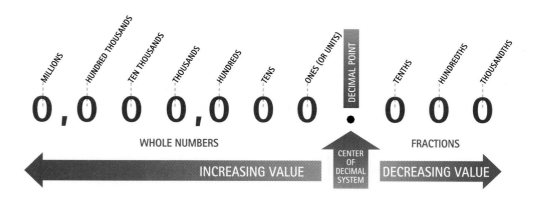

Figure 1

Notice that on the left of the decimal point are the whole numbers, and on the right the fractions. On the whole number (left) side of the scale, the measures rise increasingly in value, from ones, to tens, to hundreds, and so on to millions, which is the highest measure you will see in drug dosages. Our monetary system of dollars and cents is a decimal system, and the relative value of the whole numbers is exactly as you now know and use them: the higher the number, the higher the value.

The first key point in determining relative value of decimals is the presence of whole numbers. The higher the whole number, the higher the value.

EXAMPLE 1   10.1 is higher than 9.1

EXAMPLE 2   3.2 is higher than 2.9

EXAMPLE 3   7.01 is higher than 6.99

PROBLEM

Identify the number with the highest value in each of the following.

1.	a)	3.5	b)	2.7	c)	4.2	_____
2.	a)	6.15	b)	5.95	c)	4.54	_____
3.	a)	12.02	b)	10.19	c)	11.04	_____
4.	a)	2.5	b)	1.75	c)	0.75	_____
5.	a)	4.3	b)	2.75	c)	5.1	_____
6.	a)	6.15	b)	7.4	c)	6.95	_____

ANSWERS 1.c 2.a 3.a 4.a 5.c 6.b

If, however, the whole numbers are the same, for example **10.**2 and **10.**7, or there are no whole numbers, for example **0.**25 and **0.**35, then the fraction will determine the relative value. Let's take a closer look at the fractional side of the scale (refer to Figure 2).

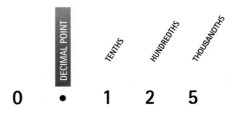

Figure 2

It is necessary to consider only three figures after the decimal point on the fractional side because drug dosages measured as decimal fractions do not contain more than three digits, for example 0.125 mg. First notice that a zero is used to replace the whole number in this decimal fraction.

If a decimal fraction is not preceded by a whole number, a zero is used in front of the decimal point to emphasize that the number is a fraction.

EXAMPLE   0.125   0.1   0.45

Look once again at Figure 2. The numbers on the right of the decimal point represent tenths, hundredths, and thousandths, in that order. When you see a decimal fraction in which the whole numbers are the same, or there are no whole numbers, stop and look closely at the number representing the **tenths**.

 The fraction with the highest number representing tenths has the higher value.

| EXAMPLE 1 | 0.3 is higher than 0.2 |

| EXAMPLE 2 | 0.41 is higher than 0.29 |

| EXAMPLE 3 | 1.21 is higher than 1.19 |

PROBLEM

Which of the following decimals has the highest value?

1. a) 0.4   b) 0.2   c) 0.5   _____
2. a) 2.73   b) 2.61   c) 2.87   _____
3. a) 0.19   b) 0.61   c) 0.34   _____
4. a) 3.5   b) 3.75   c) 3.25   _____
5. a) 0.3   b) 0.25   c) 0.4   _____
6. a) 1.35   b) 1.29   c) 1.4   _____

ANSWERS 1. c 2. c 3. b 4. b 5. c 6. c

If in decimal fractions the numbers representing the **tenths** are identical, for example, 0.25 and 0.27, then **the number representing the hundredths will determine the relative value.**

 The decimal fraction with the higher number representing hundredths will have the higher value when the tenths are identical.

| EXAMPLE 1 | 0.27 is higher than 0.25 |

| EXAMPLE 2 | 0.15 is higher than 0.1 (0.1 is the same as 0.10) |

Extra zeros on the end of decimal fractions are omitted because they can cause confusion, although they do not alter the value of the fraction (0.10 is the same as 0.1).

| EXAMPLE 3 | 2.25 is higher than 2.2 (same as 2.20) |

| EXAMPLE 4 | 9.77 is higher than 9.75 |

PROBLEM

Which of the following decimals has the highest value?

1.	a) 0.12	b) 0.15	c) 0.17	_____
2.	a) 1.21	b) 1.24	c) 1.23	_____
3.	a) 0.37	b) 0.32	c) 0.36	_____
4.	a) 3.27	b) 3.25	c) 3.21	_____
5.	a) 0.16	b) 0.11	c) 0.19	_____
6.	a) 4.23	b) 4.2	c) 4.09	_____

ANSWERS 1. c 2. b 3. a 4. a 5. c 6. a

PROBLEM

Which decimal fraction has the higher value?

a) 0.125 b) 0.25

ANSWERS The correct answer is b) 0.25. The decimal fraction which has the higher number representing the **tenths** has the higher value. 2 is higher than 1; therefore 0.25 has a higher value than 0.125. Medication errors have been made in this **identical** decimal fraction; so remember it well.

 The number of figures on the right of the decimal point is not an indication of relative value. Always look at the figure representing the tenths first, and if these are identical, the hundredths, to determine which is higher.

This completes your introduction to the relative value of decimals. The key points just reviewed will cover all situations in dosage calculations where you will have to recognize high and low values. Therefore, you are now ready to test yourself more extensively on this information.

PROBLEM

Identify the decimal with the highest value in each of the following.

1.	a) 0.25	b) 0.5	c) 0.125	_____
2.	a) 0.4	b) 0.45	c) 0.5	_____
3.	a) 7.5	b) 6.25	c) 4.75	_____
4.	a) 0.3	b) 0.25	c) 0.35	_____
5.	a) 1.125	b) 1.75	c) 1.5	_____
6.	a) 4.5	b) 4.75	c) 4.25	_____
7.	a) 0.1	b) 0.01	c) 0.04	_____
8.	a) 5.75	b) 6.25	c) 6.5	_____
9.	a) 0.6	b) 0.16	c) 0.06	_____
10.	a) 3.55	b) 2.95	c) 3.7	_____

ANSWERS 1. b 2. c 3. a 4. c 5. b 6. b 7. a 8. c 9. a 10. c

Addition and Subtraction of Decimals

There are several key points which will make addition and subtraction of decimal fractions easier and safer. Let's look at these.

 When you first write the numbers down, line up the decimal points.

EXAMPLE   To add 0.25 and 0.27

0.25   0.25
0.27 is safe   0.27 may be unsafe; it could lead to errors.

 Always add or subtract from right to left.

If you found it necessary to write the numbers down, don't confuse yourself by trying to "eyeball" the answer. Also, write any numbers carried or rewrite those reduced by borrowing, if you find this helpful.

EXAMPLE 1   When adding 0.25 and 0.27

```
  1
0.25
0.27    add the 5 and 7 first, then the 2, 2, and
0.52    the 1 you carried. Right to left.
```

EXAMPLE 2   When subtracting 0.63 from 0.71

```
  6 1
0.71    borrow 1 from 7 and rewrite as 6,
0.63    write the borrowed 1. Subtract 3 from 11.
0.08    Subtract 6 from 6. Work from right to left.
```

 Add zeros as necessary to make the fractions of equal length.

This does not alter the value of the fractions and it helps prevent confusion and mistakes.

EXAMPLE   When subtracting 0.125 from 0.25

0.25   becomes   0.250
0.125   0.125   Answer = **0.125**

If you follow these simple rules and make them a habit, you will automatically reduce calculation errors. The problems on the following page will give you an excellent opportunity to practice them.

PROBLEM

Add the following decimals.

1.	0.25 + 0.5	= _____	6.	3.7 + 1.05 + 2.2	= _____
2.	0.1 + 2.25	= _____	7.	6.42 + 13.3 + 9.55	= _____
3.	1.7 + 0.75	= _____	8.	5.57 + 4.03 + 13.02	= _____
4.	1.4 + 0.02	= _____	9.	0.33 + 8.41 + 6.09	= _____
5.	2.3 + 1.45	= _____	10.	7.44 + 3.04 + 11.31	= _____

Subtract the following decimals.

11.	1.25 - 1.125	= _____	16.	7.33 - 4.04	= _____
12.	3.2 - 0.65	= _____	17.	12.45 - 2.07	= _____
13.	2.3 - 1.45	= _____	18.	0.07 - 0.035	= _____
14.	0.02 - 0.01	= _____	19.	1.175 - 0.23	= _____
15.	5 - 2.5	= _____	20.	5.75 - 0.95	= _____

ANSWERS 1. 0.75 2. 2.35 3. 2.45 4. 1.42 5. 3.75 6. 6.95 7. 29.27 8. 22.62 9. 14.83 10. 21.79
11. 0.125 12. 2.55 13. 0.85 14. 0.01 15. 2.5 16. 3.29 17. 10.38 18. 0.035 19. 0.945 20. 4.8

Summary

This concludes the refresher on relative value, addition and subtraction of decimals. The important points to remember from this chapter are:

➡ if the decimal fraction contains a whole number, the value of the whole number is the first determiner of relative value

➡ if the fraction does not include a whole number, a zero is placed in front of the decimal point to emphasize it

➡ the number representing the tenths in a decimal fraction is the first determiner of relative value

➡ if the tenths in decimal fractions are identical, the number representing hundredths will determine relative value

➡ when adding or subtracting decimal fractions, first line up the decimal points, then add or subtract from right to left

Summary Self Test

DIRECTIONS

Choose the decimal with the highest value from each of the following.

1.	a)	2.45	b)	2.57	c)	2.19	_____
2.	a)	3.07	b)	3.17	c)	3.71	_____
3.	a)	0.12	b)	0.02	c)	0.01	_____
4.	a)	5.31	b)	5.35	c)	6.01	_____
5.	a)	4.5	b)	4.51	c)	4.15	_____
6.	a)	0.015	b)	0.15	c)	0.1	_____
7.	a)	1.3	b)	1.25	c)	1.35	_____

8. a) 0.1   b) 0.2   c) 0.25   _____

9. a) 0.125   b) 0.1   c) 0.05   _____

10. a) 13.7   b) 13.5   c) 13.25   _____

11. If you have medication tablets whose strength is 0.1 mg, and you must give 0.3 mg, you will need

     a) 1 tablet   b) less than 1 tablet   c) more than 1 tablet   _____

12. If you have tablets with a strength of 0.25 mg and you must give 0.125 mg, you will need

     a) 1 tablet   b) less than 1 tablet   c) more than 1 tablet   _____

13. If you have an order to give a dosage of 7.5 mg and the tablets have a strength of 3.75 mg, you will need

     a) 1 tablet   b) less than 1 tablet   c) more than 1 tablet   _____

14. If the order is to give 0.5 mg and the tablet strength is 0.5 mg you will give

     a) 1 tablet   b) less than 1 tablet   c) more than 1 tablet   _____

15. The order is to give 0.5 mg and the tablets have a strength of 0.25 mg. You must give

     a) 1 tablet   b) less than 1 tablet   c) more than 1 tablet   _____

DIRECTIONS

Add the following decimals.

16. $1.31 + 0.4$ = _____
17. $0.15 + 0.25$ = _____
18. $2.5 + 0.75$ = _____
19. $3.2 + 2.17$ = _____

20. $1.3 + 1.04 + 0.7$ = _____
21. $4.1 + 3.03 + 0.4$ = _____
22. $0.5 + 0.5 + 0.5$ = _____
23. $5.4 + 2.6 + 0.09$ = _____

24. You have just given 2 tablets with a dosage strength of 3.5 mg each. What was the total dosage administered?   _____

25. You are to give your patient one tablet labeled 0.5 mg and one labeled 0.25 mg. What is the total dosage of these two tablets?   _____

26. If you give two tablets labeled 0.02 mg what total dosage will you administer?   _____

27. You are to give one tablet labeled 0.8 mg and two tablets labeled 0.4 mg. What is the total dosage?   _____

28. You have two tablets, one is labeled 0.15 mg and the other 0.3 mg. What is the total dosage of these two tablets?   _____

DIRECTIONS

Subtract the following decimals.

29. $4.32 - 3.1$ = _____
30. $2.1 - 1.91$ = _____
31. $3.7 - 1.93$ = _____
32. $5.75 - 4.02$ = _____

33. $1.3 - 0.02$ = _____
34. $0.2 - 0.07$ = _____
35. $3.95 - 0.35$ = _____
36. $1.9 - 0.08$ = _____

37. Your patient is to receive a dosage of 7.5 mg and you have only one tablet labeled 3.75 mg. How many more milligrams must you give? _____

38. You have a tablet labeled 0.02 mg and your patient is to receive 0.06 mg. How many more milligrams do you need? _____

39. The tablet available is labeled 0.5 mg but you must give a dosage of 1.5 mg. How many more milligrams will you need to obtain the correct dosage? _____

40. Your patient is to receive a dosage of 1.2 mg and you have one tablet labeled 0.6 mg. What additional dosage in milligrams will you need? _____

41. You must give your patient a dosage of 2.2 mg but have only two tablets labeled 0.55 mg. What additional dosage in milligrams will you need? _____

DIRECTIONS

Determine how many tablets will be needed to give the following dosages.

42. Tablets are labeled 0.01 mg. You must give 0.02 mg. _____

43. Tablets are labeled 2.5 mg. You must give 5 mg. _____

44. Tablets are labeled 0.25 mg. Give 0.125 mg. _____

45. Tablets are 0.5 mg. Give 1.5 mg. _____

46. A dosage of 1.8 mg is ordered. Tablets are 0.6 mg. _____

47. Tablets available are 0.04 mg. You are to give 0.02 mg. _____

48. The dosage ordered is 3.5 mg. The tablets available are 1.75 mg. _____

49. Prepare a dosage of 3.2 mg using tablets with a strength of 1.6 mg. _____

50. You have tablets labeled 0.25 mg, and a dosage of 0.375 mg is ordered. _____

ANSWERS 1.b 2.c 3.a 4.c 5.b 6.b 7.c 8.c 9.a 10.a 11.c 12.b 13.c 14.a 15.c
16.1.71 17.0.4 18.3.25 19.5.37 20.3.04 21.7.53 22.1.5 23.8.09 24.7 mg 25.0.75 mg
26.0.04 mg 27.1.6 mg 28.0.45 mg 29.1.22 30.0.19 31.1.77 32.1.73 33.1.28 34.0.13 35.3.6
36.1.82 37.3.75 mg 38.0.04 mg 39.1 mg 40.0.6 mg 41.1.1 mg 42.2 tab 43.2 tab 44.1/2 tab
45.3 tab 46.3 tab 47.1/2 tab 48.2 tab 49.2 tab 50.1 1/2 tab

Multiplication and Division of Decimals

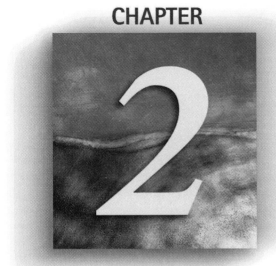

CHAPTER

Multiplication and division of decimals is a routine part of calculating drug dosages. Many clinical calculations are simple enough to do without a calculator, but there are instances where using one will save time, and be more accurate. For the purpose of understanding and review however, your instructor may wish you to do the following exercises without one. Let's begin with multiplication.

OBJECTIVES

The student will
1. define product, numerator and denominator
2. multiply decimal fractions
3. reduce fractions using common denominators
4. divide fractions and express answers to the nearest tenth, and hundredth

Multiplication of Decimals

The main precaution in multiplication of decimals is the **placement of the decimal point in the answer** (which is called the **product**).

EXAMPLE 1 0.35×0.5

Begin by lining the numbers up on the right, since this is somewhat safer; then disregard the decimals during the actual multiplication.

$$\begin{array}{r} 0.35 \\ \underline{0.5} \\ 175 \end{array}$$ Answer = **0.175**

0.35 has two numbers after the decimal, 0.5 has one. Place the decimal point three places to the left in the product. Place a zero (0) in front of the decimal to emphasize it.

 The decimal point in the product of decimal fractions is placed the same number of places to the left as the total of numbers after the decimal point in the fractions multiplied.

EXAMPLE 2
$$\begin{array}{r} 1.4 \\ \underline{0.25} \\ 70 \\ \underline{28} \\ 350 \end{array}$$ Answer = **0.35**

1.4 has one number after the decimal, 0.25 has two. Place the decimal point three places to the left in the product, and add a zero in front (0.350). Once the decimal is correctly placed the excess zero is dropped from the end of the fraction, and 0.350 becomes 0.35

If the product contains insufficient numbers for correct placement of the decimal point, add as many zeros as necessary to the left of the product to correct this.

EXAMPLE 3

$$\begin{array}{r} 0.21 \\ \underline{0.32} \\ 42 \\ \underline{63} \\ 672 \end{array}$$ Answer = **0.0672**

In this example 0.21 has two numbers after the decimal, and 0.32 also has two. However, there are only three numbers in the product, so a zero must be added to the left of these numbers to place the decimal point correctly: 672 becomes 0.0672

EXAMPLE 4

$$\begin{array}{r} 0.12 \\ \underline{0.2} \\ 24 \end{array}$$ Answer = **0.024**

There are a total of three numbers after the decimal points in 0.12 and 0.2. One zero must be added in the product to place the decimal point correctly: 24 becomes 0.024

PROBLEM

Multiply the following decimal fractions.

1. 0.45×0.2 = _____
2. 1.3×0.15 = _____
3. 3.5×1.2 = _____
4. 2.2×1.1 = _____
5. 1.3×0.05 = _____
6. 6.25×3.2 = _____

7. 0.7×0.05 = _____
8. 12.5×2.2 = _____
9. 16×0.3 = _____
10. 0.4×0.17 = _____
11. 2.14×0.9 = _____
12. 0.35×1.9 = _____

ANSWERS 1. 0.09 2. 0.195 3. 4.2 4. 2.42 5. 0.065 6. 20 7. 0.035 8. 27.5 9. 4.8 10. 0.068 11. 1.926 12. 0.665

Division of Decimals

Look at this sample division:

$$\frac{0.25}{0.125} = \frac{\text{numerator}}{\text{denominator}}$$

You may recall that the **top number**, 0.25, is called the **numerator**, while the **bottom number**, 0.125, is called the **denominator**. (If you have trouble remembering which is which think of D, for down, for denominator, the denominator is on the bottom). With this basic terminology reviewed we are now ready to look at two preliminary math steps which are used to simplify the fraction prior to final division. The first step is to eliminate the decimal points completely.

Elimination of Decimal Points

Decimal points can be eliminated from the numbers in a decimal fraction without changing its value.

 To eliminate the decimal points from decimal fractions move them the same number of places to the right in both the numerator and the denominator until they are eliminated in both. Zeros may have to be added to accomplish this.

EXAMPLE 1 $\dfrac{0.25}{0.125}$ becomes $\dfrac{250}{125}$

The decimal point must be moved three places to the right in 0.125 to make it 125. Therefore it must be moved three places in 0.25, which requires the addition of one zero to make it 250.

EXAMPLE 2 $\dfrac{0.3}{0.15}$ becomes $\dfrac{30}{15}$

The decimal point must be moved two places in 0.15 to make it 15. It must be moved two places in 0.3, which requires the addition of one zero to become 30.

EXAMPLE 3 $\dfrac{1.5}{2}$ becomes $\dfrac{15}{20}$

Move the decimal point one place in 1.5 to make it 15; add one zero to 2 to make it 20.

EXAMPLE 4 $\dfrac{4.5}{0.95}$ becomes $\dfrac{450}{95}$

Remember that moving the decimal point does not alter the value of the fraction or the answer you will obtain in the final division. It just makes the numbers easier to work with. Now try some problems on your own.

PROBLEM

Eliminate the decimal points from the following decimal fractions.

1. $\dfrac{17.5}{2}$ = _____

2. $\dfrac{0.5}{25}$ = _____

3. $\dfrac{6.3}{0.6}$ = _____

4. $\dfrac{3.76}{0.4}$ = _____

5. $\dfrac{8.4}{0.7}$ = _____

6. $\dfrac{0.1}{0.05}$ = _____

7. $\dfrac{0.9}{0.03}$ = _____

8. $\dfrac{10.75}{2.5}$ = _____

9. $\dfrac{0.4}{0.04}$ = _____

10. $\dfrac{1.2}{0.4}$ = _____

ANSWERS   1. $\dfrac{175}{20}$ 2. $\dfrac{5}{250}$ 3. $\dfrac{63}{6}$ 4. $\dfrac{376}{40}$ 5. $\dfrac{84}{7}$ 6. $\dfrac{10}{5}$ 7. $\dfrac{90}{3}$ 8. $\dfrac{1075}{250}$ 9. $\dfrac{40}{4}$ 10. $\dfrac{12}{4}$

Reduction of Fractions

Once the decimal points are eliminated the next step is to reduce the numbers as far as possible using common denominators.

 To reduce fractions divide both numbers by their highest common denominator (the highest number which will divide into both).

The **highest common denominator** is usually **2, 3, 4, 5, or multiples of these numbers**, such as 6, 8, 25, and so on.

EXAMPLE 1 $\dfrac{175}{20}$ The highest common denominator is 5

$$\dfrac{\cancel{175}}{\cancel{20}} = \dfrac{35}{4}$$

EXAMPLE 2 $\dfrac{63}{6}$ The highest common denominator is 3

$$\dfrac{\cancel{63}}{\cancel{6}} = \dfrac{21}{2}$$

EXAMPLE 3 $\dfrac{1075}{250}$ The highest common denominator is 25

$$\dfrac{\cancel{1075}}{\cancel{250}} = \dfrac{43}{10}$$

There is a second way you could have reduced the fraction in example 3, and it is equally as correct. Divide by 5, then 5 again.

$$\dfrac{\cancel{1075}}{\cancel{250}} = \dfrac{\cancel{215}}{\cancel{50}} = \dfrac{43}{10}$$

 If the highest common denominator is difficult to determine, reduce several times by using smaller common denominators.

EXAMPLE 4 $\dfrac{\cancel{376}}{\cancel{40}} = \dfrac{47}{5}$ Reduce by 8

or divide by 4, then 2 $\dfrac{\cancel{376}}{\cancel{40}} = \dfrac{\cancel{94}}{\cancel{10}} = \dfrac{47}{5}$

or divide by 2, 2, then 2 $\dfrac{\cancel{376}}{\cancel{40}} = \dfrac{\cancel{188}}{\cancel{20}} = \dfrac{\cancel{94}}{\cancel{10}} = \dfrac{47}{5}$

Remember that simple numbers are easiest to work with, and the time spent in extra reductions may be well worth the payoff in safety.

PROBLEM

Reduce the following fractions as much as possible in preparation for final division.

1. $\dfrac{84}{8}$ = _____

2. $\dfrac{20}{16}$ = _____

3. $\dfrac{250}{325}$ = _____

4. $\dfrac{96}{34}$ = _____

5. $\dfrac{175}{20}$ = _____

6. $\dfrac{40}{14}$ = _____

7. $\dfrac{82}{28}$ = _____

8. $\dfrac{100}{75}$ = _____

9. $\dfrac{50}{75}$ = _____

10. $\dfrac{60}{88}$ = _____

ANSWERS   1. $\dfrac{21}{2}$ 2. $\dfrac{5}{4}$ 3. $\dfrac{10}{13}$ 4. $\dfrac{48}{17}$ 5. $\dfrac{35}{4}$ 6. $\dfrac{20}{7}$ 7. $\dfrac{41}{14}$ 8. $\dfrac{4}{3}$ 9. $\dfrac{2}{3}$ 10. $\dfrac{15}{22}$

Reduction of Numbers Ending in Zero

There is one other type of reduction which, while not solely related to decimal fractions, is best covered at this time. This concerns reductions when both numbers in the fraction end with zeros.

EXAMPLE $\dfrac{2500}{500}$

 Fractions in which both the numerator and denominator end in a zero or zeros may be reduced by crossing off the same number of zeros in each.

EXAMPLE 1 $\dfrac{800}{250}$

In this fraction the numerator, 800, has two zeros and the denominator, 250, has one zero. The number of zeros crossed off must be the same in both numerator and denominator, so only one zero can be eliminated from each.

$$\frac{80\cancel{0}}{25\cancel{0}} = \frac{80}{25}$$

EXAMPLE 2 $\dfrac{24\cancel{00}}{20\cancel{00}} = \dfrac{24}{20}$

Two zeros can be eliminated from the denominator and numerator in this fraction.

EXAMPLE 3 $\dfrac{15\cancel{000}}{30\cancel{000}} = \dfrac{15}{30}$

In this fraction three zeros can be eliminated.

PROBLEM

Reduce the following fractions in preparation for final division.

1. $\dfrac{50}{250}$ = _____

2. $\dfrac{120}{50}$ = _____

3. $\dfrac{2500}{1500}$ = _____

4. $\dfrac{1,000,000}{750,000}$ = _____

5. $\dfrac{800}{150}$ = _____

6. $\dfrac{110}{100}$ = _____

7. $\dfrac{200,000}{150,000}$ = _____

8. $\dfrac{1000}{800}$ = _____

9. $\dfrac{60}{40}$ = _____

10. $\dfrac{150}{200}$ = _____

ANSWERS 1. $\dfrac{1}{5}$ 2. $\dfrac{12}{5}$ 3. $\dfrac{5}{3}$ 4. $\dfrac{4}{3}$ 5. $\dfrac{16}{3}$ 6. $\dfrac{11}{10}$ 7. $\dfrac{4}{3}$ 8. $\dfrac{5}{4}$ 9. $\dfrac{3}{2}$ 10. $\dfrac{3}{4}$

Expressing to the Nearest Tenth

When a fraction is reduced as much as possible it is ready for final division. This is done by dividing the numerator by the denominator. Answers are most often rounded off and expressed as decimal numbers to the nearest tenth.

 To express an answer to the nearest tenth the division is carried to hundredths (two places after the decimal). When the number representing hundredths is 5 or larger, the number representing tenths is increased by one.

EXAMPLE 1 $\dfrac{0.35}{0.4}$ = $0.35 \div 0.4 = 0.87$

Answer = **0.9**

The number representing hundredths is 7, so the number representing tenths is increased by one: 0.87 becomes 0.9

EXAMPLE 2 $\dfrac{0.5}{0.3}$ = $0.5 \div 0.3 = 1.66 =$ **1.7**

The number representing hundredths, 6, is larger than 5, so 1.66 becomes 1.7

EXAMPLE 3 $\dfrac{0.16}{0.3}$ = $0.53 =$ **0.5**

The number representing hundredths, 3, is less than 5, so the number representing tenths, 5, remains unchanged.

EXAMPLE 4 $\dfrac{0.2}{0.3}$ = $0.66 =$ **0.7**

EXAMPLE 5 An answer of 1.42 remains **1.4**

EXAMPLE 6 An answer of 1.86 becomes **1.9**

PROBLEM

Divide the following decimal numbers and express your answers to the nearest tenth.

1. $\dfrac{5.1}{2.3}$ = _____   6. $\dfrac{2.7}{1.1}$ = _____

2. $\dfrac{0.9}{0.7}$ = _____   7. $\dfrac{4.2}{5}$ = _____

3. $\dfrac{3.7}{2}$ = _____   8. $\dfrac{0.5}{2.5}$ = _____

4. $\dfrac{6}{1.3}$ = _____   9. $\dfrac{5.2}{0.91}$ = _____

5. $\dfrac{1.5}{2.1}$ = _____   10. $\dfrac{2.4}{2.7}$ = _____

ANSWERS   1. 2.2   2. 1.3   3. 1.9   4. 4.6   5. 0.7   6. 2.5   7. 0.8   8. 0.2   9. 5.7   10. 0.9

Expressing to the Nearest Hundredth

Some drugs are administered in dosages carried to the nearest hundredth. This is common in pediatric dosages, and in drugs which alter the body's vital function, for example heart rate.

 To express an answer to the nearest hundredth, the division is carried to thousandths (three places after the decimal point). When the number representing thousandths is 5 or larger, the number representing hundredths is increased by one.

EXAMPLE 1   0.736   becomes   **0.74**

The number representing thousandths, 6, is larger than 5, so the number representing hundredths, 3, is increased by 1 to become 4.

EXAMPLE 2   0.777   becomes   **0.78**

EXAMPLE 3   0.373   remains   **0.37**

The number representing thousandths, 3, is less than 5, so the number representing hundredths, 7, remains unchanged.

EXAMPLE 4   0.934   remains   **0.93**

PROBLEM

Express the following numbers to the nearest hundredth.

1. 0.175   = _____   7. 1.081   = _____

2. 0.344   = _____   8. 1.327   = _____

3. 1.853   = _____   9. 0.739   = _____

4. 0.306   = _____   10. 0.733   = _____

5. 3.015   = _____   11. 2.072   = _____

6. 2.154   = _____   12. 0.089   = _____

ANSWERS   1. 0.18   2. 0.34   3. 1.85   4. 0.31   5. 3.02   6. 2.15   7. 1.08   8. 1.33   9. 0.74   10. 0.73   11. 2.07   12. 0.09

Summary

This concludes the chapter on multiplication and division of decimals. The important points to remember from this chapter are:

➡ when decimal fractions are multiplied the decimal point is placed the same number of places to the left in the product as the total of numbers after the decimal points in the fractions multiplied

➡ zeros must be placed in front of a product if it contains insufficient numbers for correct placement of the decimal point

➡ to simplify division of decimal fractions the preliminary steps of eliminating the decimal points, and reducing the numbers by common denominators can be used

➡ when fractions are divided answers are expressed as decimal fractions to the nearest tenth, or the nearest hundredth

Summary Self Test

DIRECTIONS

Multiply the following decimals.

1. 1.49×0.05 = _____
2. 0.15×3.04 = _____
3. 0.025×3.5 = _____
4. 0.55×2.5 = _____
5. 1.31×2.07 = _____

6. 5.3×1.02 = _____
7. 0.35×1.25 = _____
8. 4.32×0.05 = _____
9. 0.2×0.02 = _____
10. 0.4×1.75 = _____

11. You are to administer four tablets with a dosage strength of 0.04 mg each. What total dosage are you giving? _____

12. You have given 2 ½ (2.5) tablets with a strength of 1.25 mg. What total dosage is this? _____

13. The tablets your patient is to receive are labeled 0.1 mg and you are to give 3 ½ (3.5) tablets. What total dosage is this? _____

14. You gave your patient 3 tablets labeled 0.75 mg each, and he was to receive a total of 2.25 mg. Did he receive the correct dosage? _____

15. The tablets available for your patient are labeled 12.5 mg, and you are to give 4 ½ (4.5) tablets. What total dosage will this be? _____

16. Your patient is to receive a dosage of 4.5 mg. The tablets available are labeled 3.5 mg, and there are 2 ½ tablets in his medication drawer. Is this a correct dosage? _____

DIRECTIONS

Divide the following fractions and express your answers to the nearest tenth.

17. $\dfrac{1.3}{0.7}$ = _____   24. $\dfrac{2,000,000}{1,500,000}$ = _____

18. $\dfrac{1.9}{3.2}$ = _____   25. $\dfrac{4.1}{2.05}$ = _____

19. $\dfrac{32.5}{9}$ = _____   26. $\dfrac{7.3}{12}$ = _____

20. $\dfrac{0.04}{0.1}$ = _____   27. $\dfrac{150,000}{120,000}$ = _____

21. $\dfrac{1.45}{1.2}$ = _____   28. $\dfrac{0.15}{0.08}$ = _____

22. $\dfrac{250}{1000}$ = _____   29. $\dfrac{2700}{900}$ = _____

23. $\dfrac{0.8}{0.09}$ = _____   30. $\dfrac{0.25}{0.15}$ = _____

DIRECTIONS

Divide the following fractions and express your answers to the nearest hundredth.

31. $\dfrac{900}{1700}$ = _____   41. $\dfrac{0.13}{0.25}$ = _____

32. $\dfrac{0.125}{0.3}$ = _____   42. $\dfrac{0.25}{0.7}$ = _____

33. $\dfrac{1450}{1500}$ = _____   43. $\dfrac{3.3}{5.1}$ = _____

34. $\dfrac{65}{175}$ = _____   44. $\dfrac{0.19}{0.7}$ = _____

35. $\dfrac{0.6}{1.35}$ = _____   45. $\dfrac{1.1}{1.3}$ = _____

36. $\dfrac{0.04}{0.12}$ = _____   46. $\dfrac{3}{4.1}$ = _____

37. $\dfrac{750}{10,000}$ = _____   47. $\dfrac{62}{240}$ = _____

38. $\dfrac{0.65}{0.8}$ = _____   48. $\dfrac{280,000}{300,000}$ = _____

39. $\dfrac{3.01}{4.2}$ = _____   49. $\dfrac{115}{255}$ = _____

40. $\dfrac{4.5}{6.1}$ = _____   50. $\dfrac{10}{14.3}$ = _____

ANSWERS   1. 0.0745   2. 0.456   3. 0.0875   4. 1.375   5. 2.7117   6. 5.406   7. 0.4375   8. 0.216
9. 0.004   10. 0.7   11. 0.16 mg   12. 3.125 mg   13. 0.35 mg   14. Yes   15. 56.25 mg   16. No   17. 1.9
18. 0.6   19. 3.6   20. 0.4   21. 1.2   22. 0.3   23. 8.9   24. 1.3   25. 2   26. 0.6   27. 1.3   28. 1.9   29. 3
30. 1.7   31. 0.53   32. 0.42   33. 0.97   34. 0.37   35. 0.44   36. 0.33   37. 0.08   38. 0.81   39. 0.72
40. 0.74   41. 0.52   42. 0.36   43. 0.65   44. 0.27   45. 0.85   46. 0.73   47. 0.26   48. 0.93   49. 0.45   50. 0.7

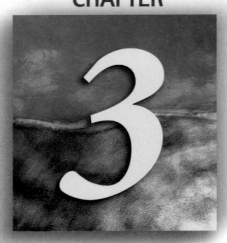

CHAPTER

Solving Common Fraction Equations

OBJECTIVES

The student will solve equations containing
1. whole numbers
2. decimal numbers

PREREQUISITES
Chapters 1 and 2

All the clinical calculations you will be doing will ultimately require that you solve an equation. A simple example is

$$\frac{1}{6} \times \frac{2}{3}$$

In this chapter the steps involved in solving equations without a calculator will be reviewed, because in many instances they will be simple enough to solve without one. Your practice will include calculating fractional answers as decimal fractions to the nearest tenth, since this is the most commonly seen clinical calculation.

Whole Number Equations

The best way to review this material is by actually working with equations. Let's start with a quick review of terminology.

EXAMPLE 1 $\frac{1}{6} \times \frac{2}{3}$

Both $\frac{1}{6}$ and $\frac{2}{3}$ are common fractions. You'll recall that **the numbers on top**, 1 and 2, are **numerators**, while those on **the bottom**, 6 and 3, are **denominators**.

Solving an equation has **four steps**, all of which you practiced in the previous two chapters:

1) elimination of decimal points (if any are present)

2) reduction of the numbers using common denominators (2, 3, 4, 5, or multiples of these numbers)

3) multiplication of the remaining numerators, then the remaining denominators

4) division of the final fraction (the numerator by the denominator) to two places after the decimal, expressing the answer to the nearest tenth.

Look again at the first example. Follow each step carefully.

EXAMPLE 1 $\dfrac{1}{6} \times \dfrac{2}{3}$

Start by reducing the fractions. Divide 2 and 6 by 2.

$$\dfrac{1}{\cancel{6}} \times \dfrac{\cancel{2}^{\,1}}{3}$$
$$\phantom{\dfrac{1}{}}_{3}$$

Next, multiply the remaining numerators ($1 \times 1 = 1$), then the remaining denominators ($3 \times 3 = 9$).

$$\dfrac{1}{9}$$

Divide the final fraction (the numerator, 1, by the denominator, 9) to two places after the decimal point.

$$1 \div 9 \;=\; 0.11 \qquad \text{Answer} = \textbf{0.1}$$

Express the answer to the nearest tenth. The number representing hundredths is 1 (less than 5), so the number representing tenths, 1, remains unchanged.

EXAMPLE 2 $\dfrac{7}{50} \times \dfrac{25}{3}$

Reduce 25 and 50 by 25; 25 becomes 1, and 50 becomes 2.

$$\dfrac{7}{\cancel{50}} \times \dfrac{\cancel{25}^{\,1}}{3}$$
$$\phantom{\dfrac{7}{}}_{2}$$

Multiply the remaining numerators, $7 \times 1 = 7$; then the denominators, $2 \times 3 = 6$.

$$\dfrac{7}{6}$$

Divide the remaining fraction (the numerator, 7, by the denominator, 6) to two places after the decimal point.

$$7 \div 6 \;=\; 1.17 \qquad \text{Answer} = \textbf{1.2}$$

The number representing hundredths, 7, is larger than 5, so the number representing tenths, 1, becomes 2.

EXAMPLE 3 $\dfrac{1}{8} \times \dfrac{4}{3}$

Reduce 4 by 4, to 1; and 8 by 4, to 2.

$$\dfrac{1}{\cancel{8}} \times \dfrac{\cancel{4}^{\,1}}{3}$$
$$\phantom{\dfrac{1}{}}_{2}$$

Multiply the numerators, $1 \times 1 = 1$; and the denominators, $2 \times 3 = 6$.

$$\frac{1}{6}$$

Divide 1 by 6 (the numerator by the denominator) to two places after the decimal point.

$$1 \div 6 = 0.17 \qquad \text{Answer} = \textbf{0.2}$$

The number representing hundredths is 7, so the number representing tenths, 1, is increased by 1, to 2.

EXAMPLE 4 $\qquad \dfrac{250}{175} \times \dfrac{150}{325}$

Reduce 250 and 175 by their highest common denominator, 25, and also 150 and 325 by 25 (or reduce twice, by 5, then 5 again).

$$\frac{\overset{10}{\cancel{250}}}{\underset{7}{\cancel{175}}} \times \frac{\overset{6}{\cancel{150}}}{\underset{13}{\cancel{325}}}$$

Multiply the remaining numerators, 10 and 6, then the remaining denominators, 7 and 13.

$$\frac{60}{91}$$

Divide the remaining fraction, 60 by 91, to two places after the decimal point.

$$60 \div 91 = 0.66 \qquad \text{Answer} = \textbf{0.7}$$

Increase the number representing tenths by 1, to 7, because the number representing hundredths is 6.

EXAMPLE 5 $\qquad \dfrac{2000}{1500} \times \dfrac{2500}{3000}$

Eliminate three zeros from 2000 and 3000, and two zeros from 1500 and 2500; reduce 25 and 15 by dividing by 5.

$$\frac{\cancel{2000}}{\underset{3}{\cancel{1500}}} \times \frac{\overset{5}{\cancel{2500}}}{\cancel{3000}}$$

Multiply the remaining numerators, 2 and 5, then the remaining denominators, 3 and 3.

$$\frac{10}{9}$$

Divide 10 by 9 to two places after the decimal point.

$$10 \div 9 = 1.11 \qquad \text{Answer} = \textbf{1.1}$$

Express the answer to the nearest tenth (the 1 remains unchanged because the number representing hundredths is less than 5).

As you can see this math is uncomplicated, and you are now ready for some problems on your own.

PROBLEM

Solve the following equations. Express fractional answers as decimal fractions to the nearest tenth.

1. $\dfrac{1}{8} \times \dfrac{6}{1}$ = _____   6. $\dfrac{2}{9} \times \dfrac{3}{5}$ = _____

2. $\dfrac{3}{5} \times \dfrac{10}{5}$ = _____   7. $\dfrac{1}{6} \times \dfrac{10}{1}$ = _____

3. $\dfrac{2}{7} \times \dfrac{8}{4}$ = _____   8. $\dfrac{7}{12} \times \dfrac{4}{10}$ = _____

4. $\dfrac{1}{50} \times \dfrac{100}{1}$ = _____   9. $\dfrac{7}{8} \times \dfrac{2}{21}$ = _____

5. $\dfrac{1}{3} \times \dfrac{4}{1}$ = _____   10. $\dfrac{1}{5} \times \dfrac{3}{1}$ = _____

ANSWERS 1. 0.8 2. 1.2 3. 0.6 4. 2 5. 1.3 6. 0.1 7. 1.7 8. 0.2 9. 0.1 10. 0.6

Decimal Fraction Equations

Equations containing decimal fractions are equally as straightforward to solve. The first step is to eliminate the decimal points.

EXAMPLE 1 $\dfrac{0.3}{1.65} \times \dfrac{2.5}{1}$

Eliminate the decimal points from the first fraction by moving it two places to the right in 1.65 and match this in the numerator by moving it two places to the right in 0.3, adding the necessary zero to make it 30 (the decimal **must** move the **same number** of places in **one numerator and one denominator**). Eliminate the decimal from the second fraction by moving it one place in 2.5, to make it 25, and by adding a zero to the 1 in the denominator to make it 10.

$$\frac{30}{165} \times \frac{25}{10}$$

Several numbers in this fraction will reduce. Do these reductions next: 30 by 10 (or cross off 1 zero in each); 25 and 165 by 5; then 33 by 3.

$$\frac{\overset{\overset{1}{\cancel{3}}}{\cancel{30}}}{\underset{\underset{11}{\cancel{33}}}{\cancel{165}}} \times \frac{\overset{5}{\cancel{25}}}{\underset{1}{\cancel{10}}}$$

Multiply the remaining numerators, $1 \times 5 = 5$; then the denominators, $11 \times 1 = 11$.

$$\frac{5}{11}$$

Divide the remaining numerator, 5, by the denominator, 11.

$$5 \div 11 = 0.45 \qquad \text{Answer} = \mathbf{0.5}$$

Express the answer to the nearest tenth; 0.45 becomes 0.5.

EXAMPLE 2 $\quad \dfrac{0.3}{1.2} \times \dfrac{2.1}{0.15}$

First eliminate the decimal points: remove them from the first fraction by moving the decimal one place to the right in both 0.3 and 1.2; remove them from the second fraction by moving the decimal two places to the right in 0.15 making it 15, and two places in 2.1 (adding a zero) to make it 210.

$$\dfrac{3}{12} \times \dfrac{210}{15}$$

These fractions will reduce several times. Do this yourself to check the examples.

$$\dfrac{\overset{1}{\cancel{3}}}{\underset{6}{\cancel{12}}} \times \dfrac{\overset{21}{\cancel{210}}}{\underset{1}{\cancel{15}}}$$

Multiply the remaining numerators, $1 \times 21 = 21$; and the remaining denominators $6 \times 1 = 6$.

$$\dfrac{21}{6}$$

Divide the remaining numerator, 21, by the remaining denominator, 6.

$$21 \div 6 = 3.50 \qquad \text{Answer} = \mathbf{3.5}$$

Eliminate the unnecessary zero and express the answer to the nearest tenth, 3.50 becomes 3.5.

EXAMPLE 3 $\quad \dfrac{0.15}{0.7} \times \dfrac{3.1}{2}$

Eliminate the decimal points by moving them two places in the first fraction: 0.15 becomes 15, and 0.7 becomes 70; and in the second fraction by moving them one place in 3.1 to make it 31, and in 2 to make it 20.

$$\dfrac{15}{70} \times \dfrac{31}{20}$$

Reduce the fractions: 15 by 5 to become 3, and 20 by 5 to become 4.

$$\dfrac{\overset{3}{\cancel{15}}}{70} \times \dfrac{31}{\underset{4}{\cancel{20}}}$$

Multiply the remaining numerators, $3 \times 31 = 93$; then the remaining denominators, $70 \times 4 = 280$.

$$\frac{93}{280}$$

Divide the final fraction, the numerator 93 by the denominator 280.

$93 \div 280 = 0.33$ Answer = **0.3**

Express the answer as a decimal fraction to the nearest tenth; 0.33 becomes 0.3.

EXAMPLE 4 $\dfrac{2.5}{1.5} \times \dfrac{1.2}{1}$

Eliminate the decimal points from 2.5 and 1.5 in the first fraction by moving them one place to the right in each; remove the decimal point in the second fraction by moving it one place to the right in 1.2, and by adding a zero to the denominator, 1, to make it 10.

$$\frac{25}{15} \times \frac{12}{10}$$

The remaining numbers will reduce several times. Do this yourself to check the example.

$$\frac{\overset{1}{\cancel{5}}\ \overset{2}{\cancel{6}}}{\underset{1}{\cancel{25}}}\times\frac{\overset{}{\cancel{12}}}{\underset{1}{\cancel{10}}}$$

$\dfrac{2}{1}$ Answer = **2**

PROBLEM

Solve the following equations. Express answers to the nearest tenth.

1. $\dfrac{2.5}{1.15} \times \dfrac{1.1}{1.3}$ = _____

2. $\dfrac{3.1}{2.7} \times \dfrac{2.2}{1.4}$ = _____

3. $\dfrac{0.05}{1.1} \times \dfrac{3}{2.1}$ = _____

4. $\dfrac{0.17}{0.3} \times \dfrac{2.5}{1.5}$ = _____

5. $\dfrac{1.75}{0.95} \times \dfrac{1.5}{2}$ = _____

6. $\dfrac{0.75}{1.15} \times \dfrac{3}{1.25}$ = _____

7. $\dfrac{10.2}{1.5} \times \dfrac{2}{5.1}$ = _____

8. $\dfrac{0.125}{0.25} \times \dfrac{2.5}{1.5}$ = _____

9. $\dfrac{0.7}{0.3} \times \dfrac{1.2}{1.4}$ = _____

10. $\dfrac{0.35}{1.7} \times \dfrac{2.5}{0.7}$ = _____

ANSWERS 1. 1.8 **2.** 1.8 **3.** 0.1 **4.** 0.9 **5.** 1.4 **6.** 1.6 **7.** 2.7 **8.** 0.8 **9.** 2 **10.** 0.7

Multiple Number Equations

Equations containing multiple numbers are equally as uncomplicated to solve.

EXAMPLE 1
$$\frac{60}{1} \times \frac{1000}{4} \times \frac{1}{1000} \times \frac{6}{1}$$

$$\frac{\overset{15}{\cancel{60}}}{1} \times \frac{\cancel{1000}}{\underset{1}{\cancel{4}}} \times \frac{1}{\underset{1}{\cancel{1000}}} \times \frac{6}{1}$$

Reduce the numbers, multiply the remaining numerators, then denominators. Divide the final fraction.

$$\frac{90}{1} \qquad \text{Answer} = \textbf{90}$$

EXAMPLE 2
$$\frac{20}{1} \times \frac{75}{1} \times \frac{1}{60}$$

$$\frac{\overset{1}{\cancel{20}}}{1} \times \frac{\overset{25}{\cancel{75}}}{1} \times \frac{1}{\underset{\underset{1}{\cancel{3}}}{\cancel{60}}}$$

Reduce the numbers; multiply the remaining numerators, then denominators. Divide the final fraction.

$$\frac{25}{1} \qquad \text{Answer} = \textbf{25}$$

EXAMPLE 3
$$\frac{1}{60} \times \frac{1}{12} \times \frac{10}{1} \times \frac{750}{1}$$

$$\frac{1}{\underset{\underset{1}{\cancel{6}}}{\cancel{60}}} \times \frac{1}{12} \times \frac{\overset{1}{\cancel{10}}}{1} \times \frac{\overset{125}{\cancel{750}}}{1}$$

Reduce the numbers; multiply the remaining numerators and denominators. Divide the final fraction; express to nearest tenth.

$$\frac{125}{12} = 10.42 \qquad \text{Answer} = \textbf{10.4}$$

EXAMPLE 4
$$\frac{2}{0.5} \times \frac{1}{1000} \times \frac{275}{1}$$

Remove the decimals.

$$\frac{20}{5} \times \frac{1}{1000} \times \frac{275}{1}$$

$$\frac{\overset{1}{\cancel{20}}}{\underset{1}{\cancel{5}}} \times \frac{1}{\underset{10}{\cancel{\underset{50}{\cancel{1000}}}}} \times \frac{\overset{\overset{11}{\cancel{55}}}{\cancel{275}}}{1}$$

Reduce; multiply numerators, then denominators. Divide final fraction; express to nearest tenth

$$\frac{11}{10} = 1.10 \qquad \text{Answer} = \mathbf{1.1}$$

EXAMPLE 5 $\qquad \frac{1}{200} \times \frac{1000}{1} \times \frac{0.5}{1}$

Remove decimal.

$$\frac{1}{200} \times \frac{1000}{1} \times \frac{5}{10}$$

$$\frac{1}{\underset{1}{\cancel{200}}} \times \frac{\overset{\overset{1}{\cancel{5}}}{\cancel{1000}}}{1} \times \frac{5}{\underset{2}{\cancel{10}}}$$

Reduce; multiply numerators, then denominators. Divide final fraction.

$$\frac{5}{2} = 2.50 \qquad \text{Answer} = \mathbf{2.5}$$

PROBLEM

Solve the following equations. Express answers to the nearest tenth.

1. $\frac{15}{1} \times \frac{350}{5} \times \frac{1}{60} = $ _____

2. $\frac{1}{30} \times \frac{60}{1} \times \frac{15}{1} = $ _____

3. $\frac{10}{1} \times \frac{2500}{24} \times \frac{1}{60} = $ _____

4. $\frac{1}{30} \times \frac{15}{1} \times \frac{100}{1} = $ _____

5. $\frac{15}{1} \times \frac{1200}{16} \times \frac{1}{60} = $ _____

ANSWERS 1. 17.5 2. 30 3. 17.4 4. 50 5. 18.8

Summary

The problems you have just practiced are representative of problems you will see in actual clinical calculations. Not complicated, not difficult. This completes the chapter on solving common fraction equations. The important points to remember are:

➡ if an equation containing decimals must be solved without the use of a calculator, start by removing any decimal points

➡ reduce the numbers in the fractions as much as possible using common denominators

➡ multiply the remaining numerators, then denominators

➡ divide the final fraction (numerator by denominator) to obtain the answer

➡ express fractional answers as decimal fractions to the nearest tenth (unless instructed otherwise)

Summary Self Test

DIRECTIONS

Solve the following equations. Express answers to the nearest tenth.

1. $\dfrac{0.8}{0.65} \times \dfrac{1.2}{1}$ = _____

2. $\dfrac{350}{1000} \times \dfrac{4.4}{1}$ = _____

3. $\dfrac{15}{1} \times \dfrac{500}{3} \times \dfrac{1}{60}$ = _____

4. $\dfrac{60}{1} \times \dfrac{500}{150} \times \dfrac{0.1}{1}$ = _____

5. $\dfrac{60}{1} \times \dfrac{250}{50} \times \dfrac{1}{1000} \times \dfrac{154}{1}$ = _____

6. $\dfrac{0.35}{1.3} \times \dfrac{4.5}{1}$ = _____

7. $\dfrac{0.4}{1.5} \times \dfrac{2.3}{1}$ = _____

8. $\dfrac{60}{1} \times \dfrac{250}{50} \times \dfrac{1}{1000} \times \dfrac{432}{1}$ = _____

9. $\dfrac{1}{75} \times \dfrac{500}{1}$ = _____

10. $\dfrac{60}{1} \times \dfrac{500}{5} \times \dfrac{1}{1000} \times \dfrac{1}{1000} \times \dfrac{3150}{1}$ = _____

11. $\dfrac{2000}{250} \times \dfrac{50}{1}$ = _____

12. $\dfrac{400}{250} \times \dfrac{250}{5}$ = _____

13. $\dfrac{10}{1} \times \dfrac{325}{1.5} \times \dfrac{1}{60}$ = _____

14. $\dfrac{60}{1} \times \dfrac{500}{400} \times \dfrac{1}{1000} \times \dfrac{400}{1}$ = _____

15. $\dfrac{60}{1} \times \dfrac{250}{8} \times \dfrac{1}{1000} \times \dfrac{5}{1}$ = _____

16. $\dfrac{60}{1} \times \dfrac{250}{50} \times \dfrac{1}{1000} \times \dfrac{216}{1}$ = _____

17. $\dfrac{60}{1} \times \dfrac{500}{2} \times \dfrac{1}{1000}$ = _____

18. $\dfrac{60}{1} \times \dfrac{500}{5} \times \dfrac{1}{1000}$ = _____

19. $\dfrac{1000}{1} \times \dfrac{50}{250} \times \dfrac{20}{1} \times \dfrac{1}{60}$ = _____

20. $\dfrac{0.15}{0.1} \times \dfrac{1.4}{1}$ = _____

21. $\dfrac{100,000}{80,000} \times \dfrac{1.2}{1}$ = _____

22. $\dfrac{1.45}{2.1} \times \dfrac{1.5}{1}$ = _____

23. $\dfrac{1500}{500} \times \dfrac{0.5}{1}$ = _____

24. $\dfrac{4}{0.375} \times 0.25$ = _____

25. $\dfrac{1}{75} \times \dfrac{1000}{1}$ = _____

26. $\dfrac{1}{90} \times \dfrac{1000}{1}$ = _____

27. $\dfrac{1}{60} \times \dfrac{1}{25} \times \dfrac{10}{1} \times \dfrac{1000}{1}$ = _____

28. $\dfrac{0.08}{0.1} \times \dfrac{1.1}{1}$ = _____

29. $\dfrac{1}{60} \times \dfrac{1}{10} \times \dfrac{10}{1} \times \dfrac{1100}{1}$ = _____

30. $\dfrac{100}{500} \times \dfrac{1}{60} \times \dfrac{30}{1}$ = _____

31. $\dfrac{20}{0.5} \times 0.3$ = _____

32. $\dfrac{40,000}{1000} \times \dfrac{30}{1}$ = _____

33. $\dfrac{0.5}{0.15} \times 0.3$ = _____

34. $\dfrac{300,000}{200,000} \times \dfrac{1.7}{1}$ = _____

35. $\dfrac{60}{1} \times \dfrac{500}{50} \times \dfrac{1}{1000} \times \dfrac{116}{1}$ = _____

36. $\dfrac{135}{100} \times \dfrac{2.5}{1}$ = _____

37. $\dfrac{1,200,000}{800,000} \times \dfrac{2.7}{1}$ = _____

38. $\dfrac{60}{1} \times \dfrac{50}{250} \times \dfrac{1}{1000} \times \dfrac{820}{1}$ = _____

39. $\dfrac{1.3}{0.75} \times \dfrac{0.9}{1}$ = _____

40. $\dfrac{15}{1} \times \dfrac{1000}{40,000} \times \dfrac{800}{1} \times \dfrac{1}{60}$ = _____

41. $\dfrac{1.5}{0.1} \times \dfrac{0.25}{1}$ = _____

42. $\dfrac{6}{900} \times \dfrac{1000}{1} \times \dfrac{0.75}{1}$ = _____

43. $\dfrac{1.5}{0.4} \times 0.35$ = _____

44. $\dfrac{1000}{1} \times \dfrac{4}{1000} \times \dfrac{42}{1}$ = _____

45. $\dfrac{1.4}{0.1} \times 0.3$ = _____

46. $\dfrac{1000}{1} \times \dfrac{250}{50} \times \dfrac{8}{1}$ = _____

47. $\dfrac{1.2}{0.1} \times 0.25$ = _____

48. $\dfrac{20}{1} \times \dfrac{1000}{60,000} \times \dfrac{1200}{1} \times \dfrac{1}{60}$ = _____

49. $\dfrac{2.2}{0.25} \times 0.6$ = _____

50. $\dfrac{60}{1} \times \dfrac{50}{250} \times \dfrac{1}{1000} \times \dfrac{450}{1}$ = _____

ANSWERS 1. 1.5 2. 1.5 3. 41.7 4. 20 5. 46.2 6. 1.2 7. 0.6 8. 129.6 9. 6.7 10. 18.9 11. 400 12. 80 13. 36.1 14. 30 15. 9.4 16. 64.8 17. 15 18. 6 19. 66.7 20. 2.1 21. 1.5 22. 1 23. 1.5 24. 2.7 25. 13.3 26. 11.1 27. 6.7 28. 0.9 29. 18.3 30. 0.1 31. 12 32. 1200 33. 1 34. 2.6 35. 69.6 36. 3.4 37. 4.1 38. 9.8 39. 1.6 40. 5 41. 3.8 42. 5 43. 1.3 44. 168 45. 4.2 46. 40,000 47. 3 48. 6.7 49. 5.3 50. 4.9

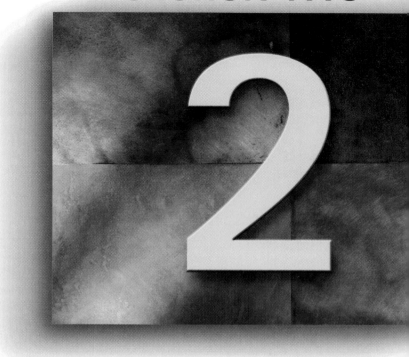

Introduction to Drug Measures

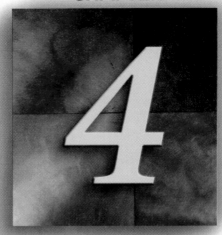

Metric, International (SI) System

OBJECTIVES

The student will

1. list the commonly used units of measure in the metric system
2. distinguish between the official abbreviations and variations in common use
3. express metric weights and volumes using correct notation rules
4. convert metric weights and volumes within the system

The major system of weights and measures used in medicine is the metric/international/SI (from the French Système International). The metric system was invented in France in 1875, and takes its name from the **meter**, a length roughly equivalent to a yard, from which all other units of measure in the system are derived. The strength of the metric system lies in its simplicity, since all units of measure differ from each other in powers of ten (10). Conversions between units in the system are accomplished by simply moving a decimal point.

While it is not necessary for you to know the entire metric system to administer medications safely, you must understand its basic structure, and become familiar with the units of measure you will be using.

Basic Units of the Metric/SI System

Three types of metric measures are in common use, those for **length**, **volume** (or capacity), and **weight**. The **basic units** or beginning points of these three measures are

length _____ **meter**   **volume** _____ **liter**   **weight** _____ **gram**

You must memorize these basic units: do so now if you do not already know them. In addition to these basic units, there are both larger and smaller units of measure for length, volume, and weight. Let's compare this concept with something familiar. The pound is a unit of weight that we use every day. A smaller unit of measure is the ounce, a larger, the ton. **However, all are units measuring weight**.

In the same way, there are smaller and larger units than the basic meter, liter, and gram. However, in the metric system there is one very important advantage: **all other units, whether larger or smaller than the basic units, have the name of the basic unit incorporated in them**. So there is never need for doubt when you see a unit of measure just what it is measuring. **Meter-length, liter-volume, gram-weight**.

PROBLEM

Identify the following metric measures with their appropriate category of weight, length, or volume.

1. milligram _____

2. centimeter _____

3. milliliter _____

4. millimeter _____

5. kilogram _____

6. microgram _____

ANSWERS   1. weight   2. length   3. volume   4. length   5. weight   6. weight

Metric/SI Prefixes

The prefixes used in combination with the names of the basic units identify the larger and smaller units of measure. The same prefixes are used with all three measures. Therefore there is a kilo**meter**, kilo**gram**, and a kilo**liter**. Prefixes also change the value of each of the basic units by the same amount. For example the prefix "kilo" identifies a unit of measure which is larger than, or multiplies the basic unit by 1000. Therefore,

1 kilometer	=	1000 meters
1 kilogram	=	1000 grams
1 kiloliter	=	1000 liters

Kilo is the only prefix you will be using which identifies a measure **larger** than the basic unit. Kilograms are frequently used as a measure for body weight, especially for infants and children.

You will see only three measures **smaller** than the basic unit in common use. The prefixes for these are:

> centi—as in centimeter
> milli—as in milligram
> micro—as in microgram

Therefore you will actually be working with only four prefixes; **kilo**, which identifies a larger unit of measure than the basics, and **centi**, **milli**, and **micro**, which identify smaller units than the basics.

Metric/SI Abbreviations

In actual use the units of measure are abbreviated. **The basic units are abbreviated to their first initial, and printed in small letters, with the exception of liter, which is capitalized.**

> gram is g   liter is L   meter is m

The abbreviations for the prefixes used in combination with the basic units are all printed using small letters.

kilo	_____	k	_____ as in kilogram	_____	kg
centi	_____	c	_____ as in centimeter	_____	cm
milli	_____	m	_____ as in milligram	_____	mg
micro	_____	mc	_____ as in microgram	_____	mcg

Micro has an additional abbreviation, the symbol μ, which is used in combination with the basic unit, as in microgram, μ**g.**

While you will see the symbol μg on drug labels for microgram, you should be aware that it has an inherent safety risk. When hand printed it is very easy for microgram (*μg*) to be mistaken for milligram (*mg*). These units differ from each other in value by 1000 (1 mg = 1000 mcg), and misreading these dosages could be critical.

To assure safety when transcribing orders by hand, always use the abbreviation mc to designate micro rather than its symbol: Example mcg.

In combination, liter remains capitalized. Therefore milliliter is mL, and kiloliter kL.

PROBLEM

Print the abbreviations for the following metric units.

1. microgram   _____
2. liter   _____
3. kilogram   _____
4. milliliter   _____
5. centimeter   _____
6. milligram   _____
7. meter   _____
8. kiloliter   _____
9. millimeter   _____
10. gram   _____

ANSWERS   1. mcg   2. L   3. kg   4. mL   5. cm   6. mg   7. m   8. kL   9. mm   10. g

Variations of Metric/SI Abbreviations

Although the metric system was invented in 1875 it was not until 1960, nearly 100 years later, that a standard system of abbreviations, the **International System of Units**, was adopted. Therefore a variety of unofficial abbreviations are still in use. Most of the variations were designed to prevent confusion with the much older apothecaries' system, which was in common use at that time in drug dosages. The major difference is that gram was abbreviated **Gm**, in an effort to differentiate it from the apothecaries' grain, **gr**. This of course led to milligram and microgram being abbreviated **mgm**, and **mcgm**. Liter was routinely abbreviated small **l**, and milliliter, **ml**. You may still see these abbreviations used, particularly ml, even on drug labels, but do not fall into the habit of using them yourself. They are officially obsolete.

Metric/SI Notation Rules

The easiest way to learn the rules of metric notations, in which a unit of measure is expressed with a quantity, is to memorize some prototypes (examples) which incorporate all the rules. Then if you get confused, you can stop and think and remember the correct way to write them. For the metric system the notations for one-half, one, and one and one-half milliliters will incorporate all the rules you must know.

Prototype Notations: **0.5 mL**   **1 mL**   **1.5 mL**

RULE 1:   **The quantity is written in Arabic Numerals, 1, 2, 3, 4, etc.**

example: 0.5   1   1.5

RULE 2: The numerals representing the quantity are placed in front of the abbreviations.

> *example:* 0.5 mL   1 mL   1.5 mL   (not mL 0.5, etc.)

RULE 3: A full space is used between the numeral and abbreviation.

> *example:* 0.5 mL   1 mL   1.5 mL   (not 0.5mL, etc.)

RULE 4: Fractional parts of a unit are expressed as decimal fractions.

> *example:* 0.5 mL   1.5 mL   (not ½ mL, 1½ mL)

RULE 5: A zero is placed in front of the decimal when it is not preceded by a whole number to emphasize the decimal point.

> *example:* 0.5 mL   (not .5 mL)

RULE 6: Unnecessary zeros are omitted so they cannot be misread and lead to medication errors.

> *example:* 0.5 mL   1 mL   1.5 mL   (not 0.50 mL, 1.0 mL, 1.50 mL)

So once again, as examples of the rules of metric notations, memorize the prototypes 0.5 mL—1 mL—1.5 mL. Just refer back to these in your memory if you get confused, and you will be able to write them correctly.

PROBLEM

Write the following metric measures using official abbreviations and notation rules.

1. two grams _____
2. five hundred milliliters _____
3. five-tenths of a liter _____
4. two-tenths of a milligram _____
5. five-hundredths of a gram _____
6. two and five-tenths kilograms _____
7. one hundred micrograms _____
8. two and three-tenths milliliters _____
9. seven-tenths of a milliliter _____
10. three-tenths of a milligram _____
11. two and four-tenths liters _____
12. seventeen and five-tenths kilograms _____
13. nine-hundredths of a milligram _____
14. ten and two-tenths micrograms _____
15. four-hundredths of a gram _____

ANSWERS 1. 2 g   2. 500 mL   3. 0.5 L   4. 0.2 mg   5. 0.05 g   6. 2.5 kg   7. 100 mcg   8. 2.3 mL   9. 0.7 mL
10. 0.3 mg   11. 2.4 L   12. 17.5 kg   13. 0.09 mg   14. 10.2 mcg   15. 0.04 g

Conversion Between Metric/SI Units

When you administer medications, you will routinely be converting units of measure within the metric system, for example g to mg, and mg to mcg. Learning the relative value of the units you will be working with is the first prerequisite to accurate conversions. There are only four metric **weights** commonly used in medicine. From **highest** to **lowest** value these are:

kg	=	kilogram
g	=	gram
mg	=	milligram
mcg	=	microgram

Only two units of **volume** are frequently used. From **highest** to **lowest** value these are:

L	=	liter
mL	=	milliliter

Each of these units differs in value from the next by 1000.

1 kg	=	1000 g
1 g	=	1000 mg
1 mg	=	1000 mcg
1 L	=	1000 mL (1000 cc)

 The abbreviations for milliliter (mL) and cubic centimeter (cc) are used interchangeably. A cc is actually the amount of physical space that a 1 mL volume occupies, but the two measures are considered identical.

Once again, from highest to lowest value the units are, for weight: kg—g—mg—mcg; for volume: L—mL (cc). Each unit differs in value from the next by 1000, and **all conversions will be between touching units of measure**, for example g to mg, mg to mcg, L to mL.

PROBLEM

Indicate if the following statements are true or false.

1.	T F	1000 cc	=	1000 L	6.	T F	1 kg	=	1000 g
2.	T F	1000 mg	=	1 g	7.	T F	1 mg	=	1000 g
3.	T F	1000 mL	=	1000 cc	8.	T F	1000 mcg	=	1 mg
4.	T F	1000 mg	=	1 mcg	9.	T F	1000 mL	=	1 L
5.	T F	1000 mcg	=	1 g	10.	T F	3 cc	=	3 mL

ANSWERS   1. F   2. T   3. T   4. F   5. F   6. T   7. F   8. T   9. T   10. T

Since the metric system is a decimal system, **conversions between the units are simply a matter of moving the decimal point**. Also because each unit of measure in common use differs from the next by 1000, if you know one conversion, you know them all.

How far do you move the decimal point? Each of the units differs from the next by 1000. There are three zeros in 1000, so **move the decimal point three places**.

Which way do you move the decimal point? If you are converting **down** the scale to a **smaller** unit of measure, for example g to mg, the quantity must get **larger**, so move the decimal three places to the **right**.

EXAMPLE 1   0.5 g = _____ mg

You are converting down the scale. Move the decimal point three places to the right. To do this, you have to add two zeros. Your answer, 500 mg, is a larger number because you moved down the scale (0.5 g = 500 mg).

EXAMPLE 2   2.5 L = _____ mL

Converting down, L to mL, move the decimal point three places to the right. Your answer will be a larger quantity (2.5 L = 2500 mL).

PROBLEM

Convert the following metric measures.

1. 7 mg   = _____ mcg
2. 1.7 L   = _____ mL
3. 3.2 g   = _____ mg
4. 0.03 kg = _____ g
5. 0.4 mg = _____ mcg

6. 1.5 mg = _____ mcg
7. 0.7 g   = _____ mg
8. 0.3 L   = _____ mL
9. 7 kg   = _____ g
10. 0.01 mg = _____ mcg

ANSWERS   1. 7000 mcg   2. 1700 mL   3. 3200 mg   4. 30 g   5. 400 mcg   6. 1500 mcg   7. 700 mg   8. 300 mL
9. 7000 g   10. 10 mcg

In metric conversions up the scale, from smaller to larger units of measure, the quantity will get smaller, for example mL to L. The decimal point moves **three places to the left.**

EXAMPLE 1   200 mL = _____ L

You are converting up the scale. Move the decimal point three places left. The quantity becomes smaller. 200 mL = 0.2 L (remember the safety feature of adding a zero in front of the decimal).

EXAMPLE 2   500 mcg = _____ mg

Move the decimal point three places to the left. The quantity becomes smaller. 500 mcg = 0.5 mg.

PROBLEM

Convert the following metric measures.

1. 3500 mL = _____ L
2. 520 mg   = _____ g
3. 1800 mcg = _____ mg
4. 750 cc   = _____ L
5. 150 mg   = _____ g

6. 250 mcg = _____ mg
7. 1200 mg = _____ g
8. 600 mL   = _____ L
9. 100 mg   = _____ g
10. 950 mcg = _____ mg

ANSWERS   1. 3.5 L   2. 0.52 g   3. 1.8 mg   4. 0.75 L   5. 0.15 g   6. 0.25 mg   7. 1.2 g   8. 0.6 L   9. 0.1 g
10. 0.95 mg

Common Errors in Metric/SI Dosages

Most errors in metric dosages occur when a dosage or calculation contains a decimal. So let's take a close look at some basic safety rules which can reduce the possibility of error.

The first way to prevent errors is to make sure orders are interpreted and transcribed correctly. Doctors do not always write orders in the safest manner, and you must learn to question everything that looks suspicious. A common error is **failure to write a zero in front of the decimal point** in decimal fractions, for example .2 mg instead of 0.2 mg. This makes the decimal easy to miss. This error can be eliminated by strict adherence to the rule of placing a zero in front of decimal fractions. Regardless of the presence of a zero in a written order, make sure one is added when it is transferred to a medication administration record or patient chart.

 Fractional dosages in the metric system must be transcribed with a zero in front of the decimal point to draw attention to it.

The next most common error is **to include zeros where they should not be**, for example .20 mg. An order written like this can easily be misread as 20 mg. Or, consider a dosage written 2.0 mg. The same potential for error exists. There is an unnecessary zero included in the order.

 Unnecessary zeros must be eliminated when metric dosages are transcribed.

The third error to watch for is in **calculations where decimal fractions are involved**. The presence of a decimal point in a calculation should raise a warning flag to slow down and double check all math. Use your reasoning powers. If you misplace a decimal point, you are going to get an answer a minimum of ten times too much, or too little. Learn to question quantities that seem unreasonable. A 1 mL dosage makes sense if you are calculating an IM injection. A 0.1 mL or 10 mL (or a 10 tab) dosage does not, and this is the type of error you might see. Be alert when assessing answers, and determine if they seem reasonable.

 Question answers to calculations which seem unreasonably large or small.

The final error to be aware of is in **conversions within the metric system**. Errors in conversions can be eliminated by thinking **three**. All conversions between the g, mg and mcg measures used in dosages are accomplished by moving the decimal point **three** places. Always, and forever. There are not many things you can use the words "always" and "forever" for, but conversions between these units of measure in the metric system is one of those rare instances.

 Conversions between g, mg, mcg units of measure in metric dosages require moving the decimal point three places.

If you are constantly mindful of these problem areas you can be an outstandingly safe clinical practitioner.

Summary

This concludes your refresher on the metric system. The important points to remember from this chapter are:

➡ the meter, liter, and gram are the basic units of metric measures

➡ larger and smaller units than the basics are identified by the use of prefixes

➡ the larger unit you will be seeing is the kilo, whose prefix is k

➡ the smaller units you will be seeing are milli—m, micro—mc, and centi—c

➡ each prefix changes the value of the basic unit by the same amount

➡ converting from one unit to another within the system is accomplished by moving the decimal point

➡ when you convert down the scale to smaller units of measure the quantity will get larger

➡ when you convert up the scale to larger units of measure the quantity will get smaller

➡ fractional dosages are transcribed with a zero in front of the decimal point

➡ unnecessary zeros are eliminated from dosages

➡ conversions between g, mg, mcg, and mL, L all require moving the decimal point three places

Summary Self Test

DIRECTIONS

List the basic units of measure of the metric system and indicate what type of measure they are used for.

1. _____   _____

   _____   _____

   _____   _____

DIRECTIONS

Which of the following are official metric/SI abbreviations?

2. a) L   e) mg
    b) g   f) kg
    c) kL   g) ml
    d) mgm   h) G

   _____

DIRECTIONS

Express the following measures using official metric abbreviations and notation rules.

3. six-hundredths of a milligram _____

4. three hundred and ten milliliters _____

5. three-tenths of a kilogram _____

6. four-tenths of a cubic centimeter _____

7. one and five-tenths grams _____

8. one-hundredths of a gram _____

9. four thousand milliliters _____

10. one and two-tenths milligrams _____

DIRECTIONS

List the four commonly used units of weight and the two of volume, from highest to lowest value.

11. _____   _____

    _____   _____

    _____

    _____

DIRECTIONS

Convert the following metric measures.

12. 160 mg = _____ g	27. 300 mg = _____ g
13. 10 kg = _____ g	28. 2.5 mg = _____ mcg
14. 1500 µg = _____ mg	29. 1 kL = _____ L
15. 750 mg = _____ g	30. 3 L = _____ cc
16. 200 mL = _____ L	31. 10 cc = _____ mL
17. 0.3 g = _____ mg	32. 0.7 mg = _____ mcg
18. 0.05 g = _____ mg	33. 4 g = _____ mg
19. 0.15 g = _____ mg	34. 1000 mL = _____ L
20. 1.2 L = _____ mL	35. 2.5 mL = _____ cc
21. 15 mL = _____ cc	36. 1000 mg = _____ g
22. 2 mg = _____ mcg	37. 0.2 mg = _____ mcg
23. 900 mcg = _____ mg	38. 2000 g = _____ kg
24. 2.1 L = _____ mL	39. 1.4 g = _____ mg
25. 475 mL = _____ L	40. 2.5 L = _____ cc
26. 0.9 cc = _____ mL	

ANSWERS 1. gram-weight; liter-volume; meter-length   2. a, b, c, e, f   3. 0.06 mg   4. 310 mL   5. 0.3 kg
6. 0.4 cc   7. 1.5 g   8. 0.01 g   9. 4000 mL   10. 1.2 mg   11. kg, g, mg, mcg; L, mL   12. 0.16 g   13. 10,000 g
14. 1.5 mg   15. 0.75 g   16. 0.2 L   17. 300 mg   18. 50 mg   19. 150 mg   20. 1200 mL   21. 15 cc   22. 2000 mcg
23. 0.9 mg   24. 2100 mL   25. 0.475 L   26. 0.9 mL   27. 0.3 g   28. 2500 mcg   29. 1000 L   30. 3000 cc   31. 10 mL
32. 700 mcg   33. 4000 mg   34. 1 L   35. 2.5 cc   36. 1 g   37. 200 mcg   38. 2 kg   39. 1400 mg   40. 2500 cc

Additional Drug Measures: Unit, Percentage, Milliequivalent, Ratio, Apothecary, Household

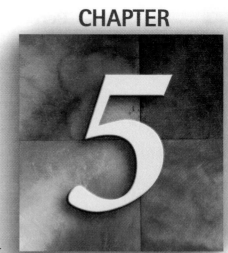

CHAPTER

5

W hile metric measures predominate in medications there are several other measures frequently used, particularly in parenteral solutions, which are important for you to know. In addition you must be able to recognize several measures in the apothecaries' and household systems, since you may occasionally see these.

OBJECTIVES

The student will recognize dosages
1. measured in units
2. measured as percentages
3. using ratio strengths
4. in milliequivalents
5. in apothecary measures
6. in household measures

International Units (U)

A number of drugs are measured in International Units. Insulin, penicillin, and heparin are commonly seen examples. A unit measures a drug in terms of its action, not its physical weight. Units are abbreviated U, and are written using Arabic numerals in front of the symbol, with a space between, for example 2000 U, or 1,000,000 U. Commas are not normally used in a quantity unless it has at least five numbers, for example 45,000 U.

PROBLEM

Express the following unit dosages using their official abbreviation.

1. two hundred and fifty thousand units _____
2. ten units _____
3. five thousand units _____
4. forty four units _____
5. forty thousand units _____
6. one million units _____
7. one thousand units _____
8. twenty five hundred units _____
9. thirty four units _____
10. one hundred units _____

ANSWERS 1. 250,000 U 2. 10 U 3. 5000 U 4. 44 U 5. 40,000 U 6. 1,000,000 U 7. 1000 U 8. 2500 U 9. 34 U 10. 100 U

Percentage (%) Measures

Percentage strengths are used extensively in intravenous solutions, and somewhat less commonly for a variety of other medications, including eye and topical (for external use) ointments. Percentage (%) means parts per hundred. The higher the percentage strength, the stronger the solution or ointment.

 In solutions percent represents the number of grams of drug per 100 mL/cc of solution.

EXAMPLE 1   100 mL of a 1% solution will contain 1 gram of drug

EXAMPLE 2   100 mL of a 2% solution will contain 2 grams of drug

EXAMPLE 3   50 mL of a 1% solution will contain 0.5 grams of drug

EXAMPLE 4   200 mL of a 2% solution will contain 4 grams of drug

PROBLEM

1. How many grams of drug will 100 mL of a 10% solution contain?   _____

2. How many grams of drug will 50 mL of a 10% solution contain?   _____

3 How many grams of drug will 200 mL of a 10% solution contain?   _____

4. A 500 cc IV bag is labeled 5% Dextrose in Water. How many grams of dextrose will it contain?   _____

5. A 1000 cc IV bag has a solution strength of 10%. How many grams of drug does this represent?   _____

6. An IV of 200 cc 5% Dextrose will contain how many grams of dextrose?   _____

7. If 350 cc of a 10% Dextrose IV are infused, how many grams will the patient receive?   _____

8. An IV of 5% Dextrose is discontinued after only 150 cc have infused. How many grams of dextrose is this?   _____

9. A drug is diluted in 100 cc of a 5% Dextrose IV fluid. How many grams of dextrose does this contain?   _____

10. A full 1000 cc IV of 5% Dextrose will contain how much dextrose?   _____

ANSWERS   1. 10 grams   2. 5 grams   3. 20 grams   4. 25 grams   5. 100 grams   6. 10 grams   7. 35 grams   8. 7.5 grams   9. 5 grams   10. 50 grams

Milliequivalent (mEq) Measures

Milliequivalents (**mEq**) is an expression of the number of grams of a drug contained in 1 mL of a normal solution. This is a definition which may be quite understandable to a pharmacist or chemist, but you need not memorize it. Milliequivalent dosages are written using Arabic numbers, with the abbreviation following, for example 30 mEq. You will see milliequivalents used in a variety of oral and parenteral solutions, potassium chloride being a common example.

Express the following milliequivalent dosages using correct abbreviations.

1. sixty milliequivalents   _____
2. fifteen milliequivalents   _____
3. forty milliequivalents   _____
4. one milliequivalent   _____
5. fifty milliequivalents   _____
6. eighty milliequivalents   _____
7. fifty five milliequivalents   _____
8. seventy milliequivalents   _____
9. thirty milliequivalents   _____
10. twenty milliequivalents   _____

ANSWERS 1. 60 mEq 2. 15 mEq 3. 40 mEq 4. 1 mEq 5. 50 mEq 6. 80 mEq 7. 55 mEq 8. 70 mEq 9. 30 mEq 10. 20 mEq

Ratio Measures

Ratio strengths are used primarily in solutions. They represent parts of drug per parts of solution, for example 1 : 1000 (one part drug to 1000 parts solution).

EXAMPLE 1   A 1 : 100 strength solution has 1 part drug in 100 parts solution

EXAMPLE 2   A 1 : 5 solution contains 1 part drug in 5 parts solution

EXAMPLE 3   A solution which is 1 part drug in 2 parts solution would be written 1 : 2

The **more solution** a drug is dissolved in the **weaker the strength** becomes. For example, a ratio strength of 1 : 10 (1 part drug to 10 parts solution) is much stronger than a 1 : 100 (1 part drug in 100 parts solution).

Ratio strengths are always expressed in their simplest terms. For example 2 : 10 would be incorrect, since it can be reduced to 1 : 5. Dosages expressed using ratio strengths are not common, but you do need to know what they represent.

Express the following solution strengths as ratios.

1. 1 part drug to 200 parts solution   _____
2. 1 part drug to 4 parts solution   _____
3. 1 part drug to 7 parts solution   _____

Identify the strongest solution in each of the following.

4. a) 1 : 20   b) 1 : 200   c) 1 : 2   _____
5. a) 1 : 50   b) 1 : 20   c) 1 : 100   _____
6. a) 1 : 1000   b) 1 : 5000   c) 1 : 2000   _____

ANSWERS 1. 1 : 200 2. 1 : 4 3. 1 : 7 4. c 5. b 6. a

Apothecary and Household Measures

The apothecaries' and household are the oldest of the drug measurement systems. Apothecary measures are seldom used today, but you must be aware of their existence, just in case one is. Apothecary dosages are also rarely seen on medication labels, other than for older drugs such as phenobarbital and aspirin. Even if a drug label does contain an apothecary dosage it will always be in conjunction with the metric dosage equivalent.

There is only one apothecary measure for weight, the grain; and three for volume (liquids), the minim, dram and ounce. Their abbreviations/symbols are:

WEIGHT	VOLUME		
grain gr	minim	m	min
	dram	ℨ	dr
	ounce	℥	oz

You may have difficulty remembering the difference between the symbols for dram and ounce. So let's take a minute to clarify these. **An ounce equals 30 mL**, or a full medication cup in case it's easier for you to relate to that. It is the larger of the two measures and the symbol is likewise larger, having an extra loop on top. In fact it almost looks like oz written carelessly ℥. **A dram equals 4 mL**. It just covers the bottom of a medication cup and is therefore very small compared with an ounce. Its symbol is also smaller ℨ. It is important not to confuse these symbols because the large difference in measures, 30 mL for ounce as opposed to 4 mL for dram could make errors very serious.

Once again: ounce = ℥ = 30 mL

dram = ℨ = 4 mL

A **minim** is approximately equal in size to a **drop**, so it is a very small measure.

1 minim = m or min = 1 drop

Three **household** measures still occasionally used are:

tablespoon—T or tbs   teaspoon—t or tsp   drop—gtt

Memorize these if you are not already familiar with them. Be careful not to confuse the single letter abbreviations for table and teaspoon. A tablespoon is larger (15 mL) and is printed with a capital T; the teaspoon, which is smaller (5 mL), is printed with a small t.

Once again: tablespoon = T or tbs = 15 mL

teaspoon = t or tsp = 5 mL

PROBLEM

Write the symbols and/or abbreviations for the following measures.

1. minim _____ _____

2. teaspoon _____ _____

3. ounce _____ _____

4. grain _____

5. dram _____ _____

6. drop _____

7. tablespoon _____ _____

ANSWERS 1. min, m   2. t, tsp   3. ℥, oz   4. gr   5. ʒ, dr   6. gtt   7. T, tbs

Apothecary/Household Notations

The best overall description of apothecary notations is that they are the exact opposite of metric notations. The symbol/abbreviation is placed in front of the quantity, which may be expressed in Arabic numbers, for example gr 2, or Roman numerals, for example gr II. Do you need a refresher in Roman Numerals? One to ten they are: I, II, III, IV, V, VI, VII, VIII, IX, X. In both systems fractional dosages may be expressed as common fractions, for example gr 1/2, except that the symbol s̄s̄ may also be used for one half, gr s̄s̄. All, or none of these rules may be followed, so if you do see an apothecary notation don't expect consistency.

Apothecary/Household to Metric/SI Equivalents Table

When an order is written in apothecary or household measures it will have to be converted to metric, because few drug labels contain apothecary or household dosages. There are two recommended ways to do this. The first is to use an **Equivalents Table**. Most medication rooms/carts should have one. So let's begin by looking at the Equivalents Table in Figure 3. Notice that **liquid** equivalents are on the **left**, and **weights** on the **right**.

APOTHECARY / HOUSEHOLD / METRIC EQUIVALENTS								
Liquid				**Weight**				
oz	mL	min	mL	gr	mg	gr	mg	
1 = 30		45 = 3		15 = 1000		1/4 = 15		
½ = 15		30 = 2		10 = 600		1/6 = 10		
		15 = 1		7½ = 500		1/8 = 7.5		
dr	mL	12 = 0.75		5 = 300		1/10 = 6		
2½ = 10		10 = 0.6		4 = 250		1/15 = 4		
2 = 8		8 = 0.5		3 = 200		1/20 = 3		
1¼ = 5		5 = 0.3		2½ = 150		1/30 = 2		
1 = 4		4 = 0.25		2 = 120		1/40 = 1.5		
		3 = 0.2		1½ = 100		1/60 = 1		
1 min = 1 gtt		1½ = 0.1		1 = 60		1/100 = 0.6		
1T = 15 mL		1 = 0.06		3/4 = 45		1/120 = 0.5		
1t = 5 mL		¾ = 0.05		1/2 = 30		1/150 = 0.4		
		½ = 0.03		1/3 = 20		1/200 = 0.3		
						1/250 = 0.25		

Figure 3

The numbers on this equivalents table, as on most equivalents tables, are small and close together. This contributes to the most common error in the use of equivalents tables, which is to misread from one column to another. For example, if you are converting gr ⅛ to mg, it is not impossible to incorrectly read one line above the correct equivalent, 10 mg, or one line below, 6 mg. To eliminate this possibility **always use a guide to read from one column to the other**. Use any straight edge available and you will see immediately that gr ⅛ is equivalent to 7.5 mg. Very simple, very safe.

PROBLEM

Use the equivalents table in Figure 3 to determine the following equivalent measures.

1. gr ¼   = _____ mg
2. 30 mL   = oz _____
3. 100 mg = gr _____
4. gr ⅙   = _____ mg
5. 60 mg   = gr _____
6. 4 mL   = dr _____
7. gr 7½   = _____ mg
8. oz ½   = _____ mL
9. 300 mg = gr _____
10. 15 mg   = gr _____
11. gr ¹⁄₁₀₀ = _____ mg
12. 0.4 mg = gr _____
13. 2 min   = _____ gtt
14. 30 mg   = gr _____
15. 10 mL   = _____ t
16. 2 T   = _____ mL

ANSWERS 1. 15 mg 2. oz 1 3. gr 1 ½ 4. 10 mg 5. gr 1 6. dr 1 7. 500 mg 8. 15 mL 9. gr 5 10. gr ¼
11. 0.6 mg 12. gr 1/150 13. 2 gtt 14. gr ½ 15. 2 t 16. 30 mL

The Apothecary/Metric Conversion Clock

The second way to remember conversions is to visualize an "apothecary/metric clock." Because 60 mg equal gr 1, and there are 60 minutes in one hour, mg can be used to represent minutes, and fractions of the hour to represent gr. Refer to Figure 4 to see how this works for conversions.

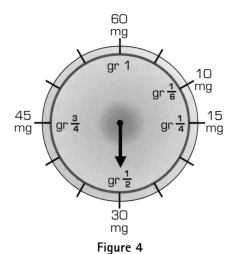

Figure 4

As you can see on this "clock," 60 mg (representing 60 minutes) equals gr 1 (1 hour). It then follows that 30 mg equals gr ½, 10 mg = gr ⅙ and so on. Two hours (gr 2) = 120 mg, and gr 5 = 300 mg. One additional equivalent to remember which does not correspond exactly to the clock is gr 15, which equals 1000 mg (1 gram).

A few moments ago you also learned that 1 oz = 30 mL, 1 dr = 4 mL, 1 T = 15 mL, 1 tsp = 5 mL. Use these equivalents now in the problems on the next page.

PROBLEM

Convert the following to equivalent measures.

1. gr ¾   = _____ mg   6. 300 mg   = gr _____

2. gr ¼   = _____ mg   7. gr ⅙   = _____ mg

3. ½ oz   = _____ mL   8. 10 mL   = _____ t

4. gr 15   = _____ mg   9. dr 1   = _____ mL

5. 8 mL   = dr _____   10. 2 T   = _____ mL

ANSWERS   1. 45 mg   2. 15 mg   3. 15 mL   4. 1000 mg   5. dr 2   6. gr 5   7. 10 mg   8. 2 t   9. 4 mL   10. 30 mL

Summary

This concludes your introduction to the additional measures you will see used in dosages, and in solutions. The important points to remember are:

➡ **international units, abbreviated U, measure a drug by its** action rather than weight

➡ **percentage (%) strengths are used in solutions and ointments**

➡ **percent represents grams of drug per 100 mL of solution**

➡ **the higher the percentage strength, the stronger the solution**

➡ **milliequivalent is abbreviated mEq, and is a frequently used** measure in solutions

➡ **ratio strengths represent parts of drug per parts of solution**

➡ **apothecary measures are so infrequently used that they should be** immediately converted to metric measures to prevent medication errors

➡ **to convert apothecary or household measures to metric, use an** Equivalents Table, or the metric "clock"

➡ **the larger ℥ symbol represents ounce, the smaller ʒ dram**

➡ **T or tbs is the abbreviation for tablespoon (15 mL); t or tsp for** teaspoon (5 mL)

Summary Self Test

DIRECTIONS

Express the following dosages using official symbols/abbreviations.

1. three hundred thousand units   _____

2. forty five units   _____

3. ten percent   _____

4. two and a half percent   _____

5. forty milliequivalents   _____

6   a one in two thousand ratio   _____

7. two ounces   _____

8. three drams   _____

9. one tablespoon   _____

10. seven and one half grains   _____

11. five teaspoons   _____

12. the metric clock equivalent to 60 mg   _____

13. ten units   _____

14. a one in two ratio   _____

15. five percent   _____

16. twenty milliequivalents   _____

17. fourteen units   _____

18. twenty percent   _____

19. two million units   _____

20. one hundred thousand units   _____

ANSWERS 1. 300,000 U 2. 45 U 3. 10 % 4. 2.5 % 5. 40 mEq 6. 1 : 2000 7. 2 oz, ℥ II (varies) 8. ℥ III, 3 dr (varies) 9. 1 T, 1 tbs (varies) 10. gr VII s̄s̄ or gr 7 $^1/_2$ 11. 5 tsp, 5 t (varies) 12. gr I 13. 10 U 14. 1 : 2 15. 5 % 16. 20 mEq 17. 14 U 18. 20% 19. 2,000,000 U 20. 100,000 U

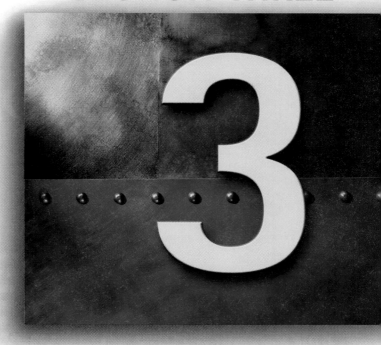

SECTION THREE

Reading Medication Labels and Syringe Calibrations

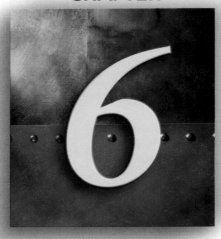
Reading Oral Medication Labels

OBJECTIVES

The student will
1. identify scored tablets, unscored tablets, and capsules
2. read drug labels to identify trade and generic names
3. locate dosage strengths and calculate simple dosages
4. measure oral solutions using a medicine cup

Medication labels contain a variety of information which ranges from simple to complex. In this chapter you will be introduced to labels of oral medications which are generally the least complicated. With this instruction, you will be able to locate drugs and calculate simple dosages without confusion, as well as understand the more complicated labels presented in later chapters.

We will begin with labels for solid drug preparations. These include tablets; scored tablets (which contain an indented marking to make breakage for partial dosages possible); enteric coated tablets (which delay absorption until the drug reaches the small intestine); capsules (powdered or oily drugs in a gelatin cover); and sustained or controlled release capsules (action spread over a prolonged period of time, for example 12 hours). See illustrations in Figure 5.

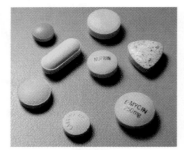

Tablets

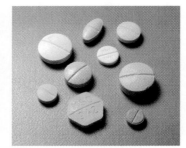

Scored Tablets

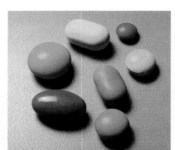

Enteric Coated Tablets

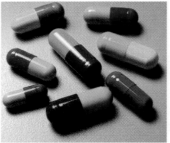

Capsules

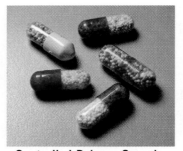

Controlled Release Capsules

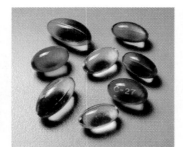

Gelatin Capsules

Figure 5

Tablet and Capsule Labels

The most common type of label you will see in the hospital setting is the **unit dosage label**, in which each tablet or capsule is packaged separately.

EXAMPLE 1

Look at the Lanoxin® label in Figure 6, which is a unit dosage label. The first thing to notice is that this drug has two names. The first, Lanoxin, is its **trade name**, which is identified by the ® registration symbol. Trade names are usually capitalized and printed first on the label. The name in smaller print, digoxin, is the **generic or official name** of the drug. Each drug has only one official name, but may have several trade names, each for the exclusive use of the company which manufactures it. It is important to remember, however, that most labels do contain **both** names, because drugs may be ordered by either name depending on hospital policy or physician preference. You will frequently need to cross check trade and generic names for accurate drug identification.

Next on the label is the **dosage strength**, 250 mcg (written with its SI symbol, μg) or 0.25 mg. The dosage is often representative of the **average dosage strength, the dosage given to the average patient at one time**. This label also identifies the manufacturer of this drug, Burrough Wellcome Co.

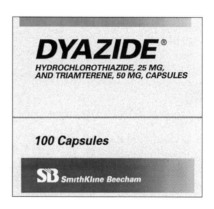

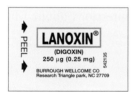

Figure 6   Figure 7

EXAMPLE 2

The Dyazide® label in Figure 7 is **not** a unit dosage label. Notice the "100 Capsules" labeling near the center, which indicates that this package contains 100 capsules. All multiple tablet/capsule packages will list the actual number of drugs they contain, and this must not be confused with the dosage strength. **The dosage strength will have units of measure incorporated with it, for example mg.** Dyazide® actually contains two drugs: hydrochlorothiazide 25 mg, and triamterene 50 mg. These are the generic names, and **each has the dosage incorporated with the name.** It is not uncommon for tablets or capsules to contain more than one drug, and when this is the case, dosages are usually ordered by trade name, in this case Dyazide®, and number of capsules to be administered.

Tablets and capsules which contain more than one drug are ordered by trade name and number of tablets or capsules to be given, rather than by dosage.

EXAMPLE 3

The label in Figure 8 bears only one name, phenobarbital, which is actually the generic name of the drug. This labeling is common with drugs which have been in use for many years. The official (generic) name was so well established that drug manufacturers did not try to promote their own trade names. Also notice that immediately after the drug name are the initials **U.S.P.** This is the abbreviation for **U**nited **S**tates **P**harmacopeia, one of the two official national listings of drugs. The other is the **National Formulary, N.F.** You will see U.S.P. and N.F. on drug labels, and must not confuse this with other initials which identify additional drugs, or specific action of drugs in a preparation.

Next, notice that this label gives the dosage strength of phenobarbital in both metric and apothecaries' units of measure, 15 mg and gr 1/4. Finally, on the right of the label, printed sideways, are the letters "EXP." This represents "expiration," the last date when the drug should be used. Make a habit of checking the expiration dates on labels.

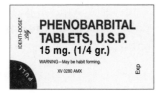

Figure 8

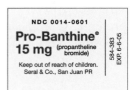

Figure 9

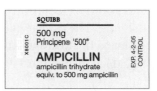

Figure 10

PROBLEM

Refer to the label in Figure 9 and answer the following questions about this drug.

1. What is the generic name? _____

2. What is the trade name? _____

3. What is the dosage strength? _____

4. What is the expiration date? _____

ANSWERS   1. propantheline bromide   2. Pro-Banthine®   3. 15 mg   4. 6-6-05 (2005)

PROBLEM

Refer to the label in Figure 10 and answer the following questions about this drug.

1. What is the generic name? _____

2. What is the trade name? _____

3. What is the dosage strength? _____

4. What is the expiration date? _____

ANSWERS   1. ampicillin trihydrate   2. Principen®   3. 500 mg (If you said the dosage strength was 500 you were only half right. Dosage strengths must **always** be expressed with a unit of measure, in this case mg, 500 mg).
4. expires 4-2-05 (2005)

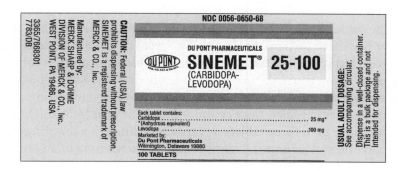

Figure 11

While most drugs are available in the unit dosage format, you may see packages or bottles containing multiple capsules or tablets. The labels are larger, and contain more information. Refer to the Sinemet® label in Figure 11.

Sinemet® is another example of a combined drug tablet. The generic names of the drugs it contains are carbidopa and levodopa. These are listed on the label in several places: directly under the trade name, then with the **amount** of each drug in the fine print at the bottom of the label. Also notice the yellow box to the right of the trade name, which contains the numbers 25–100. This again is the amount of carbidopa–25 mg, and levodopa–100 mg. Contrast this with the Sinemet® labels in Figures 12 and 13.

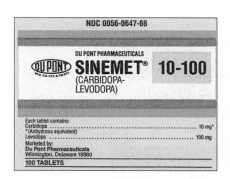

Figure 12

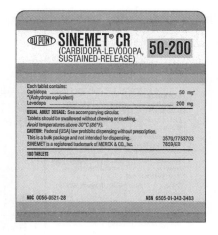

Figure 13

In Figure 12 the dosage strengths are different. A blue box to the right of the trade name identifies the strengths of carbidopa and levodopa as 10 mg and 100 mg, actually a lower dosage. And finally, Figure 13 is a label for Sinemet® **CR**, a **c**ontrolled **r**elease or sustained release tablet, with yet another dosage strength (in the pink box) of 50–200, carbidopa 50 mg, levadopa 200 mg.

 Extra initials after a drug name identify additional drugs in the preparation, or a special drug action.

Unlike the previous combined drug tablet discussed, an order for Sinemet® **must** include the dosage, since it is available in several strengths.

Tablet/Capsule Dosage Calculation

When the time comes for you to administer medications, you will have to read a medication record or Kardex to prepare the dosage. This will tell you the name and amount of drug to be given, but **it will not tell you how many tablets or capsules contain this dosage**. This you must calculate yourself. However, this is not difficult. Most tablets/capsules are prepared in average dosage strengths, and most orders will involve giving one half to three tablets (or one to three capsules, since capsules cannot be broken in half). **Learn to question orders for more than three tablets or capsules.** Although a few drugs require multiple tablets, most do not, and an unusual number could be a warning of an error in prescribing, transcribing, or your calculations.

 Regardless of the source of an error, if you give a wrong drug or dosage you are legally responsible for it.

Let's look at some sample orders and do some actual dosage calculations. Assume that both tablets in our problems are scored and can be broken in half.

PROBLEM

Refer to the Thorazine® label in Figure 14 and answer the following questions.

1. What is the dosage strength? _____

2. If you have an order for 100 mg, give _____

3. If you have an order for 150 mg, give _____

4. If 300 mg are ordered, give _____

5. What is the generic name of this drug? _____

6. What is the total number of tablets in this package? _____

NSN 6505-00-763-5748
Store at controlled room temperature (59° to 86°F).
Dispense in a tight, light-resistant container.
Each tablet contains chlorpromazine hydrochloride, 100 mg.
Dosage: This strength tablet is for use only in severe neuropsychiatric conditions. See accompanying prescribing information.
Important: Use safety closures when dispensing this product unless otherwise directed by physician or requested by purchaser.
Caution: Federal law prohibits dispensing without prescription
Manufactured by
SmithKline Beecham Pharmaceuticals
Philadelphia, PA 19101
Marketed by SCIOS NOVA INC.

100mg
NDC 0007-5077-20

THORAZINE®
CHLORPROMAZINE HCl
TABLETS

100 Tablets

SB SmithKline Beecham

Figure 14

ANSWERS 1. 100 mg   2. 1 tab   3. 1½ tab   4. 3 tab   5. chlorpromazine HCl   6. 100 tab

PROBLEM

Refer to the Cardizem® label in Figure 15 and answer the following questions.

1. What is the dosage strength?   _____

2. If 15 mg is ordered, give   _____

3. If 60 mg is ordered, give   _____

4. If 30 mg is ordered, give   _____

5. What is the generic name of this drug?   _____

6. What is the total number of tablets in this package?   _____

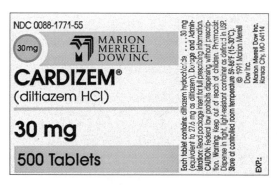

Figure 15

ANSWERS   1. 30 mg   2. ½ tab   3. 2 tab   4. 1 tab   5. diltiazem HCl   6. 500 tablets

It is not uncommon to have a drug **ordered** in one unit of metric measure, for example mg, and discover that it is **labeled** in another measure, for example g. It will then be necessary to **convert the units to calculate the dosage**. This is not difficult because conversions will always be between touching units of measure: g and mg, or mg and mcg. Converting is a matter of moving the decimal point three places.

EXAMPLE 1

Refer to the Tigan® label in Figure 16. A dosage of 0.25 g has been ordered. The label reads 250 mg. Convert the g to mg and you can mentally verify that these dosages are identical. Give 1 capsule.

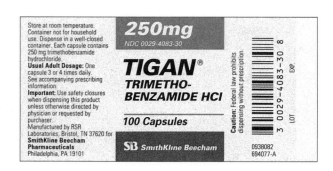

Figure 16

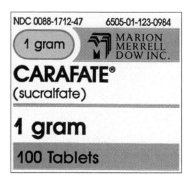

Figure 17

EXAMPLE 2

Refer to the Carafate® label in Figure 17. Carafate® 2000 mg is ordered. The label reads 1 gram. You must give 2 tablets. (1 tab = 1000 mg, so 2000 mg requires 2 tab).

PROBLEM

Locate the appropriate labels for the following dosages, and indicate how many tablets or capsules are needed to give them.

1. Achromycin® V 1 g _____ cap

2. Catapres® 100 mcg _____ tab

3. Tagamet® 0.8 g _____ tab

4. Mevacor® 20 mg _____ tab

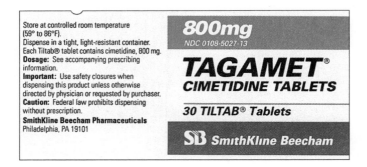

Store at controlled room temperature (59° to 86°F).
Dispense in a tight, light-resistant container.
Each Tiltab® tablet contains cimetidine, 800 mg.
Dosage: See accompanying prescribing information.
Important: Use safety closures when dispensing this product unless otherwise directed by physician or requested by purchaser.
Caution: Federal law prohibits dispensing without prescription.
SmithKline Beecham Pharmaceuticals
Philadelphia, PA 19101

800mg
NDC 0108-5027-13

TAGAMET®
CIMETIDINE TABLETS

30 TILTAB® Tablets

SB SmithKline Beecham

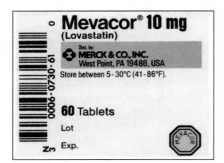

○ **Mevacor® 10 mg**
(Lovastatin)

Dist. by:
MERCK & CO., INC.
West Point, PA 19486, USA
Store between 5 - 30°C (41 - 86°F).

0006-0730-61

60 Tablets

Lot

Z m Exp.

Catapres® .1
(clonidine HCl USP) 0.1 mg
LOT.
EXP.
Boehringer Ingelheim Ltd.
Ridgefield, CT 06877

PEEL TO OPEN

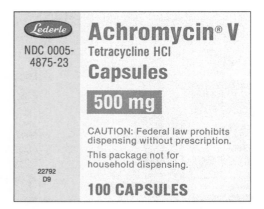

Lederle **Achromycin® V**
NDC 0005-4875-23
Tetracycline HCl
Capsules

500 mg

CAUTION: Federal law prohibits dispensing without prescription.

This package not for household dispensing.

22792
D9

100 CAPSULES

ANSWERS   1. 2 cap   2. 1 tab   3. 1 tab   4. 2 tab

PROBLEM

Locate the appropriate labels for the following drug orders and indicate the number of tablets/capsules which will be required to administer the dosages ordered. Assume that all tablets are scored. Notice that both generic and trade names are used for the orders, and a label may be used in more than one problem.

1. isosorbide dinitrate 80 mg   _____ tab

2. sulfasalazine 0.5 g   _____ tab

3. sulfasalazine 1 g   _____ tab

4. hydrochlorothiazide 25 mg   _____ tab

5. chlordiazepoxide HCl 50 mg   _____ cap

6. Stelazine® 7.5 mg   _____ tab

7. Minipress® 2 mg   _____ cap

8. phenytoin Na 90 mg   _____ cap

9. diphenhydramine HCl 100 mg _____ cap

10. allopurinol 450 mg   _____ tab

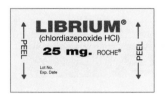

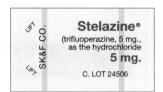

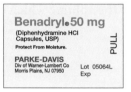

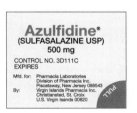

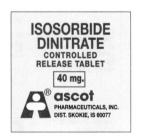

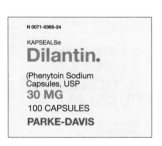

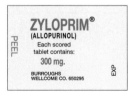

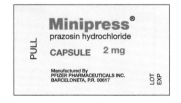

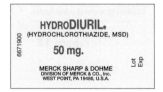

ANSWERS   1. 2 tab   2. 1 tab   3. 2 tab   4. ½ tab   5. 2 cap   6. 1½ tab   7. 1 cap   8. 3 cap   9. 2 cap   10. 1½ tab

Oral Solution Labels

In liquid drug preparations, the weight of the drug is contained in a certain **volume of solution**, most frequently mL or cc's. Let's review dosages in some solid and liquid drug preparations to illustrate the difference.

EXAMPLE 1 **Solid:** 250 mg in **1 tablet**   **Liquid:** 250 mg in **5 mL**

EXAMPLE 2 **Solid:** 100 mg in **1 capsule**   **Liquid:** 100 mg in **10 mL**

Solution strength can also be expressed in ounces, drams, teaspoons, or tablespoons, but these measures are less common. Let's look at some solution labels so that you can become familiar with them.

EXAMPLE 3

Refer to the Tegopen® label in Figure 18. The information it contains will be familiar. Tegopen® is the trade name, cloxacillin sodium is the generic or official name. The dosage strength is **125 mg per 5 mL. As with solid drugs, the medication record will tell you the dosage of the drug to be administered, but rarely will it specify the volume which contains this dosage.**

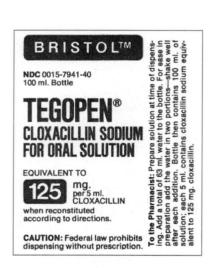

Figure 18   Figure 19

PROBLEM

Refer to the cloxacillin label in Figure 18 again, and calculate the following dosages.

1. The order is for cloxacillin Na soln. 125 mg. Give _____

2. The order is for Tegopen® soln. 0.25 g. Give _____

ANSWERS 1. 5 mL 2. 10 mL If you did not express your answers as mL they are incorrect. Numbers have no meaning unless they are expressed with a unit of measure, in this case mL.

Refer to the Elixophyllin® label in Figure 19 on the previous page, and calculate the following dosages.

1. The order is for theophylline soln. 160 mg. Give _____

2. The order is for Elixophyllin soln. 40 mg. Give _____

3. Theophyllin soln. 80 mg has been ordered. Give _____

ANSWERS 1. 30 mL 2. 7.5 mL 3. 15 mL   Your answers are incorrect unless they include mL as the unit of measure.

PROBLEM

Refer to the solution labels in Figures 20 and 21 and calculate the following dosages.

1. Prozac® soln. 10 mg   _____

2. cefaclor susp. 187 mg   _____

3. Ceclor® susp. 374 mg   _____

4. fluoxetine HCl soln. 30 mg   _____

5. Prozac® soln. 40 mg   _____

6. fluoxetine HCl soln. 20 mg   _____

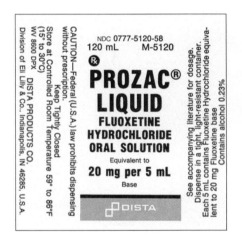

Figure 20

Figure 21

ANSWERS 1. 2.5 mL 2. 5 mL 3. 10 mL 4. 7.5 mL 5. 10 mL 6. 5 mL

Measurement of Oral Solutions

Oral solutions can be measured using a **calibrated medicine cup** such as the one shown in Figure 22. Notice that it contains calibrations in mL (cc), tbs, tsp, dr, and oz. To pour accurately hold the cup at eye level, then line up the measure you need and pour.

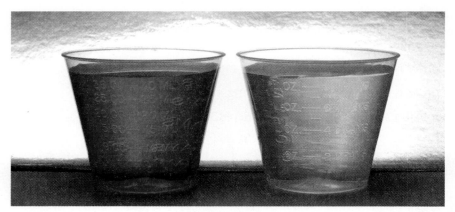

Figure 22

Solutions can also be measured using specially calibrated **oral syringes** such as those illustrated in Figures 23 and 24. Oral syringes have safety features built into their design to prevent their being mistaken for hypodermic syringes. One of these features is color, as illustrated in Figure 23 (hypodermic syringes are not colored, although their packaging and needle covers may be, to aid in identification). A second feature is the syringe tip, which is a different size and shape, and is often off center (termed **eccentric**). Figure 24 illustrates an eccentric oral syringe tip.

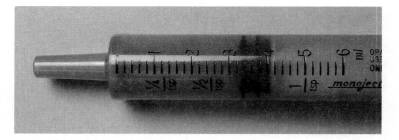

Figure 23

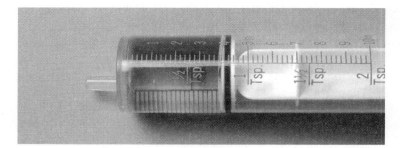

Figure 24

Hypodermic syringes (without a needle) can also be used to measure and administer oral dosages. The main concern with correct syringe identification is that oral syringes, which are **not sterile**, not be confused and used for hypodermic medications, which **are** sterile. This mistake has been made, in spite of the fact that hypodermic needles do not fit correctly on oral syringes. The precaution, therefore, does need to be stressed.

Oral solutions may also be ordered as drops (gtt), and when this is the case the dropper is usually attached to the bottle stopper. It is also common for medicine droppers to be calibrated, for example in mL, or by actual dosage, 125 mg, 250 mg, etc.

Summary

This concludes the chapter on reading oral medication labels. The following are important points to remember:

➡ most labels contain both generic and trade names

➡ dosages are clearly printed on the label, except for preparations containing multiple drugs, which will list the name and dosage of all ingredients

➡ multiple dosage medications will be ordered by trade name and number of tablets/capsules to be given

➡ the letters U.S.P. (United States Pharmacopeia) and N.F. (National Formulary) on drug labels identify their official generic listings

➡ additional letters which follow a drug name are used to identify additional drugs in the preparation, or a special action of the drug

➡ most dosages of oral medications will involve giving one half to three tablets (1–3 capsules, which cannot be broken in half)

➡ check drug expiration dates before use

➡ drug expiration dates are often printed on each label

➡ oral solution dosages are measured in cc's, oz, tsp, tbs, or gtt

➡ for accurate measurement oral solutions are poured at eye level when a medicine cup is used

➡ liquid medications may be measured and administered with an oral syringe, or hypodermic syringe (without the needle)

➡ care must be taken not to use oral syringes for hypodermic medication preparation because these are not sterile

Summary Self Test

Page 62

Summary Self Test

DIRECTIONS

Locate the appropriate label for each of the following drug orders, and indicate the number of tablets/capsules or mL/cc which will be required to administer them. Assume that all tablets are scored, and can be broken in half.

PART I

1. Glucotrol® 15 mg   _____

2. ciprofloxacin HCl 0.5 g   _____

3. verapamil HCl 240 mg   _____

4. Trental® 200 mg   _____

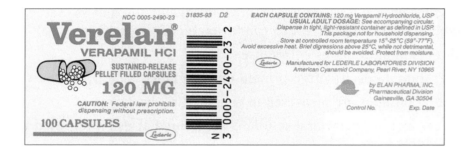

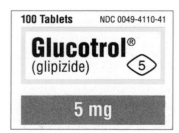

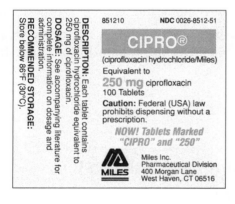

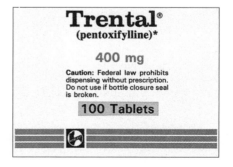

5. Theo-24® 200 mg   _____

6. amoxicillin susp 250 mg   _____

7. Coumadin® 4 mg   _____

8. Calan® SR 240 mg   _____

9. Myambutol® 300 mg   _____

10. phenobarbital 30 mg   _____

11. ZIAC™ 5 mg   _____

12. lithium 600 mg   _____

13. timolol maleate 40 mg   _____

14. captopril 12.5 mg   _____

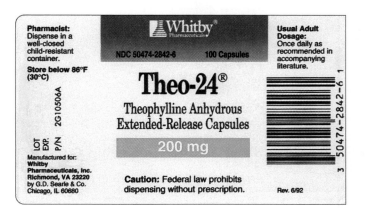

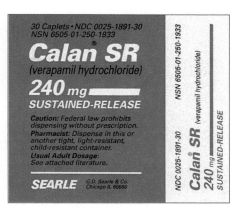

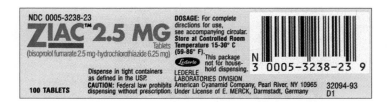

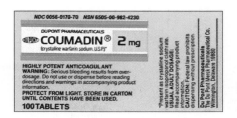

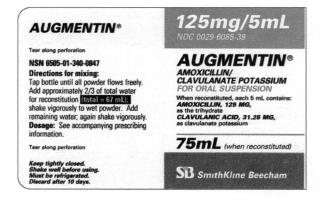

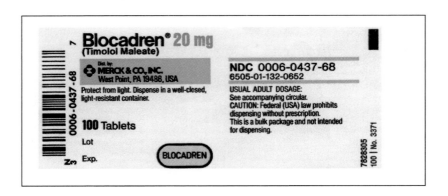

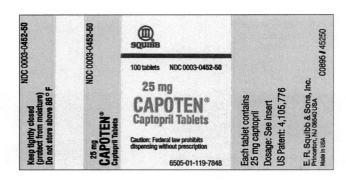

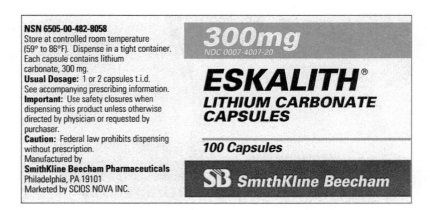

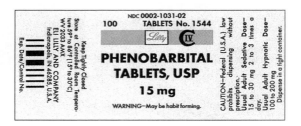

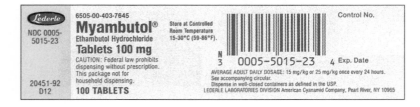

PART III

15. acetaminophen 650 mg   _____

16. Aldactone® 75 mg   _____

17. meclizine HCl 50 mg   _____

18. Reglan® 15 mg   _____

19. propranolol HCl 30 mg   _____

20. metoprolol tartrate 0.15 g   _____

21. nifedipine 10 mg   _____

22. furosemide 10 mg   _____

23. Lasix® 30 mg   _____

24. dexamethasone 3 mg   _____

25. Tenormin® 150 mg   _____

26. terbutaline 2.5 mg   _____

27. Procan® SR 0.75 g   _____

28. Synthroid® 225 mcg   _____

29. DiaBeta® 5 mg   _____

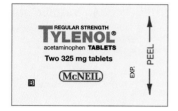

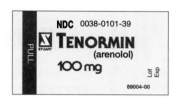

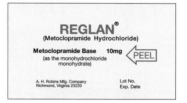

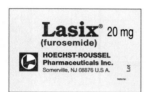

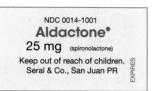

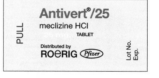

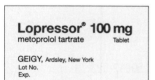

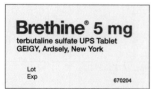

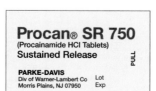

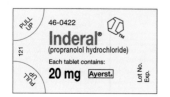

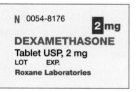

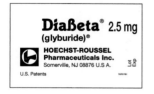

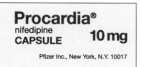

PART IV

30. erythromycin susp 0.25 g _____

31. Percocet® 2 tab _____

32. Flagyl® 0.75 g _____

33. piroxicam 40 mg _____

34. Vasotec® 5mg _____

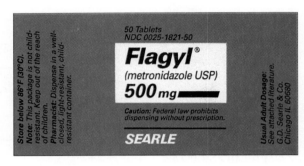

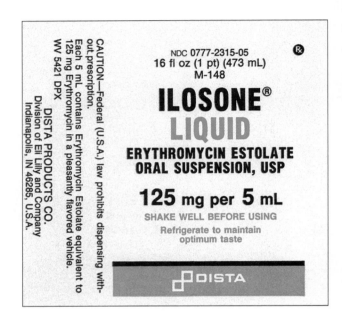

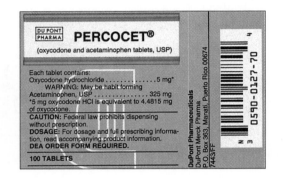

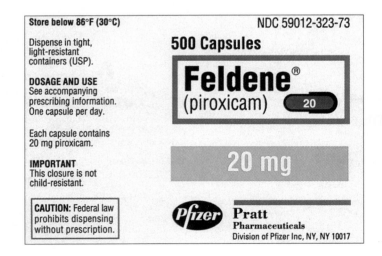

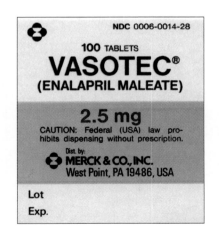

PART V

35. cefaclor oral susp 0.5 g _____

36. spironolactone 100 mg _____

37. Trimox® 0.5 g _____

38. Augmentin® 0.75 g _____

39. Proventil® syrup 4 mg _____

40. Dilantin® 60 mg _____

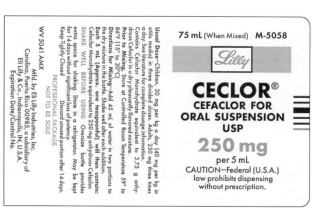

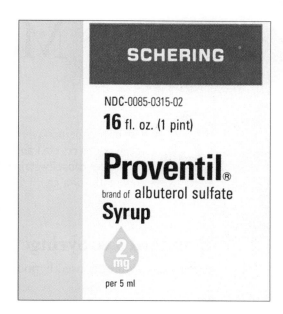

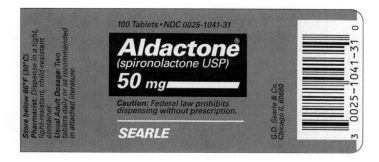

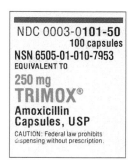

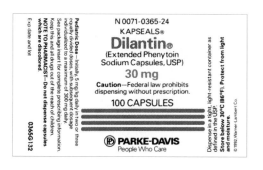

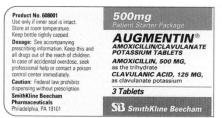

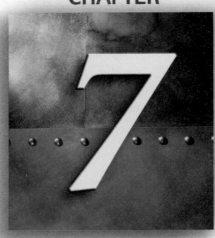

Hypodermic Syringe Measurement

A variety of hypodermic syringes are in common use. Syringes have different capacities (3 cc, 6 cc, 20 cc, etc.) and different calibrations, but **all are calibrated in cc's.** The smaller capacity syringes are further divided into tenths, or two-tenths, or hundredths of a cc.

Standard 3 cc Syringe

The most commonly used hypodermic syringe is the 3 cc size illustrated in Figure 25.

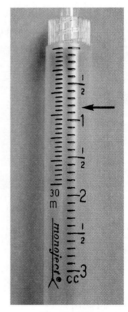

Figure 25

One of the most important things to notice on a syringe is whether or not it still contains the now largely obsolete minim scale of the apothecary system. Notice the minim scale on the left of the 3 cc syringe in Figure 25. It has recently been reported that most incorrect dosage measurements occur from misreading the minim scale rather than the metric scale, which is on the right of the barrel.

If a syringe contains a minim scale care must be taken not to mistake it for the metric scale.

Look at the calibrations on the right side, for metric (cc) measures. **The first thing to notice about any syringe is exactly how many calibrations there are in each 1 cc.** On this 3 cc syringe there are ten calibrations in each cc, which indicates that the syringe is calibrated in tenths. Larger calibrations identify the 0, 1/2 (0.5), and full cc measures. The shorter calibrations between these identify the tenths. For example the arrow in Figure 25 identifies 0.8 cc.

PROBLEM

Use decimal numbers, for example 2.2 cc, to identify the measurements indicated by the arrows on the standard 3 cc syringes in Figure 26.

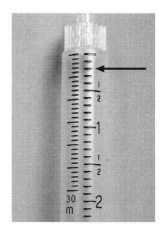 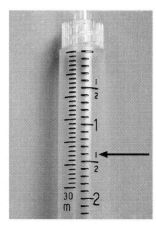 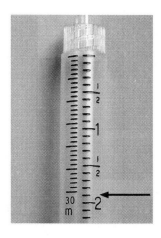

Figure 26

1. _____   2. _____   3. _____

ANSWERS   1. 0.2 cc   2. 1.4 cc   3. 1.9 cc

Did you have difficulty with the 0.2 cc calibration in problem 1? Remember that **the first long calibration on all syringes is zero**. It is slightly longer than the 0.1 cc and subsequent one tenth calibrations. Be careful not to mistakenly count it as 0.1 cc.

You have just been looking at photos of syringe barrels only. Next look at the assembled syringes in Figure 27. Notice that the black suction tip of the plunger has two widened areas in contact with the barrel, which look like two distinct rings. **Calibrations are read from the front, or top ring.** Do not become confused by the second, bottom ring, or by the raised middle section of the suction tip.

PROBLEM

What dosages are measured by the three assembled syringes in Figure 27?

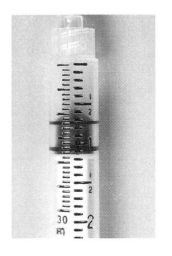
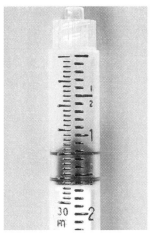
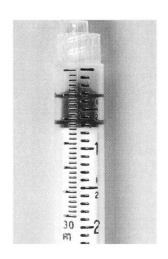

Figure 27

1. _____

2. _____

3. _____

ANSWERS   1. 0.7 cc   2. 1.2 cc   3. 0.3 cc

PROBLEM

Draw an arrow or shade in the following syringe barrels to indicate the required dosages. Have your instructor check your accuracy.

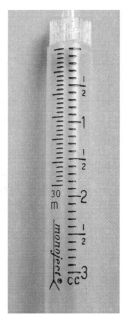
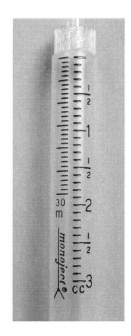
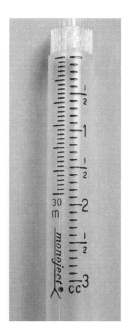

1. 1.3 cc   2. 2.4 cc   3. 0.9 cc

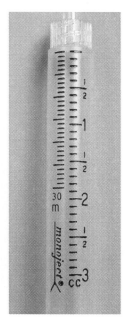   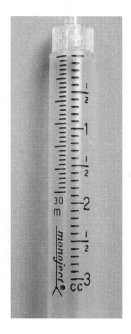   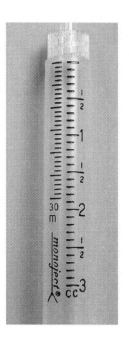

4. 2.5 cc   5. 1.7 cc   6. 2.1 cc

PROBLEM

Identify the dosages measured on the following 3 cc syringes.

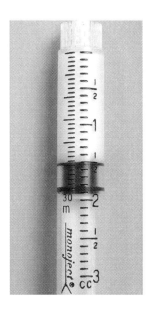   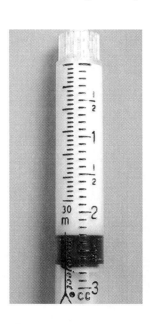   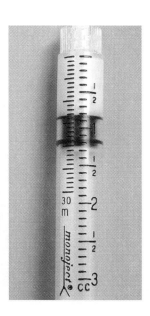

1. _____   2. _____   3. _____

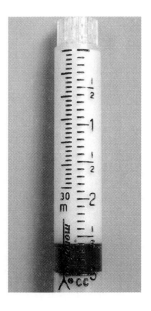 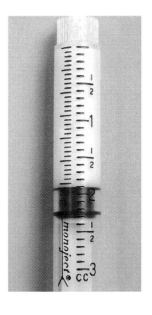 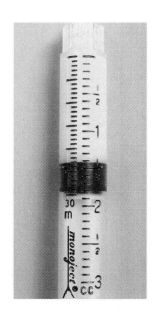

4. _____ 5. _____ 6. _____

ANSWERS 1. 1.5 cc 2. 2.3 cc 3. 0.8 cc 4. 2.6 cc 5. 1.9 cc 6. 1.4 cc

Safety Syringes

A number of new "safety" syringes have been developed in recent years in an effort to reduce the danger of accidental contaminated needle sticks. Several of these syringes are shown in Figure 28. Take a few minutes to read the description of each, as you will in all probability be using them in the clinical setting.

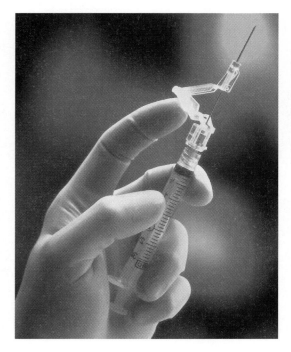

Becton Dickinson's (B-D) "SafetyGlide"™ syringe contains a protective needle guard, which can be activated by a single finger to cover and seal the needle after injection.

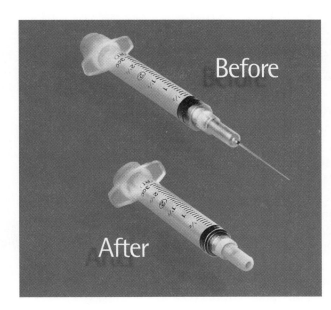

Retractable Technologies "VanishPoint"® needle automatically retracts into the syringe barrel after injection.

Sherwood-Davis & Geck "Monoject® Safety Syringe" contains a protective sheath, which can be used to protect its sterility for transport for injection, and be locked into place to provide a permanent shield for disposal following injection.

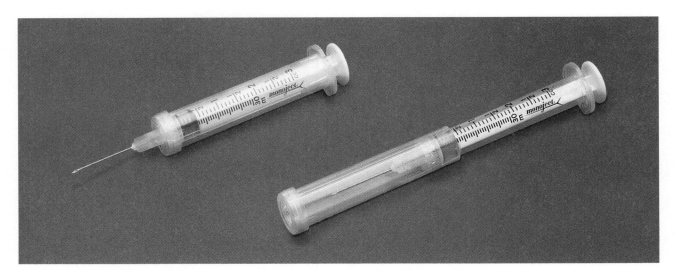

Figure 28

Tuberculin Syringe

When dosages of **small volumes** are necessary they are measured in **hundredths**, rather than tenths, for example 0.27 cc, and 0.64 cc. Pediatric dosages sometimes require measurement in hundredths, as does heparin. A special 1 cc syringe calibrated in hundredths, called the tuberculin (TB), is used for these measurements. Refer to Figure 29.

Once again **first notice there is a 30 minim scale on the left of the barrel**. Then take a close look at the metric scale on the right. As you can see the calibrations are very small and close together. This mandates particular care and an unhurried approach when dosages are measured using this syringe. Notice that the total capacity of the syringe is 1.00 (1 cc), and that **longer calibrations identify zero, and each successive .05 cc**. Also notice that only alternate tenths are numbered: .20, .40, .60 etc., and that the actual calibration which identifies these falls between the 2 and 0, the 4 and 0, and so on. The shorter calibrations measure hundredths. Spend some time examining the calibrations to be sure you understand them. For example, the syringe in Figure 29 measures 0.63 cc.

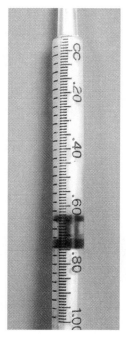

Figure 29

PROBLEM

Identify the measurements on the six tuberculin syringes shown below and on the next page.

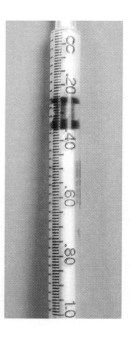
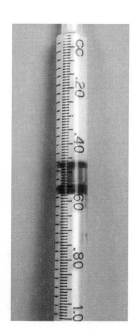
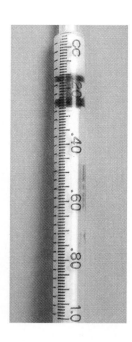

1. _____   2. _____   3. _____

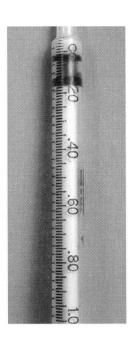

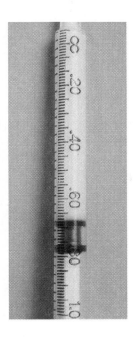

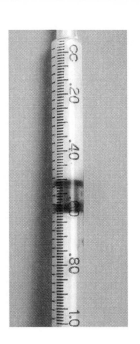

4. _____

5. _____

6. _____

ANSWERS   1. 0.24 cc   2. 0.46 cc   3. 0.15 cc   4. 0.06 cc   5. 0.67 cc   6. 0.50 cc

PROBLEM

Draw an arrow or shade in the barrel to identify the dosages indicated on the following TB syringes. Have your instructor check your answers.

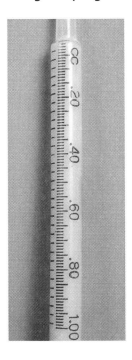

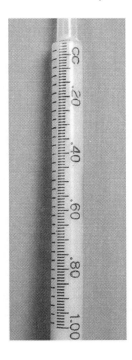

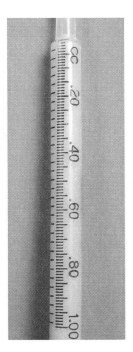

1. 0.28 cc

2. 0.61 cc

3. 0.45 cc

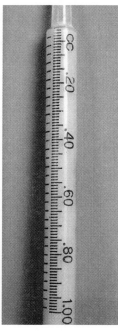
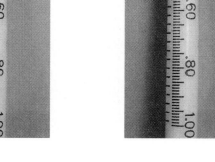
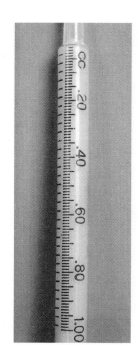

4. 0.12 cc   5. 0.97 cc   6. 0.70 cc

Tubex® and Carpuject® Cartridges

Tubex® and Carpuject® are the trade names of the two most widely used **injection cartridges**. These cartridges come **pre-filled** with sterile medication and are **clearly labeled to identify both drug and dosage**. The cartridges are designed to slip into **plastic injectors**, which provide the plunger for the actual injection. Refer to the Tubex® cartridge in Figure 30, and the Carpuject® cartridge in Figure 31.

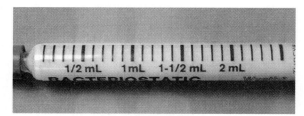

Figure 30

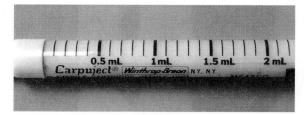

Figure 31

Both cartridges have a volume of 2.5 mL. They are calibrated in tenths, and each 0.5 (1/2) mL has a heavier calibration, which is also numbered. The cartridges are routinely overfilled with 0.1 mL to 0.2 mL of medication to allow for manipulation of the syringe to expel air from the needle prior to injection. The cartridges are designed with sufficient capacity to allow for addition of a second (compatible) drug when combined dosages are ordered.

PROBLEM

Identify the dosages measured on the following cartridges.

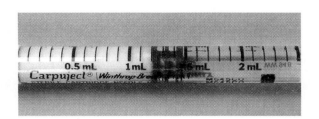

1. _____

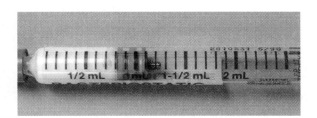

2. _____

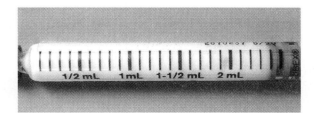

3. _____

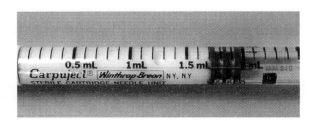

4. _____

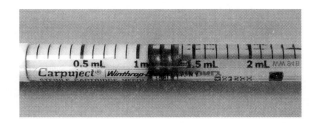

5. _____

6. _____

PROBLEM

Shade in the cartridges to indicate the following dosages. Have your instructor check your answers.

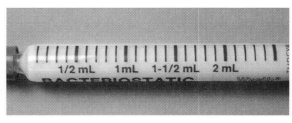

1. 2.5 mL

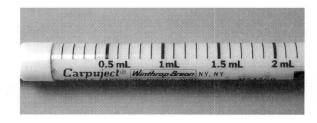

2. 1.4 mL

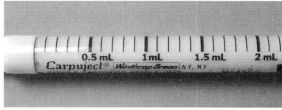

3. This cartridge is pre-filled with 1 mL of medication, and you are to add 0.8 mL of a second drug.
   Total Volume _____

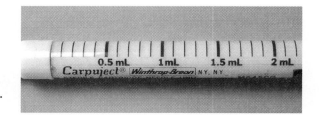

4. The cartridge contains 0.8 mL, and you must add an additional 0.8 mL.
   Total Volume _____

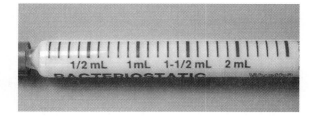

5. The cartridge contains 1.5 mL, and you are to add another 1 mL.
   Total Volume _____

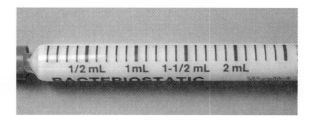

6. The cartridge contains 1 mL, and you must add an additional 1.2 mL.
   Total Volume _____

ANSWERS 3. 1.8 mL 4. 1.6 mL 5. 2.5 mL 6. 2.2 mL

5, 6, 10 and 12 cc Syringes

When volumes larger than 3 cc are required a 5, 6, 10 or 12 cc syringe may be used. Refer to Figure 32 and examine the calibrations between each numbered cc to determine how these syringes are calibrated.

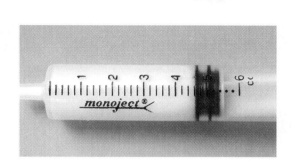
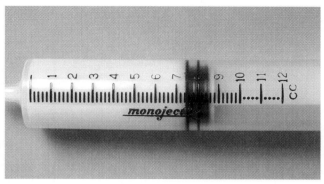

Figure 32

As you have discovered, the calibrations divide each cc of these syringes into **five**, so that **each shorter calibration actually measures two tenths, 0.2 cc.** The 6 cc syringe on the left measures 4.6 cc, and the 12 cc syringe on the right measures 7.4 cc. These syringes are most often used to measure whole rather than fractional cc's, but in your practice readings we will include a full range of measurements.

PROBLEM
What dosages are measured on the following syringes?

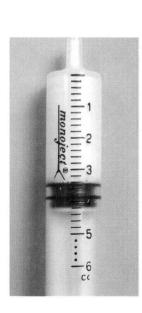
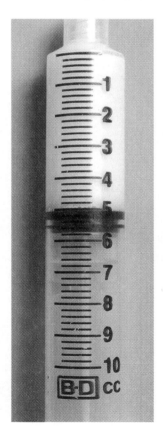
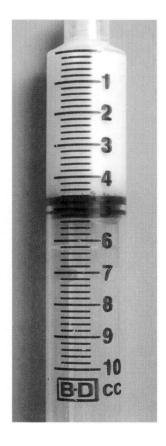

1. _____   2. _____   3. _____

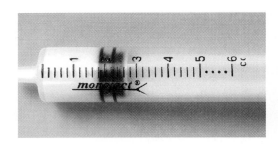

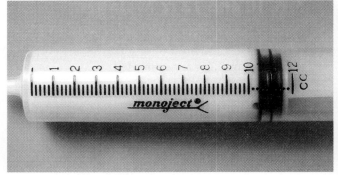

4. _____

5. _____

ANSWERS   1. 3.4 cc   2. 5 cc   3. 4.6 cc   4. 1.8 cc   5. 10.4 cc

PROBLEM

Measure the dosages indicated on the six syringes shown below and on the next page. Have an instructor check your accuracy.

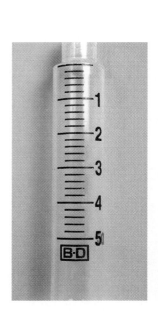

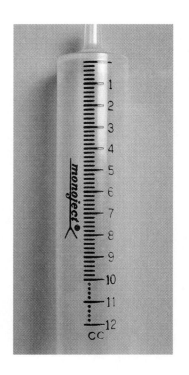

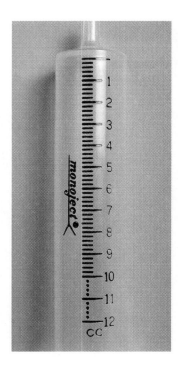

1. 1.4 cc

2. 3.2 cc

3. 6.8 cc

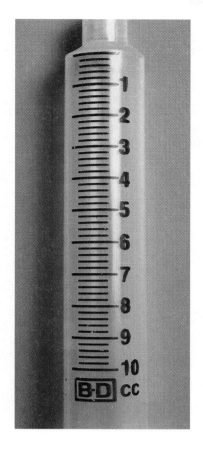

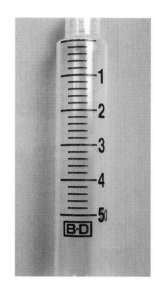

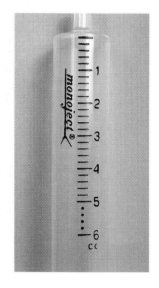

4. 9.4 cc

5. 3 cc

6. 5.6 cc

20 cc and Larger Syringes

Examine the 20 cc syringe in Figure 33 and determine how it is calibrated.

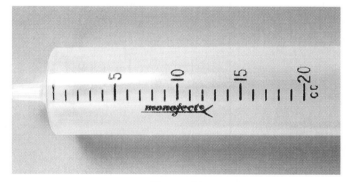

Figure 33

As you can see, this syringe is calibrated in **1 cc increments**, with larger calibrations identifying the 0, 5, 10, 15 and 20 cc volumes. Syringes with a 50 cc capacity are also calibrated in full cc measures. These syringes are used only for measurement of large volumes.

PROBLEM

What dosages are measured on the following 20 cc syringes?

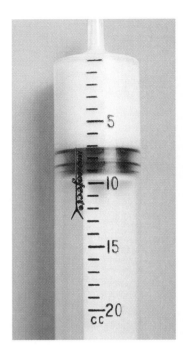
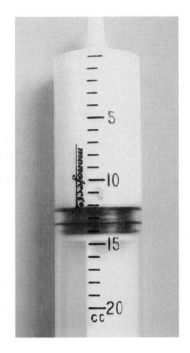
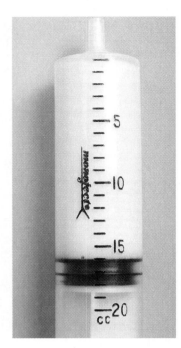

1. _____   2. _____   3. _____

PROBLEM

Shade in or draw arrows on the three syringe barrels shown below and on the next page, to identify the volumes listed. Have your answers checked by your instructor.

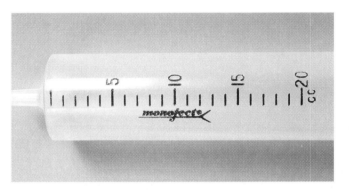

1. 11 cc

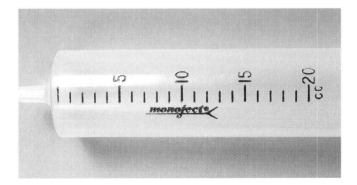

2. 18 cc

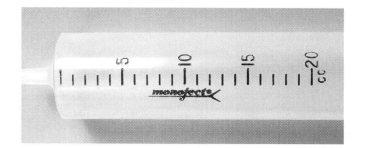

3. 9 cc

Summary

This concludes your introduction to syringe calibrations. The important points to remember from this chapter are:

➡ 3 cc syringes are calibrated in tenths

➡ TB syringes are calibrated in hundredths

➡ care must be taken not to misread the minim scale on 3 mL and TB syringes as the metric scale

➡ 5, 6, 10 and 12 cc syringes are calibrated in fifths (two tenths)

➡ syringes larger than 12 cc are calibrated in full cc measures

➡ the first long calibration on all syringes indicates zero

➡ pre-filled cartridges such as the Tubex® and Carpuject® are overfilled with 0.1 to 0.2 mL of medication to allow for air expulsion from the needle

➡ pre-filled cartridges are sufficiently large to allow for the addition of a second compatible drug

➡ all syringe calibrations must be read from the top, or front ring of the plunger's suction tip

Summary Self Test

DIRECTIONS

Identify the dosages measured on the following syringes and cartridges.

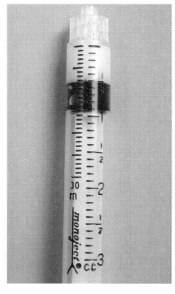

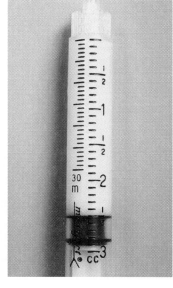

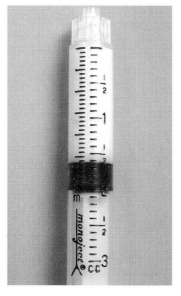

1. _____

2. _____

3. _____

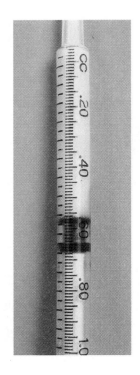

4. _____

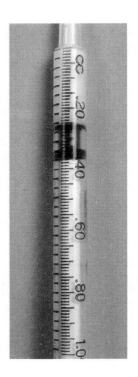

5. _____

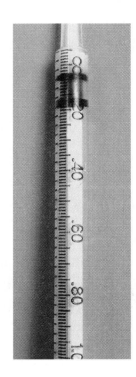

6. _____

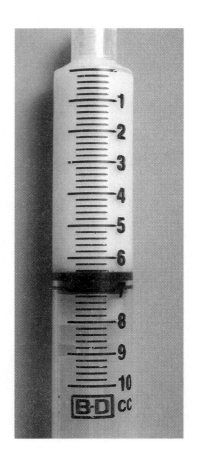

7. _____

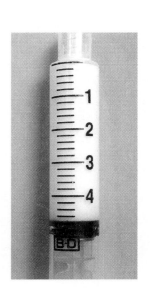

8. _____

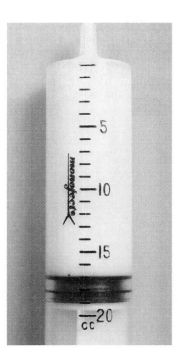

9. _____

10. _____

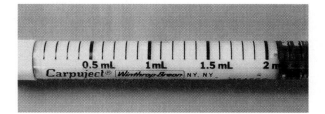

11. _____

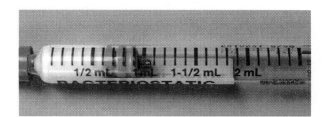

DIRECTIONS

Draw arrows or shade the barrels on the following syringes/cartridges to measure the indicated dosages. Have your answers checked by your instructor.

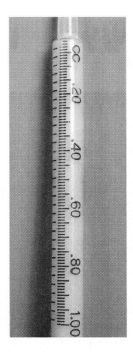

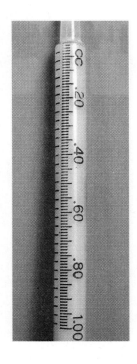

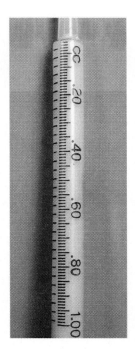

12. 0.52 cc   13. 0.31 cc   14. 0.94 cc

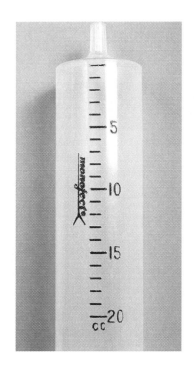

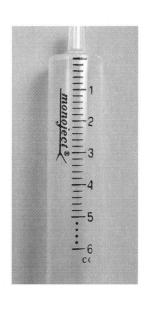

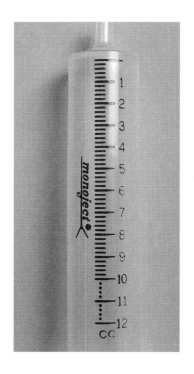

15. 13 cc

16. 1.2 cc

17. 7.6 cc

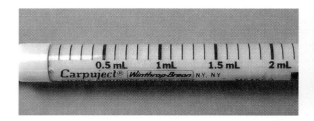

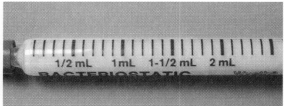

18. 1.1 mL

19. 0.7 mL

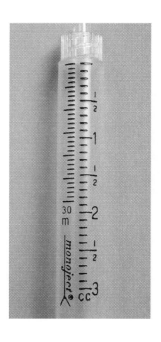

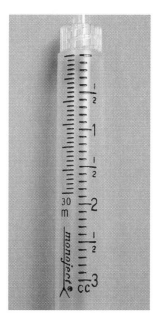

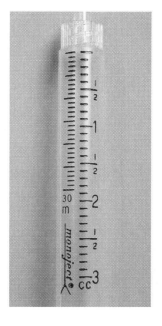

20. 1.7 cc

21. 2.2 cc

22. 0.9 cc

Reading Parenteral Medication Labels

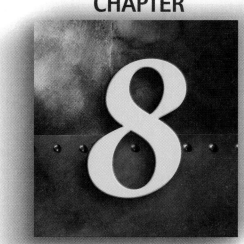

Parenteral medications are administered by injection, the intravenous (IV), intramuscular (IM), and subcutaneous (s.c.) being the most frequently used routes. The labels of oral and parenteral solutions are very similar, but the volume of the average parenteral dosage is much smaller. Intramuscular and subcutaneous solutions in particular are manufactured so that the **average adult dosage will be contained in a volume of between 0.5 and 3 mL.** Volumes larger than 3 mL are difficult for a single injection site to absorb. The 0.5–3 mL volume can be used as a guideline for accuracy of calculations in IM and s.c. dosages. Excessively larger or smaller volumes would need to be questioned, and calculations rechecked.

Intravenous medication administration is usually a two step procedure: the dosage is prepared first, then may be further diluted in IV fluids prior to administration. In this chapter we will be concerned only with the first step of IV drug preparation, which is accurate measurement of the prescribed dosage.

Parenteral drugs are packaged in a variety of single use glass ampules, single and multiple use rubber stoppered vials, and increasingly, in pre-measured syringes and cartridges. See Figure 34.

OBJECTIVES

The student will
1. read parenteral solution labels and identify dosage strengths
2. measure parenteral dosages in metric, milliequivalent, unit, percentage, and ratio strengths using 3 cc, TB, 6 cc, 12 cc, and 20 cc syringes

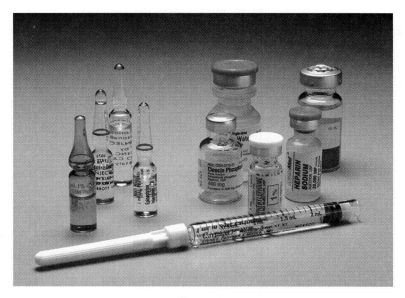

Figure 34
Ampules, vials, and pre-filled cartridge

Reading Metric/SI Solution Labels

We will begin by looking at parenteral solution labels on which the dosages are expressed in metric dosages.

EXAMPLE 1

Refer to the Vistaril® label in Figure 35. The immediate difference you will notice between this and oral solution labels is the **size**. Ampules and vials are small and their labels are small, which requires that they be **read with particular care**. The information, however, is similar to oral labels. Vistaril® is the trade name of the drug; hydroxyzine hydrochloride is the generic name. The dosage strength is 50 mg per mL (in red rectangular area). The total vial contents are 10 mL (in black, upper left). Calculating dosages is not usually complicated. For example if a dosage of Vistaril® 100 mg is ordered you would give 2 mL; if 50 mg are ordered give 1 mL; for 25 mg give 0.5 mL.

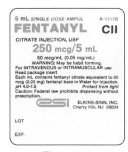

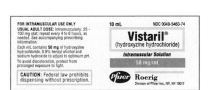

Figure 35   Figure 36   Figure 37

EXAMPLE 2

The Nebcin® (tobramycin) label in Figure 36 has a dosage strength of 80 mg per 2 mL. To prepare an 80 mg dosage you would draw up 2 mL; 40 mg requires 1 mL; and 60 mg would be 1.5 mL.

EXAMPLE 3

The fentanyl citrate solution in Figure 37 has a dosage strength of 250 mcg/5 mL. To prepare a 0.25 mg (250 mcg) dosage you will need 5 mL; for a 0.125 mg dosage 2.5 mL. Once again these simple dosages can be calculated mentally.

PROBLEM

Refer to the Garamycin® label in Figure 38 and answer the following questions.

1. What is the total volume of this vial? _____

2. What is the dosage strength? _____

3. If gentamicin 80 mg were ordered, how many mL would this be? _____

4. If gentamicin 60 mg were ordered, how many mL would this be? _____

5. How many mL would you need to prepare a 20 mg dosage? _____

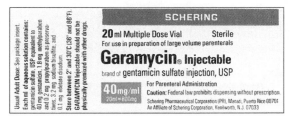

Figure 38

ANSWERS   1. 20 mL   2. 40 mg/mL   3. 2 mL   4. 1.5 mL   5. 0.5 mL

Percent (%) and Ratio Solution Labels

Drugs labeled as **percentage solutions** often express the drug strength in **metric measures in addition to percentage strength**. Refer to the lidocaine label in Figure 39. Notice that this is a 2% solution, and the vial which contains it has a total volume of 5 mL. Also notice that the dosage strength is listed in metric measures: 20 mg/mL. Lidocaine is most often ordered in mg, for example 20 mg requires 1 mL, 10 mg would require 0.5 mL, and 30 mg would require 1.5 mL. However, lidocaine is also used as a local anesthetic and a doctor may request, for example, that you prepare 3 mL of 2% lidocaine, which requires no calculation at all, but simply locating the correct percentage strength, and drawing up 3 mL.

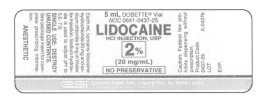

Figure 39

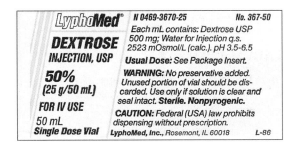

Figure 40

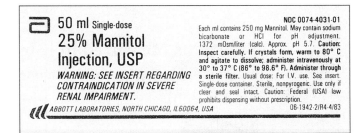

Figure 41

PROBLEM

Refer to the dextrose label in Figure 40 and answer the following questions.

1. What is the percentage strength of this dextrose solution? _____

2. How many mL does the vial contain? _____

3. If you are asked to prepare 20 mL of a 50% dextrose solution, how much will you draw up in the syringe? _____

4. The dosage also appears on this label in metric measures. What is the metric dosage strength of this solution? _____

5. If you are asked to prepare 25 g of dextrose from this vial, what volume will you draw up? _____

Refer to the Mannitol label in Figure 41 and answer the following questions.

6. What is the percentage strength of this solution? _____

7. How many mL does this preparation contain? _____

8. What is the metric dosage strength of this solution? _____

9. If you were asked to prepare a 1 g dosage, what volume would this require? _____

ANSWERS   1. 50%   2. 50 mL   3. 20 mL   4. 25 g/50 mL   5. 50 mL   6. 25%   7. 50 mL   8. 250 mg/mL   9. 4 mL

Parenteral medications expressed in **ratio strengths** are not common, and **when they are ordered it will be by number of cc/mL**. Labels may also contain metric weights.

PROBLEM

Refer to the epinephrine label in Figure 42 and answer the following questions.

1. What is the ratio strength of this solution? _____

2. What volume is this contained in? _____

3. What is the metric dosage strength of this solution? _____

> **1 mL ampule**
>
> **epinephrine HCl**
>
> **1 : 1000**
>
> contains 1 mg epinephrine as
> the hydrochloride in each 1 mL

Figure 42

ANSWERS   1. 1 : 1000   2. 1 mL   3. 1 mg/mL

Solutions Measured in International Units (U)

A number of drugs are measured in **International Units**. The next two labels will introduce you to U labels.

PROBLEM

Refer to the heparin label in Figure 43 and answer the following questions.

1. What is the total volume of this vial? _____

2. What is the dosage strength? _____

3. If a volume of 1.5 mL is prepared, how many units will this be? _____

4. How many mL will you need to prepare a dosage of 55,000 U? _____

5. If 0.25 mL of this medication is prepared, what dosage will this be? _____

Refer to the oxytocin label in Figure 44 and answer the following questions.

6. What is the dosage strength of this solution? _____

7. If a dosage of 10 U is ordered, what volume will you need? _____

8. If a dosage of 5 U is ordered, what volume will you prepare? _____

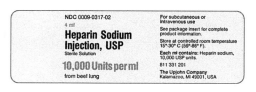

Figure 43

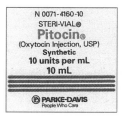

Figure 44

Refer to the insulin label in Figure 45 and answer the following questions.

9. What is the dosage strength of this insulin? _____

10. If 50 U of regular insulin was ordered, how many cc would this require? _____

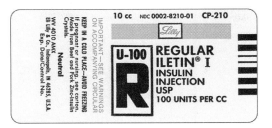

Figure 45

ANSWERS 1. 4 mL 2. 10,000 U/mL 3. 15,000 U 4. 5.5 mL 5. 2500 U 6. 10 U per mL 7. 1 mL 8. 0.5 mL
9. 100 U per cc 10. 0.5 cc

Solutions Measured as Milliequivalents (mEq)

The next four labels will introduce you to milliequivalent (mEq) dosages. Refer to the calcium gluconate label in Figure 46 and notice that this solution has a dosage strength of 0.465 mEq/mL. If a dosage of 0.465 mEq were ordered, you would draw up 1 mL in the syringe.

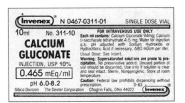

Figure 46

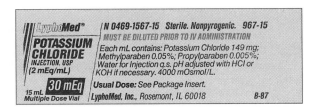

Figure 47

PROBLEM

Refer to the potassium chloride label in Figure 47 and answer the following questions.

1. What is the total volume and total dosage strength of this vial? _____

2. What is the dosage in mEq per mL? _____

3. If you are asked to prepare 30 mEq for addition to an IV, what volume would you draw up? _____

Refer to the potassium chloride label in Figure 48 and answer the following dosage questions. Notice that this label lists the strength of potassium chloride in mg as well as mEq. All of the questions can be answered by careful reading of the label.

4. What is the strength of this solution in mEq per mL? _____

5. If you were asked to prepare 40 mEq for addition to an IV solution, what volume would you draw up in the syringe? _____

6. What is the strength of this solution expressed in mg per mL? _____

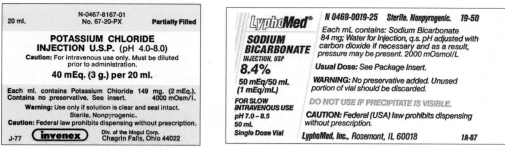

Figure 48   Figure 49

Refer to the sodium bicarbonate label in Figure 49. Notice that this solution lists the drug strength in mEq, percentage, and mg. Read the label very carefully and locate the answers to the following questions.

7. What is the dosage strength expressed in mEq/mL? _____

8. What is the total volume of the vial, and how many mEq does this volume contain? _____

9. What is the strength per mL expressed as mg? _____

10. If you were asked to prepare 10 mL of an 8.4% sodium bicarbonate solution, what volume would you draw up in a syringe? _____

ANSWERS 1. 15 mL/30 mEq   2. 2 mEq/mL   3. 15 mL   4. 2 mEq/mL   5. 20 mL   6. 149 mg   7. 1 mEq/mL
8. 50 mL/50 mEq   9. 84 mg/mL   10. 10 mL

Summary

This concludes the introduction to parenteral solution labels. The important points to remember from this chapter are:

→ the most commonly used parenteral administration routes are IV, IM, and s.c.

→ the labels of most parenteral solutions are quite small and must be read with particular care

→ the average IM and s.c. dosage will be contained in a volume of between 0.5 and 3 mL. This volume can be used as a guideline to accuracy of calculations

→ IV medication preparation is usually a two step procedure: measurement of the dosage, then dilution according to manufacturers' recommendations or doctors' order

→ parenteral drugs may be measured in metric, ratio, percentage, unit, or mEq dosages

→ if dosages are ordered by percentage or ratio strength, they are usually specified in cc/mL to be administered

→ most IM and s.c. dosages are prepared using a 3 cc syringe, or 1 cc tuberculin syringe

Summary Self Test

DIRECTIONS

Read the parenteral drug labels provided to measure the following dosages. Then indicate on the syringe provided exactly how much solution you will draw up to obtain these dosages. Have your answers checked by your instructor to be sure you have measured the dosages correctly.

Dosage Ordered   **mL/cc Needed**

1. Depo-Provera® 0.2 g   _____

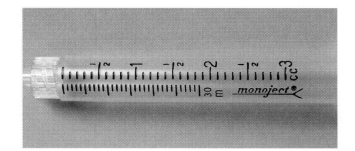

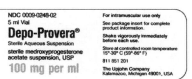

2. furosemide 10 mg   _____

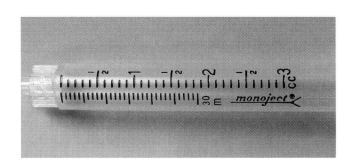

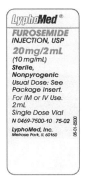

3. heparin 2,500 U   _____

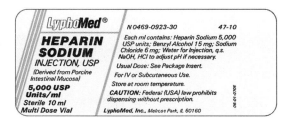

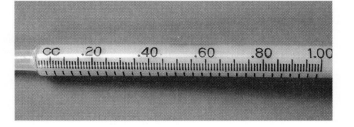

Dosage Ordered	mL/cc Needed

4. Cleocin® 0.9 g _____

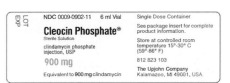

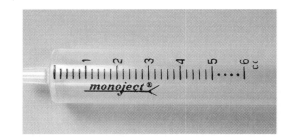

5. atropine 0.2 mg _____

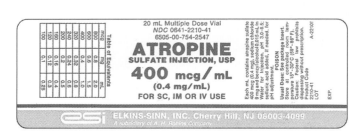

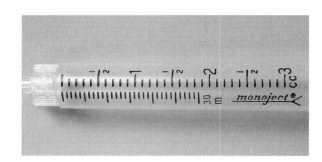

6. hydroxyzine HCl 25 mg _____

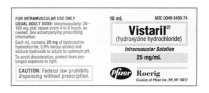

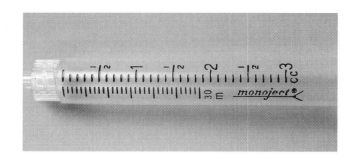

7. Robinul® 100 mcg _____

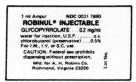

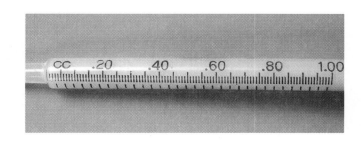

Dosage Ordered	mL/cc Needed

8. Tigan® 200 mg _____

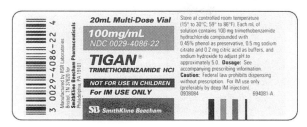

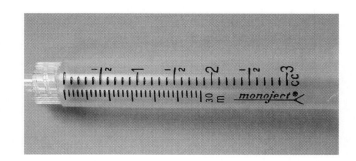

9. aminophylline 0.25 g _____

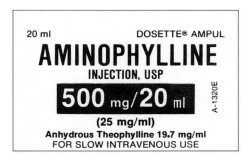

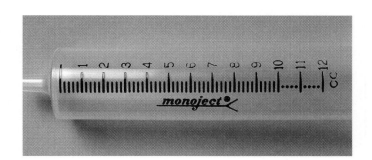

10. cyanocobalamin 1000 mcg _____

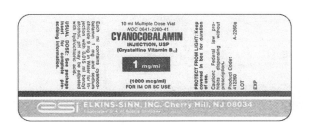

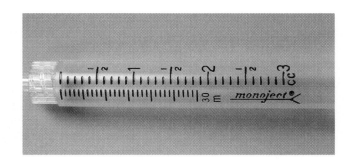

11. tobramycin 30 mg _____

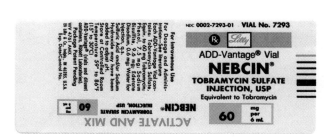

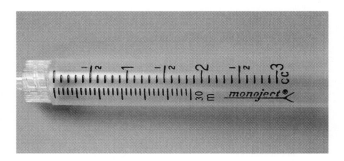

Dosage Ordered	mL/cc Needed

12. amikacin 100 mg   _____

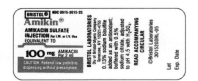

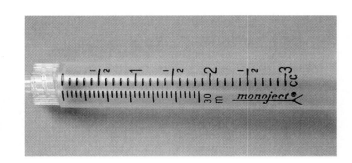

13. Zantac® 75 mg   _____

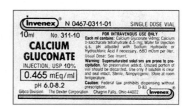

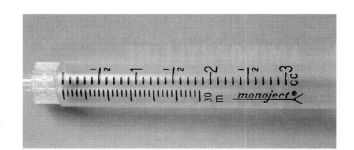

14. calcium gluconate 0.93 mEq   _____

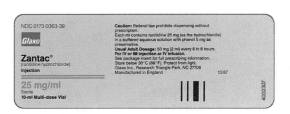

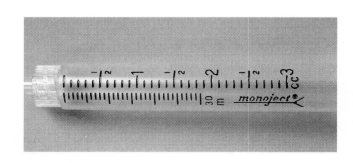

15. diazepam 7.5 mg   _____

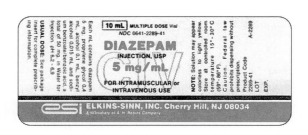

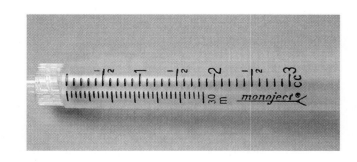

Dosage Ordered	mL/cc Needed

16. heparin 1000 U _____

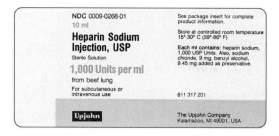

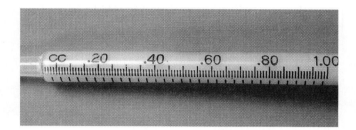

17. perphenazine 2.5 mg _____

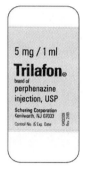

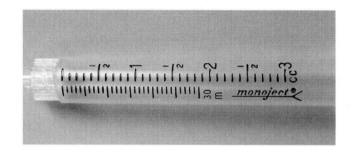

18. phenytoin Na 0.15 g _____

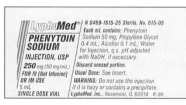

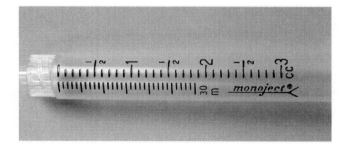

19. medroxyprogesterone 1 g _____

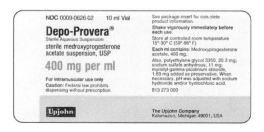

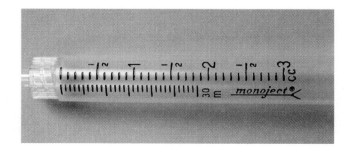

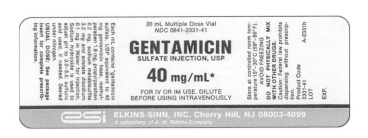

Dosage Ordered   **mL/cc Needed**

20. gentamicin 60 mg   _____

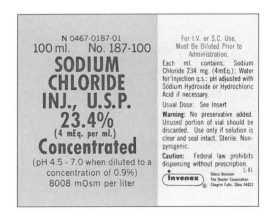

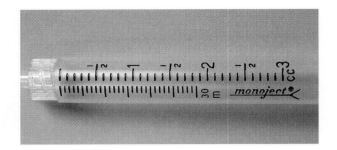

21. lidocaine HCl 50 mg   _____

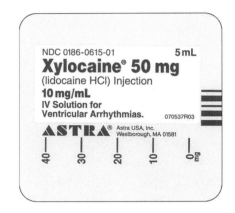

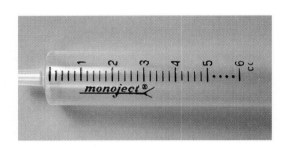

22. sodium chloride 40 mEq   _____

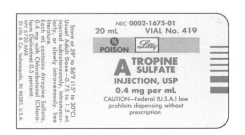

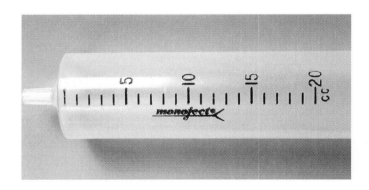

23. atropine 0.4 mg   _____

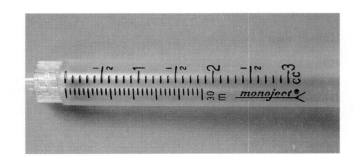

24. meperidine 50 mg   _____

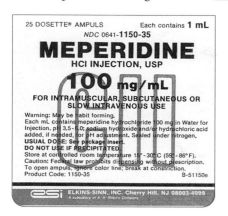

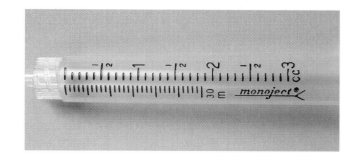

25. cimetidine 150 mg   _____

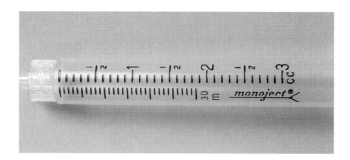

26. clindamycin 0.3 g   _____

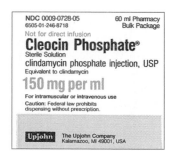

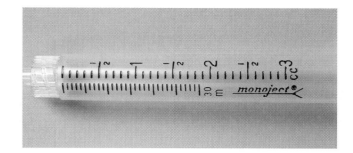

27. morphine sulfate 15 mg   _____

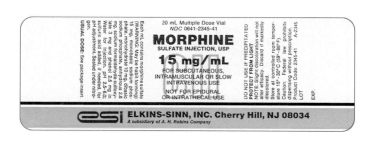

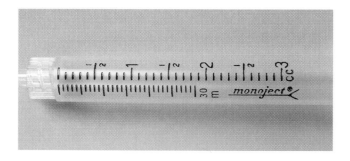

Dosage Ordered	mL/cc Needed

28. Compazine® 10 mg _____

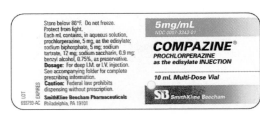

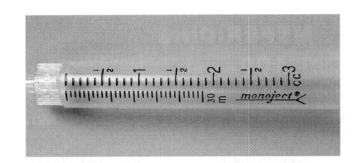

29. nitroglycerin 10 mg _____

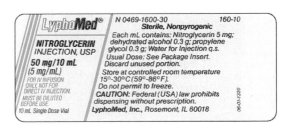

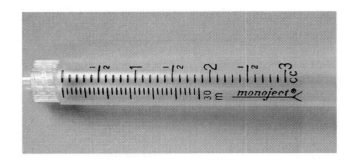

30. doxorubicin HCl 20 mg _____

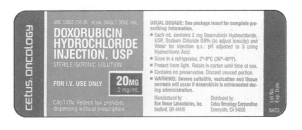

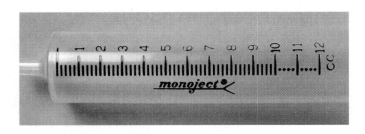

31. meperidine 50 mg _____

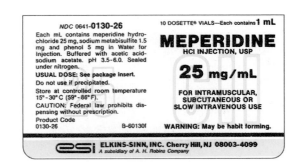

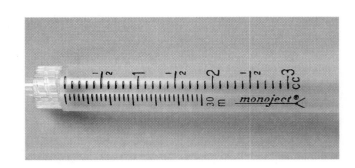

Dosage Ordered	mL/cc Needed

32. methadone HCl 15 mg _____

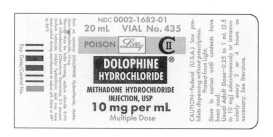
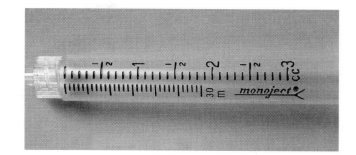

33. Celestone® 12 mg _____

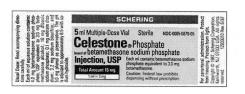
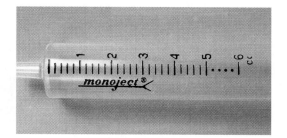

34. naloxone 0.8 mg _____

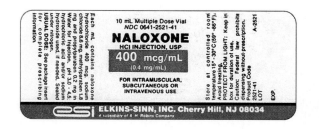
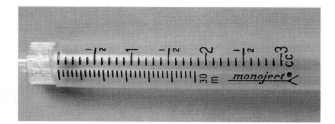

35. dexamethasone 2 mg _____

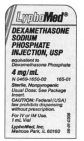
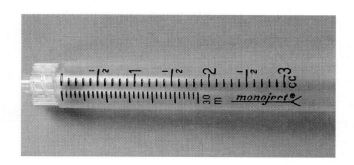

Dosage Ordered	mL/cc Needed

36. chlorpromazine 50 mg _____

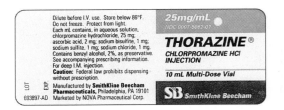

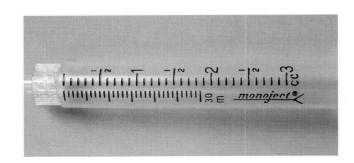

37. Pronestyl® 0.5 g _____

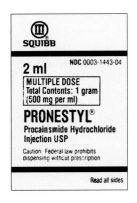

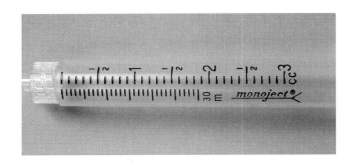

38. Ergotrate® maleate 0.2 mg _____

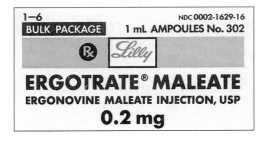

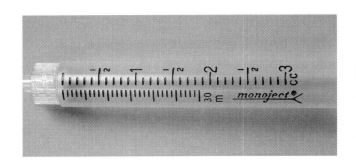

39. morphine 15 mg _____

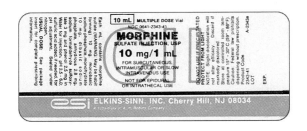

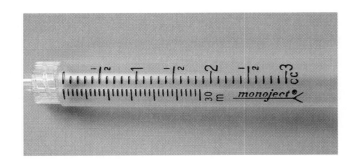

Dosage Ordered	mL/cc Needed

40. Betalin® 0.2 mg _____

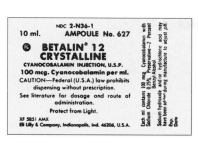

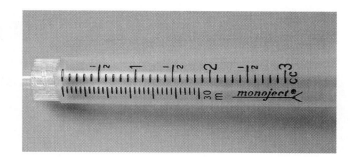

41. Cogentin 1000 mcg _____

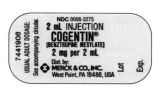

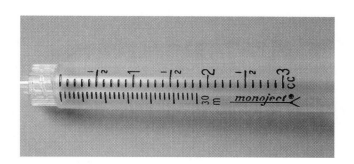

42. Aldomet 125 mg _____

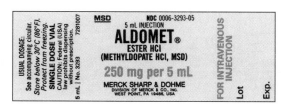

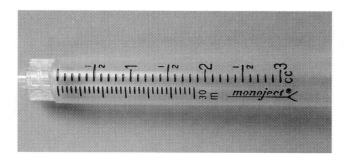

ANSWERS 1. 2 mL 2. 1 mL 3. 0.5 mL 4. 6 mL 5. 0.5 mL 6. 1 cc 7. 0.5 mL 8. 2 mL 9. 10 mL
10. 1 mL 11. 3 mL 12. 2 mL 13. 3 mL 14. 2 mL 15. 1.5 mL 16. 1 mL 17. 0.5 mL 18. 3 mL 19. 2.5 mL
20. 1.5 mL 21. 5 mL 22. 10 mL 23. 1 mL 24. 0.5 mL 25. 1 mL 26. 2 mL 27. 1 mL 28. 2 mL 29. 2 mL
30. 10 mL 31. 2 mL 32. 1.5 mL 33. 4 mL 34. 2 mL 35. 0.5 mL 36. 2 mL 37. 1 mL 38. 1 mL 39. 1.5 mL
40. 2 mL 41. 1 mL 42. 2.5 mL

Reconstitution of Powdered Drugs

The student will
1. prepare solutions from powdered drugs using directions printed on vial labels
2. prepare solutions from powdered drugs using drug literature or inserts
3. determine expiration dates and times for reconstituted drugs
4. calculate simple dosages from reconstituted drugs

Many drugs are shipped in powdered form because they retain their potency only a short time in solution. Reconstitution of these drugs is often the responsibility of hospital pharmacies, but this does not eliminate the need to know how to read and follow reconstitution directions, and how to label drugs with an expiration date and time once they have been reconstituted. The drug label, or instructional package insert, will give specific directions for reconstitution of the drug. Reading these requires care, and this chapter will take you step by step through the entire process.

Reconstitution of a Single Strength Solution

Let's start with the simplest type of reconstitution instructions, for a single strength solution. Examine the label for the oxacillin 2 g vial in Figure 50.

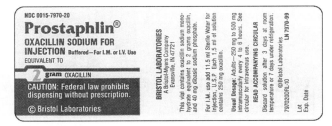

NDC 0015-7970-20

Prostaphlin®
OXACILLIN SODIUM FOR
INJECTION Buffered—For I.M. or I.V. Use
EQUIVALENT TO

2 gram OXACILLIN

CAUTION: Federal law prohibits dispensing without prescription.

© Bristol Laboratories

BRISTOL LABORATORIES
A Bristol-Myers Company
Evansville, IN 47721

This vial contains oxacillin sodium mono-hydrate equivalent to 2 grams oxacillin, and 40 mg dibasic sodium phosphate.

For I.M. use add 11.5 ml Sterile Water for Injection, U.S.P. Each 1.5 ml of solution contains 250 mg oxacillin.

Usual Dosage: Adults—250 mg to 500 mg intramuscularly every 4 to 6 hours. See circular for intravenous use.

READ ACCOMPANYING CIRCULAR

Discard solution after 3 days at room temperature or 7 days under refrigeration.

©Bristol Laboratories

797020DRL-10   LN 7970-99

Lot
Exp. Date

Figure 50

The first step in reconstitution is to locate the directions. They are on this label at the right side, printed sideways. Notice that the instructions read "for IM use add 11.5 mL sterile water." This would be done using a sterile syringe and aseptic technique. The vial is then rotated and upended until **all the medication is dissolved**.

Next, notice the information which relates to the length of time the reconstituted solution may be stored. You are instructed to "discard solution after 3 days at room temperature, or 7 days under refrigeration."

 The person who reconstitutes a drug is responsible for labeling it with the date and time of expiration, and with her/his name or initials.

Let's assume this oxacillin solution was mixed at 2 p.m. on January 3rd. What expiration information would you print on the vial if it is stored in the refrigerator? "Exp (expires) Jan 10th 2 p.m.," which is 7 days from the time mixed. If it is stored at room temperature it must be labeled "Exp Jan 6th 2 p.m.," which is 3 days.

Once the solution is prepared and labeled with your name or initials and the expiration date, you can concentrate on the dosage strength. Notice that the label indicates that "Each 1.5 mL of solution contains 250 mg oxacillin." There is a total dosage of 2 g in this vial, or eight dosages of 250 mg at 1.5 mL each, for a total volume of 12 mL. You added only 11.5 mL to the vial to reconstitute the drug, and the reason for the increased volume is that the powder itself occupies space. **The total volume of the prepared solution will always exceed the volume of the diluent you add**, because it consists of the diluent plus the powder volume. Refer to the dosage strength again, which is 250 mg per 1.5 mL. If a 250 mg dosage is ordered, you would prepare 1.5 mL; for a 0.5 g dosage prepare 3 mL.

PROBLEM

Another medication prepared in powdered form is Kefzol® (cefazolin Na). Refer to the label in Figure 51 and answer the following questions about this medication.

1. How much diluent is added to the vial for reconstitution? _____

2. What type of diluent is used? _____

3. What is the dosage strength per mL of the prepared solution? _____

4. If the order is for 450 mg, what volume must you give? _____

5. What is the dosage strength of the total vial? _____

6. How many mL is the total solution after reconstitution? _____

7. How long will the drug retain its potency at room temperature? _____

8. If the drug is reconstituted at 0800 on Oct 3rd and stored at room temperature, what expiration date will you print on the label? _____

ANSWERS   1. 2 mL   2. sterile water, or 0.9% sodium chloride   3. 225 mg per mL   4. 2 mL   5. 500 mg   6. 2.2 mL   7. 24 hr   8. 0800 Oct 4th.

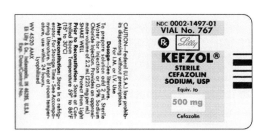

Figure 51

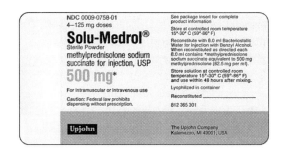

Figure 52

PROBLEM

Read the Solu-Medrol® label in Figure 52 and answer the following questions.

1. What volume of diluent must be used to reconstitute this vial? _____

2. What kind of diluent is specified? _____

3. How long will the reconstituted solution retain its potency at room temperature? _____

4. If the Solu-Medrol® is reconstituted at 11 a.m. Feb 26th, what expiration date and time will you print on the label? _____

5. What else will you print on the label? _____

6. What will be the dosage strength per mL of this reconstituted solution? _____

7. If a dosage of 125 mg of methylprednisolone is ordered, how much solution will you prepare? _____

ANSWERS   1. 8 mL   2. Bacteriostatic Water with Benzyl Alcohol   3. 48 hours   4. Exp 11 a.m. Feb 28th
5. your name or initials   6. 62.5 mg per mL   7. 2 mL

Reconstitution of Multiple Strength Solutions

Some powdered drugs offer a choice of dosage strengths. When this is the case you must choose the strength most appropriate for the dosage ordered. For example, refer to the penicillin label in Figure 53. The dosage strengths which can be obtained are listed on the right.

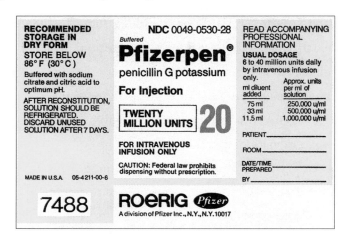

Figure 53

Notice that three dosage strengths are listed: 250,000 U, 500,000 U and 1,000,000 U per mL. If the dosage ordered is 500,000 U, the most appropriate strength to mix would be 500,000 U per mL. Read across from this strength, and determine how much diluent must be added to obtain it. The answer is 33 mL. If the dosage ordered is 1,000,000 U, what would be the most appropriate strength to prepare, and how much diluent would this require? The answer is 1,000,000 U/mL, and 11.5 mL.

Notice that this label does not tell you what type of diluent to use. **When information is missing from the label, look for it on the package information insert which comes with the drug.** Don't start guessing. All the information you need is in print somewhere, just take your time and locate it.

 A multiple strength solution such as this one requires that you add one additional piece of information to the label after you reconstitute it: the dosage strength you have just mixed.

PROBLEM

Refer to the Pfizerpen® label in Figure 53 to answer these additional questions.

1. If you add 75 mL of diluent to prepare a solution of penicillin, what dosage strength will you print on the label? _____

2. Does this prepared solution require refrigeration? _____

3. If you reconstitute it on June 1st at 2 p.m., what expiration date will you print on the label? _____

4. What is the total dosage strength of this vial? _____

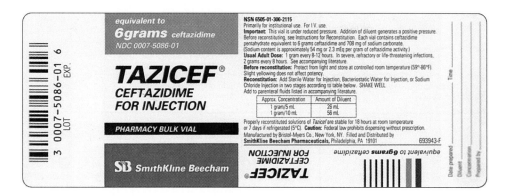

Figure 54

Refer to the Tazicef® label in Figure 54 and answer the following questions.

5. What is the total strength of ceftazidime in this vial? _____

6. What kind of diluent is recommended for reconstitution? _____

7. If you wish to prepare a 1 g/10 mL strength, how much diluent will you add to the vial? _____

8. How much diluent will you add for a 1 g/5 mL strength? _____

9. What is the expiration time for this drug if it is stored at room temperature? _____

10. If you reconstitute this drug at 0915 on April 17th and store it under refrigeration, what will you print on the label? _____

ANSWERS 1. 250,000 U/mL 2. Yes 3. Exp 2 p.m. June 8th 4. twenty million units 5. 6 grams 6. Sterile Water; Bacteriostatic Water; Sodium Chloride 7. 56 mL 8. 26 mL 9. 18 hours 10. Exp 0915 April 24th

Reconstitution from Package Insert Directions

If the label does not contain reconstitution directions, you must obtain these from the information insert which accompanies the vial. The labels for Claforan® in Figures 55 and 56 fall into this category. Refer to these now, and to the portion of the package insert directions reproduced in Figure 57. Notice that the insert instructions are for three vial strengths: 1 g, 2 g and 500 mg, but that only the labels for the 1 g and 2 g vials are included.

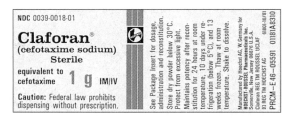

Figure 55

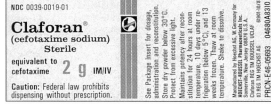

Figure 56

```
Preparation of Solution: Claforan for IM or IV administration should be reconstituted as follows
```

Strength	Amount of Diluent To Be Added (mL)	Approximate Withdrawable Volume (mL)	Approximate Average Concentration (mg/mL)
Intramuscular			
500 mg vial	2	2.2	230
1 g vial	3	3.4	300
2 g vial	5	6.0	330
Intravenous			
500 mg vial	10	10.2	50
1 g vial	10	10 4	95
2 g vial	10	11.0	180

Shake to dissolve, inspect for particulate matter and discoloration prior to use. Solutions of Claforan range from light yellow to amber, depending on concentration. diluent used. and length and condition of storage
For intramuscular use: Reconstitute with Sterile Water for Injection or Bacteriostatic Water for Injection as described above.

Figure 57

PROBLEM

Read the Claforan® labels and package insert provided and answer the questions below on dosage strength and diluent quantities which pertain to them.

Vial Strength	Amount of Diluent	Dosage Strength of Prepared Solution
1. cefotaxime 1 g (prepare for IM injection)	a) _____	b) _____
2. cefotaxime 2 g (prepare for IM injection)	a) _____	b) _____
3. cefotaxime 1 g (prepare for IV administration)	a) _____	b) _____
4. cefotaxime 2 g (prepare for IV administration)	a) _____	b) _____

5. What diluent is recommended for IM reconstitution? _____

6. How long will the solution retain its potency after reconstitution? _____

ANSWERS   1. a) 3 mL b) 300 mg/mL   2. a) 5 mL b) 330 mg/mL   3. a) 10 mL b) 95 mg/mL   4. a) 10 mL b) 180 mg/mL   5. Sterile Water or Bacteriostatic Water   6. 24 hours at room temperature; 10 days if refrigerated below 5°C; 13 weeks frozen

PROBLEM

Refer to the Tazicef® label and insert, on the next page, and answer the following questions.

1. How much diluent must be added to this vial for IV reconstitution? _____

2. What kind of diluent must be used? _____

3. If you reconstitute the drug at 3 p.m. on May 24th and the solution is stored at room temperature, what expiration information will you print on the label? _____

4. What expiration information will you print if the solution is refrigerated? _____

5. What is the concentration per mL of this solution? _____

6. What is the dosage of the total vial? _____

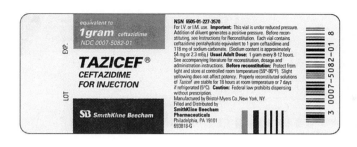

RECONSTITUTION
Single Dose Vials:
For I.M. injection, I.V. direct (bolus) injection, or I.V. infusion, reconstitute with Sterile Water for Injection according to the following table. The vacuum may assist entry of the diluent. SHAKE WELL.

Table 5

Vial Size	Diluent to Be Added	Approx. Avail. Volume	Approx. Avg. Concentration
Intramuscular or Intravenous Direct (bolus) Injection			
1 gram	3.0 ml.	3.6 ml.	280 mg./ml.
Intravenous Infusion			
1 gram	10 ml.	10.6 ml.	95 mg./ml.
2 gram	10 ml.	11.2 ml.	180 mg./ml.

Withdraw the total volume of solution into the syringe (the pressure in the vial may aid withdrawal). The withdrawn solution may contain some bubbles of carbon dioxide.

NOTE: As with the administration of all parenteral products, accumulated gases should be expressed from the syringe immediately before injection of 'Tazicef'.

These solutions of 'Tazicef' are stable for 18 hours at room temperature or seven days if refrigerated (5°C.). Slight yellowing does not affect potency.

For I.V. infusion, dilute reconstituted solution in 50 to 100 ml. of one of the parenteral fluids listed under COMPATIBILITY AND STABILITY.

ANSWERS   **1.** 10 mL   **2.** Sterile Water   **3.** Exp 9 a.m. May 25th   **4.** Exp 3 p.m. May 31st   **5.** 95 mg/mL   **6.** 1 gram

---

Summary

This concludes the chapter on reconstitution of powdered drugs. The important points to remember from this chapter are:

➡ if the label does not contain reconstitution directions these may be found on the vial package insert

➡ the type and amount of diluent to be used for reconstitution must be exactly as specified in the instructions

➡ if directions are given on labels for both IM and IV reconstitution, be careful to read the correct set for the solution you are preparing

➡ the person who reconstitutes a powdered drug must initial the vial and print the expiration date on the label, unless all the drug is used immediately

➡ if a multiple strength solution is prepared the strength of the reconstituted drug also must be printed on the label

---

Summary Self Test

DIRECTIONS

Refer to the nafcillin Na label on page 110, and answer the following questions about reconstitution.

1. What is the total dosage of this vial?   _____

2. What volume of diluent must be used for reconstitution?   _____

3. What will be the dosage strength of 1 mL of reconstituted solution?   _____

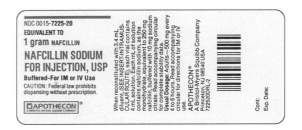

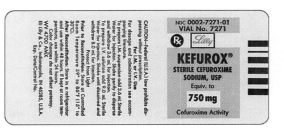

DIRECTIONS

Refer to the Kefurox® label and answer the following questions.

4. What is the total dosage of this vial?   _____

5. How much diluent will you add for IM preparation?   _____

6. How much diluent is recommended for IV preparation?   _____

7. What kind of diluent is to be used?   _____

8. How long will the solution retain its potency if stored at room temperature?   _____

9. If you reconstitute the cefuroxime at 0730 on Nov 1st and it is refrigerated for reuse, what expiration information will you print on the label?   _____

SQUIBB

1 box • 10 vials   NDC 0003-1476-10

250 mg per vial
VELOSEF®
Cephradine for Injection USP

E. R. Squibb & Sons, Inc.
Princeton, NJ 08540
Made in USA

VELOSEF®
Cephradine for Injection USP
Each vial contains 250 mg cephradine with 79 mg anhydrous sodium carbonate; total sodium content is approximately 34 mg (1.5 mEq)
For intramuscular or intravenous use
To prepare IM solution add 1.2 mL sterile diluent. To prepare IV solution add 5 mL sterile diluent. Use solution within 2 hours if stored at room temperature. Solution retains full potency for 24 hours when stored at 5° C.
See insert for detailed information
Usual adult dosage: 500 mg to 1 gram qid—See insert
Caution: Federal law prohibits dispensing without prescription
Store at room temperature; avoid excessive heat
Protect from light   US Patent 3,940,483   M5366F / D7610

DIRECTIONS

Refer to the Velosef® label and answer the following questions.

10. What is the dosage strength of this vial?   _____

11. What volume of diluent must you add to prepare the solution for IM use?   _____

    For IV use?   _____

12. How long will this reconstituted cephradine retain its potency at room temperature?   _____

NDC 0206-8620-11

ZOSYN™

40.5 GRAM

Sterile Piperacillin
Sodium and
Tazobactam
Sodium

Lederle

PHARMACY BULK VIAL

Each vial provides sterile piperacillin sodium and tazobactam sodium cryodesiccated powders equivalent to 36 grams of piperacillin, 4.5 grams of tazobactam and 84.54 mEq (1,944 mg) of sodium.
CAUTION: Federal law prohibits dispensing without prescription.

For IV Use

Contains no preservative.
Reconstitute with exactly 152 mL of a suitable diluent to achieve a concentration of 200 mg/mL of piperacillin and 25 mg/mL of tazobactam. Discard any unused portion after 24 hours if stored at room temperature or after 48 hours if refrigerated.
See package circular for complete directions for use.

Prior to Reconstitution: Store at Controlled Room Temperature 15-30°C (59-86°F). **After Reconstitution: DO NOT FREEZE RECONSTITUTED SOLUTION** See package circular for stability of reconstituted solution.

Control No. _____ Exp. Date _____
Date Prepared _____
Diluent Used _____
Prepared by _____

32324-93 D1
LEDERLE PIPERACILLIN, INC.
Carolina, Puerto Rico 00987

DIRECTIONS

Refer to the Zosyn™ label and answer the following questions.

13. How much diluent is used to reconstitute this solution?   _____

14. What is the total strength of the vial?   _____

15. What is the strength of this Zosyn™ solution per mL?   _____

16. How long will the solution retain its potency at room temperature?   _____

    If refrigerated?   _____

SQUIBB® MARSAM™

1 box • 10 vials   **NDC 0003-0668-05**

5,000,000 units per vial
PENICILLIN G SODIUM
for INJECTION USP

Caution: Federal law prohibits dispensing without prescription

PENICILLIN G SODIUM for INJECTION USP

Each vial provides 5,000,000 units penicillin G sodium with approx. 140 mg citrate buffer (composed of sodium citrate and not more than 4.6 mg citric acid). One million units penicillin contains approx. 2.0 mEq sodium.
Sterile • For intramuscular or intravenous drip use
Usual dosage: See insert
PREPARATION OF SOLUTION: Add 23 mL, 18 mL, 8 mL, or 3 mL diluent to provide 200,000 u, 250,000 u, 500,000 u, or 1,000,000 u per mL, respectively.
Sterile solution may be kept in refrigerator 1 week without significant loss of potency.
Store at room temperature prior to constitution
© 1986 Squibb-Marsam, Inc.

For information contact:
Squibb-Marsam, Inc., Cherry Hill, NJ 08034

Made by Glaxochem, Ltd., Greenford, Middlesex, England.
Filled in Italy by Squibb S.p.A. Dist. by
E. R. Squibb & Sons, Inc., Princeton, NJ 08540   C5277 / 66805

DIRECTIONS

Refer to the penicillin G Na label and answer the following questions.

17. How much diluent must be added to obtain a 250,000 U/mL concentration?   _____

    To obtain a 1,000,000 U/mL concentration?   _____

18. The type of diluent is not specified. Where would you find this information?   _____

19. If this solution is reconstituted at 8:10 p.m. Nov 30th, and stored under refrigeration, what expiration information will you print on the label?   _____

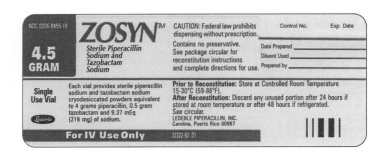

Intravenous Administration
Reconstitute ZOSYN per gram of piperacillin with 5 mL of a suitable diluent from the list provided below. Shake well until dissolved. Single dose vials should be used immediately after reconstitution. Discard any unused portion after 24 hours if stored at room temperature, or after 48 hours if stored at refrigerated temperature [2 to 8°C (36 to 46°F)]. It may be further diluted to the desired final volume with the diluent.

Compatible Intravenous Diluents
0.9% Sodium Chloride for Injection
Sterile Water for Injection
Dextran 6% in Saline
Dextrose 5%
Potassium Chloride 40 mEq
Bacteriostatic Saline/Parabens
Bacteriostatic Water/Parabens
Bacteriostatic Saline/Benzyl Alcohol
Bacteriostatic Water/Benzyl Alcohol
LACTATED RINGERS SOLUTION IS NOT COMPATIBLE WITH ZOSYN
Intermittent Intravenous Infusion - Reconstitute as previously described with 5 mL of an acceptable diluent per 1 gram of piperacillin and then further dilute in the desired volume (at least 50 mL). Administer by infusion over a period of at least 30 minutes. During the infusion it is desirable to discontinue the primary infusion solution.

DIRECTIONS

Refer to the 4.5 g Zosyn™ label and insert, and answer the following questions. Read all information very carefully.

20. How much diluent will be required to reconstitute this medication? _____

21. How many different diluents are listed as being acceptable for reconstitution? _____

22. The package insert specifically lists the name of an IV solution which may not be used as a diluent. Which solution is this? _____

23. Almost all IV medications are further diluted in IV fluids for administration. What does the package insert say about this in regards to administration of Zosyn™? _____

24. The infusion time is also specified on the insert literature. What is it? _____

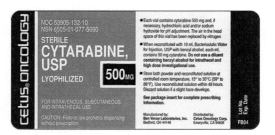

DIRECTIONS

Refer to the cytarabine label and answer the following questions.

25. What is the strength of this medication? _____

26. What diluent must be used for reconstitution? _____

    How much? _____

27. There is a special precaution on the label about a diluent not to be used. What is it? _____

28. How long does the reconstituted cytarabine solution retain its potency at room temperature? _____

DIRECTIONS

Refer to the Fortaz® label and answer the following questions.

29. What type of diluent is recommended for reconstitution? _____
    How much? _____

30. If this drug is reconstituted at 0200 on March 23rd and stored at room temperature, what expiration information will you print on the label? _____

31. If it is stored under refrigeration, what date and time will you print? _____

32. What is the dosage strength of this vial of ceftazidime? _____

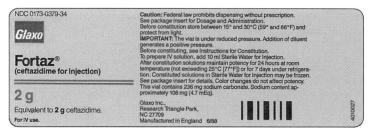

DIRECTIONS

Refer to the vancomycin HCl label and insert preparation directions and answer the following questions.

33. What is the total strength of this vial? _____

34. What is the dosage strength per mL? _____

35. How much diluent must be added to reconstitute this powdered medication? _____

36. What type of diluent? _____

37. How must the reconstituted solution be stored? _____

38. If you reconstituted this medication at 1:15 p.m. on April 15th, what information will you print on the label? _____

39. Prior to IV administration this solution must be further diluted. What minimum amount of additional diluent will be required? _____

40. What time factor is mentioned regarding the IV administration of this drug? _____

PREPARATION AND STABILITY
At the time of use, reconstitute by adding either 10 mL of Sterile Water for Injection to the 500-mg vial or 20 mL of Sterile Water for Injection to the 1-g vial of dry, sterile vancomycin powder. Vials reconstituted in this manner will give a solution of 50 mg/mL. FURTHER DILUTION IS REQUIRED.
After reconstitution, the vials may be stored in a refrigerator for 14 days without significant loss of potency. Reconstituted solutions containing 500 mg of vancomycin must be diluted with at least 100 mL of diluent. Reconstituted solutions containing 1 g of vancomycin must be diluted with at least 200 mL of diluent. The desired dose, diluted in this manner, should be administered by intermittent intravenous infusion over a period of at least 60 minutes.

ANSWERS 1. 1 g   2. 3.4 mL   3. 250 mg   4. 750 mg   5. 3.6 mL   6. 9 mL   7. Sterile Water   8. 24 hours   9. Exp 0730 Nov 3rd   10. 250 mg   11. 1.2 mL; 5 mL   12. 2 hours   13. 152 mL   14. 40.5 g   15. 200 mg   16. 24 hours; 48 hours   17. 18 mL; 3 mL   18. package insert information sheet   19. Exp 8:10 p.m. Dec 7th   20. 22.5 mL (5 mL/g)   21. 9   22. Lactated Ringers soln   23. dilute in at least 50 mL of additional fluid   24. at least 30 min   25. 500 mg   26. Bacteriostatic Water; 10 mL   27. No diluents containing benzyl alcohol   28. 48 hr   29. Sterile Water; 10 mL   30. Exp 0200 March 24th   31. Exp 0200 March 30th   32. 2 g   33. 500 mg   34. 50 mg/mL   35. 10 mL   36. Sterile Water   37. under refrigeration   38. Exp 1:15 p.m. April 29th   39. 100 mL   40. minimum of 60 min

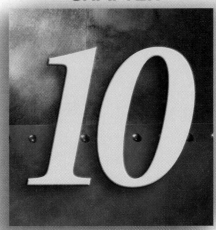

CHAPTER

Measuring Insulin Dosages

OBJECTIVES

The student will
1. distinguish between insulins of animal and human origin
2. discuss the difference between rapid, intermediate and long acting insulins
3. read insulin labels to identify origin and type
4. read calibrations on U–100 insulin syringes
5. measure single insulin dosages
6. measure combined insulin dosages

nsulin dosages are measured in units (U), with the 100 U per cc (U -100) strength being used almost exclusively. Dosages are measured using special insulin syringes which are calibrated to match the dosage strength of insulin being used. For example U -100 syringes are used to prepare U -100 strength dosages. This chapter will show you a variety of U -100 syringes to illustrate how to measure dosages. However, let's begin with an introduction to the types of insulin in use.

Types of Insulin

Insulins are classified by **origin** (animal or human) and by **action** (rapid, intermediate or long acting). The origin or source of insulins is printed on every label, and it is important to know where to locate this information as physicians may specify origin when writing insulin orders. Notice the small print on the Regular insulin label in Figure 58 which identifies its pork (animal) origin, and the Regular insulin label in Figure 59 which identifies its human (recombinant DNA) origin. Also notice how similar these labels are. Careful reading of insulin labels is essential for correct identification. Insulins prepared in multiple use vials are routinely labeled with each patient's name. However this does not eliminate the need to read the label carefully prior to dosage preparation.

Next look at the labels in Figures 60 and 61. Both of these insulins are of human origin

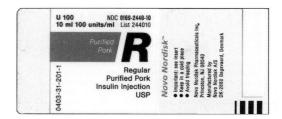

Figure 58

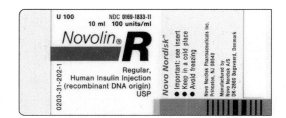

Figure 59

and use the trade name Humulin®. Then notice the initials which follow the trade name: L (Lente®) and U (Ultralente®). These identify the type of insulin by action time. There are three basic action times of insulins. Regular and Semilente® have the most rapid action, beginning in ½ hr, peaking in 2½–5 hr, and ending in 8 hr. In the intermediate range are the Lente® and NPH insulins, beginning in 1½–2½ hr, peaking in 4–15 hr, and ending in 16–24 hr. Among the long acting insulins are the Ultralente® whose action begins in 4 hr, peaks in 10–30 hr, and ends in 36 hr. Another commonly used insulin is the "70/30." This is a combination of 70% NPH and 30% Regular. Insulin types and dosages are prescribed to correlate with life style, diet and activity schedule.

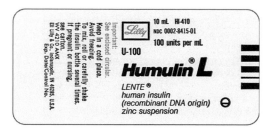

Figure 60

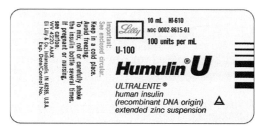

Figure 61

PROBLEM

Identify the type, and origin of each of the insulins from the following six labels.

	Type of Insulin	Origin
1.	_____	_____
2.	_____	_____
3.	_____	_____
4.	_____	_____
5.	_____	_____
6.	_____	_____

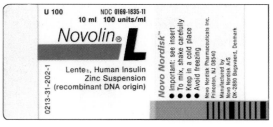

Label 1

Label 2

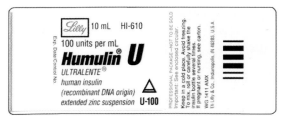

Label 3

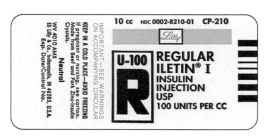

Label 4

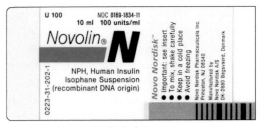

Label 5

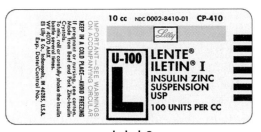

Label 6

ANSWERS 1. Lente®; human   2. NPH; beef and pork   3. Ultralente®; human   4. Regular; beef and pork
5. NPH; human   6. Lente®; beef and pork

U-100 Insulin and Syringes

Refer back to each of the labels you have just read and you will notice that **all have a U-100 strength** (100 U per cc/mL).

 To prepare U-100 insulin dosages you must use a U-100 calibrated syringe.

Refer to the U-100 syringe pictured in Figure 62 and you will notice that it is very small. In order to read the calibrations and number of units it is necessary to **rotate insulin syringes from side to side**. To make it possible for you to practice measuring insulin dosages in this chapter, the syringe calibrations have been flattened out. These are the identical calibrations which appear on the syringes, so your dosage practice will be authentic.

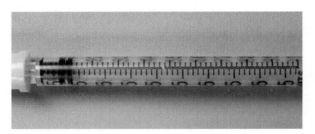

Figure 62

The designation U-100 means that the insulin dosage strength is 100 U per cc. Insulin syringes are calibrated to this 100 U/cc dosage, but they do not all have a 1 cc capacity. There are actually several sizes (capacities) of U-100 syringes in use. The easiest of these to read and use are the Lo-Dose® syringes.

Lo-Dose® Syringes

Lo-Dose® syringes have a capacity of 30 or 50 U. Lo-Dose® insulin syringes do exactly what their name implies: they measure low dosages, but on an enlarged and easier to read scale. This larger scale is an important safety feature for diabetic patients, who frequently have vision problems, as well as for ease of use by medical personnel.

Refer to the calibrations on the 50 U (½ cc) Lo-Dose® capacity syringes in Figure 63 on the next page. Notice that each calibration measures 1 U, and that each 5 U increment is numbered.

PROBLEM

Refer to the syringe calibrations for the 50 U Lo-Dose® syringes below and identify the dosages indicated by the shaded areas.

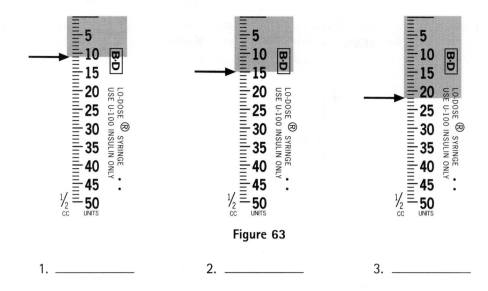

Figure 63

1. _____   2. _____   3. _____

PROBLEM

Use the U–100 Lo-Dose® calibrations in Figure 64 to shade in the following dosages. Have your instructor check your accuracy.

Figure 64

1. 33 U   2. 38 U   3. 18 U

1 cc Capacity Syringes

There are two 1 cc U-100 insulin syringes in common use. Refer to the first of these in Figure 65. Notice the 100 U capacity, and that, in contrast to the Lo-Dose® syringes, only each 10 U increment is numbered: 10, 20, 30, etc. Next notice the number of calibrations in each 10 U increment, which is five, indicating that **this syringe is calibrated in 2 U increments. Odd numbered units are measured between the even calibrations.** For example the shading on syringe 4 identifies 85 U.

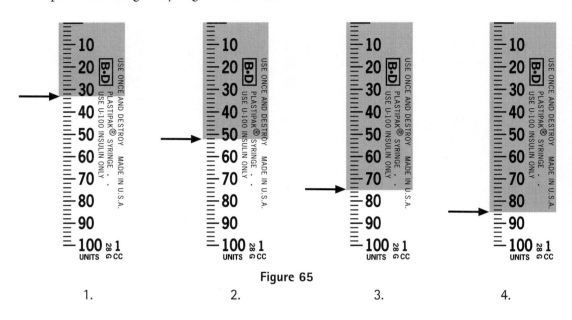

Figure 65

1.   2.   3.   4.

PROBLEM

Identify the dosages indicated on the 1 cc U–100 syringes in Figure 65.

1. _____   2. _____   3. _____   4. _____.

ANSWERS   1. 33 U   2. 52 U   3. 75 U   4. 85 U

PROBLEM

Shade in the syringes in Figure 66 to measure the following dosages.

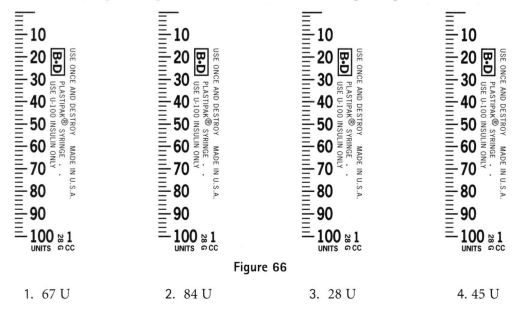

Figure 66

1. 67 U   2. 84 U   3. 28 U   4. 45 U

The second type of 1 cc U-100 syringe is illustrated in Figure 67. Notice that this syringe has a **double scale, the odd numbers are on the left, and the even are on the right**. Each 5 U increment is numbered, but on **opposite sides** of the syringe. This syringe does have a calibration for each 1 U increment, but in order to count every one to measure a dosage the syringe would have to be rotated back and forth, which could cause confusion. There is a safer way to read the calibrations. To measure uneven numbered dosages, for example 7, 13, 27, etc., use the uneven (left) scale only; for even numbered dosages such as 6, 10, 56, etc., use the even (right) scale only. **Count each calibration (on one side only) as 2 U, because that is what it is measuring.**

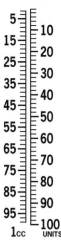

Figure 67

To prepare an 89 U dosage start at 85 U on the uneven left scale, count the first calibration above this as 87 U, the next as 89 U (**each calibration on the same side measures 2 U**).

EXAMPLE 2

To measure a 26 U dosage, use the even numbered right side calibrations. Start at 20 U, move up one calibration to 22 U, another to 24 U, and one more to 26 U (**each calibration is 2 U**).

PROBLEM

Identify the dosages measured on the 1 cc U-100 syringes provided.

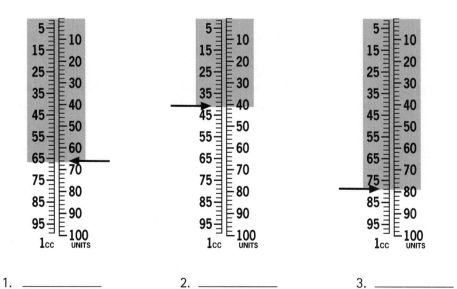

1. _____   2. _____   3. _____

ANSWERS   1. 66 U   2. 41 U   3. 79 U

PROBLEM

Shade in each U–100 syringe provided to identify the following dosages.

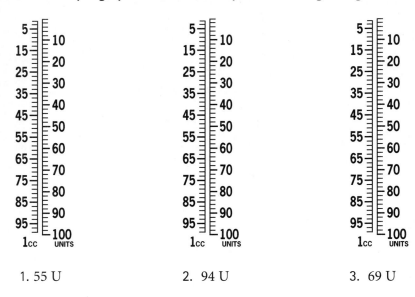

1. 55 U   2. 94 U   3. 69 U

Combining Insulin Dosages

Insulin dependent individuals must have at least one, and sometimes several subcutaneous injections of insulin per day. In order to reduce the number of injections as much as possible, it is common to combine two insulins in a single syringe, for example a short acting with either an intermediate or long acting insulin.

 When two insulins are combined in the same syringe, the regular (shortest acting) insulin is drawn up first.

Both insulins will be withdrawn from sealed 10 mL vials, which requires that an amount of air equal to the insulin to be withdrawn be injected into each vial as a preliminary step. This keeps the pressure inside the vials equalized. An additional step concerns preparation of the insulin itself. Regular insulin does not need to be mixed prior to withdrawal, but intermediate and long acting insulins precipitate out. They need to be rotated and mixed before withdrawal from the vial. **The smallest capacity syringe possible should be selected to prepare the dosage,** as the enlarged scale is easier to read and therefore more accurate.

The actual step by step procedure for combining insulins is as follows:

EXAMPLE 1

A dosage of 10 U of Regular and 48 U of NPH insulin has been ordered.

STEP 1: Locate the correct insulins and rotate the NPH until it is thoroughly mixed.

STEP 2: Use an alcohol wipe to cleanse both vial tops.

STEP 3: The combined dosage (10 U + 48 U = 58 U) requires the use of a 1 cc U-100 syringe. Draw up 48 U of air and insert the needle into the NPH vial. Keep the needle tip above the insulin and inject the air.

STEP 4: Draw up 10 U of air and inject this into the Regular insulin vial. Draw up the 10 U of Regular insulin.

STEP 5: Insert the needle back into the NPH vial and draw up 48 U of NPH insulin. This will require that you draw the plunger back until the total insulin in the syringe is 58 U (10 U Regular + 48 U NPH). Withdraw the needle and administer the insulin promptly so that the NPH does not have time to precipitate out.

EXAMPLE 2

The order is to give 16 U of Regular insulin and 22 U of Lente® insulin.

STEP 1: Locate the correct insulins and rotate the Lente® to mix it.

STEP 2: Cleanse both vial tops.

STEP 3: Use a 50 U capacity syringe (16 U + 22 U = 38 U). Draw up 22 U of air. Insert the needle into the Lente® vial. Keep the needle tip above the insulin as you inject the air into the vial.

STEP 4: Draw up 16 U of air and inject it into the Regular insulin vial. Draw up the 16 U of Regular insulin.

STEP 5: Insert the needle back into the Lente® vial and draw up Lente® insulin until the syringe capacity is 38 U (16 U Regular + 22 U Lente®). Administer the dosage promptly.

PROBLEM

For each of the following combined insulin dosages, indicate the total volume of the combined dosage, and the smallest capacity syringe you can use to prepare it (30 U, 50 U and 100 U capacity syringes are available).

	Total Volume	Syringe Size
1. 28 U Regular, 64 U NPH	_____	_____
2. 16 U Ultralente®, 6 U Regular	_____	_____
3. 33 U Regular, 41 U Lente®	_____	_____
4. 21 U Regular, 52 U NPH	_____	_____
5. 13 U Regular, 27 U Ultralente®	_____	_____

ANSWERS 1. 92 U; 100 U 2. 22 U; 30 U 3. 74 U; 100 U 4. 73 U; 100 U 5. 40 U; 50 U

Summary

This concludes the chapter on measuring insulin dosages. The important points to remember from this chapter are:

➡ insulin labels must be read very carefully as they all look very similar

➡ U–100 insulins are measured using U–100 calibrated syringes

➡ the smallest capacity syringe possible is used to increase accuracy of dosage preparation

➡ calibrations on 30 U and 50 U syringes are in 1 U increments

➡ calibrations on 100 U syringes may be in 1 U or 2 U increments

➡ when insulin dosages are combined the Regular insulin is drawn up first

➡ the intermediate and long acting insulins precipitate out and must be thoroughly mixed before measurement, and administered promptly after measurement

---

Summary Self Test

DIRECTIONS

Use the syringe calibrations provided to measure the following dosages. For combined insulin dosages, use arrows to indicate the exact calibration to be used for each insulin ordered. Have your instructor check your answers.

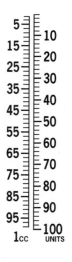

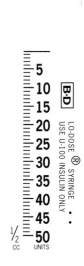

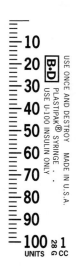

1. 37 U Regular

2. 17 U Regular
    12 U Lente®

3. 48 U NPH

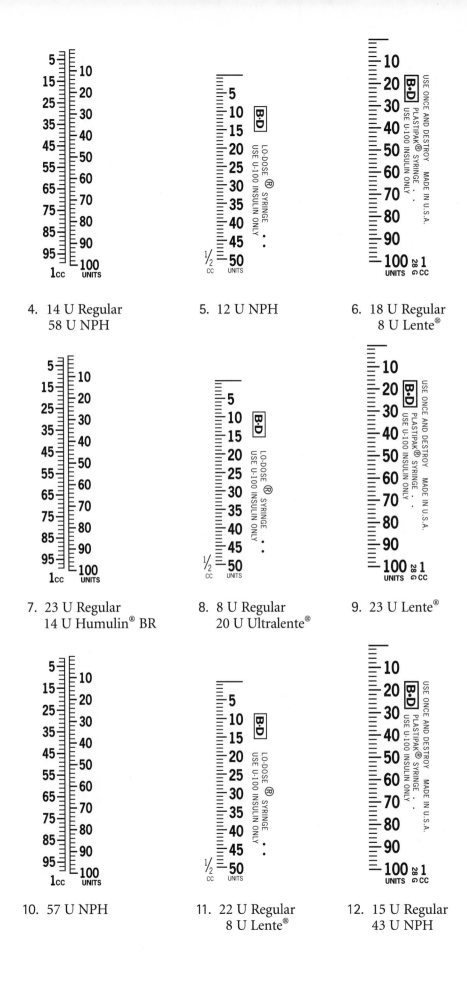

4. 14 U Regular
   58 U NPH

5. 12 U NPH

6. 18 U Regular
   8 U Lente®

7. 23 U Regular
   14 U Humulin® BR

8. 8 U Regular
   20 U Ultralente®

9. 23 U Lente®

10. 57 U NPH

11. 22 U Regular
    8 U Lente®

12. 15 U Regular
    43 U NPH

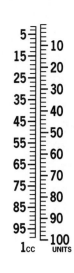
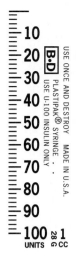

13. 24 U Regular
    27 U Lente®

14. 33 U Regular
    10 U Humulin® L

15. 55 U Regular

DIRECTIONS

Identify the dosages measured on the following syringes.

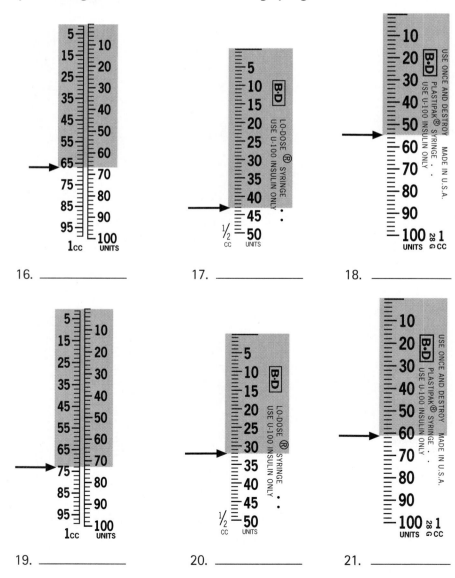

16. _____

17. _____

18. _____

19. _____

20. _____

21. _____

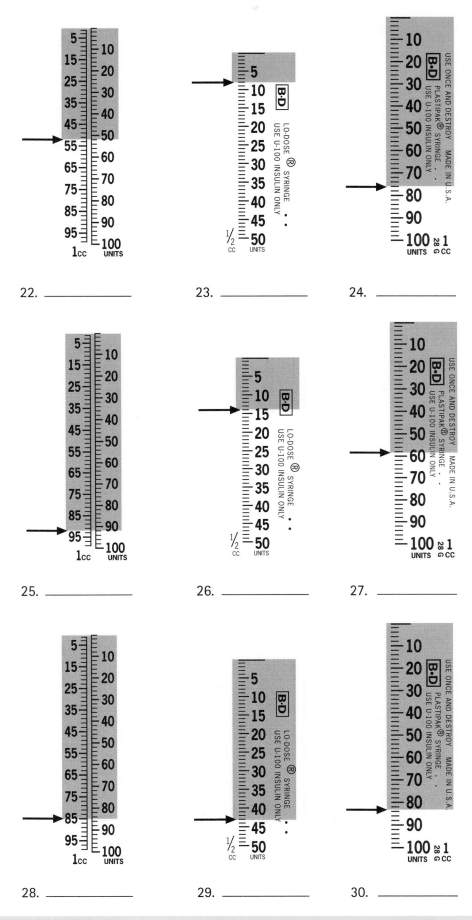

22. _____

23. _____

24. _____

25. _____

26. _____

27. _____

28. _____

29. _____

30. _____

ANSWERS   16. 67 U   17. 43 U   18. 54 U   19. 73 U   20. 32 U   21. 61 U   22. 52 U   23. 8 U   24. 76 U
25. 92 U   26. 14 U   27. 58 U   28. 85 U   29. 43 U   30. 83 U

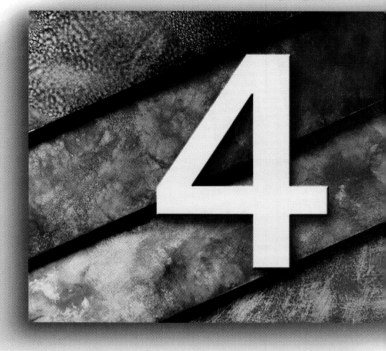

Dosage Calculations

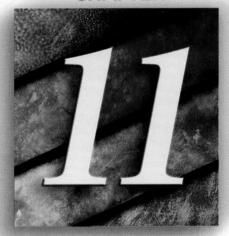

Dosage Calculation Using Ratio and Proportion

OBJECTIVES
The student will
1. define ratio
2. define proportion
3. solve dosage problems using ratio and proportion
4. assess answers obtained to determine if they are logical

PREREQUISITES
Chapters 1–8

Ratios

A **ratio** consists of **two numbers which have a significant relationship to each other**. Earlier in the text you learned how to read the dosage on drug labels. Each of these dosages was expressed as a ratio: a certain weight (strength) of drug in a tablet (tab), capsule (cap), or a certain volume of solution, most commonly mL/cc. For example 50 mg per mL, 100 mcg per tab, 1000 U per mL.

There are **two ways to express (write)** a ratio. The numbers can be **separated by a colon**, or **written as a common fraction**. For example

Separated by a colon		As a common fraction
50 mg : 1 mL	or	$\dfrac{50 \text{ mg}}{1 \text{ mL}}$
100 mcg : 1 tab	or	$\dfrac{100 \text{ mcg}}{1 \text{ tab}}$
1000 U : 1 mL	or	$\dfrac{1000 \text{ U}}{1 \text{ mL}}$

While it is more common to see ratios written with the quantity of drug first as in the above examples, it is equally correct to reverse this order and express the quantity or volume first, as follows

1 mL : 50 mg	or	$\dfrac{1 \text{ mL}}{50 \text{ mg}}$
1 tab : 100 mcg	or	$\dfrac{1 \text{ tab}}{100 \text{ mcg}}$
1 mL : 1000 U	or	$\dfrac{1 \text{ mL}}{1000 \text{ U}}$

 A ratio consists of two numbers which have a significant relationship to each other. It can be expressed with the numbers separated by a colon, or as a common fraction.

PROBLEM

Express the following dosages as ratios using whichever form of ratio you prefer, either common fraction, or separated by a colon. Include the units of measure as well as the numerical value when you write the ratios.

1. An injectable solution which contains 100 mg in each 1.5 mL _____

2. An injectable solution which contains 250 mg in each 0.7 mL _____

3. A tablet which contains 0.4 mg of drug _____

4. Two tablets which contain 450 mg of drug _____

ANSWERS   1. 1.5 mL : 100 mg; 100 mg : 1.5 mL; $\frac{1.5\ mL}{100\ mg}$; $\frac{100\ mg}{1.5\ mL}$ 2. 250 mg : 0.7 mL; 0.7 mL : 250 mg; $\frac{250\ mg}{0.7\ mL}$; $\frac{0.7\ mL}{250\ mg}$ 3. 1 tab : 0.4 mg; 0.4 mg : 1 tab; $\frac{1\ tab}{0.4\ mg}$; $\frac{0.4\ mg}{1\ tab}$ 4. 2 tab : 450 mg; 450 mg : 2 tab; $\frac{2\ tab}{450\ mg}$; $\frac{450\ mg}{2\ tab}$.   If you did not include the units of measure your answers are incorrect.

To complete the balance of this chapter you will need to choose the style of ratio (and proportion) you prefer to use. If you wish to express ratios as a common fraction, for example, $\frac{1\ mL}{50\ mg}$, turn now to page 134 under the heading "Ratio and Proportion Expressed Using Common Fractions." If you prefer ratios separated by a colon continue on this page.

Ratio and Proportion (R&P) Expressed Using Colons

While a ratio is an expression of a significant relationship between two numbers, **a proportion** takes this one step further, and is used **to show the relationship between two ratios**. In a proportion the ratios may be separated by an **equal (=) sign**, or by a **double colon (::)**. For example,

$$1 : 50 = 2 : 100 \qquad \text{or} \qquad 1 : 50 :: 2 : 100$$

The equal (=) sign will be used for all examples of proportion in this text, but you may use the double colon (::) if you prefer this alternate format.

 A true proportion contains two ratios which are equal.

The previous example is a true proportion.

$$1 : 50 = 2 : 100$$

This is a simple comparison, and by using our previous drug strength examples we can mentally verify that the ratios are equal, and that the proportion is true.

EXAMPLE 1   1 **tab** : 50 mg = 2 **tab** : 100 mg

If 1 tablet contains 50 mg, 2 tablets will contain 100 mg.

EXAMPLE 2   1 **mL** : 50 mg = 2 **mL** : 100 mg

If 1 mL contains 50 mg, 2 mL will contain 100 mg.

You can also prove mathematically that these ratios are equal, and that the proportion is true. Look again at example 1.

$$1 \text{ tab} : 50 \text{ mg} = 2 \text{ tab} : 100 \text{ mg}$$

The numbers on the **ends** of the proportion (1, 100) are called the **extremes**, while those in the **middle** (50, 2) are called the **means**.

In a true proportion the product of the means equals the product of the extremes.

If you multiply the means, then the extremes, their products (answers) will be equal.

EXAMPLE 1   1 tab : 50 mg = 2 tab : 100 mg

extremes
1 : 50 = 2: 100
means

$$50 \times 2 = 100 \times 1$$
$$100 = 100$$

The product of the means, 100, equals the product of the extremes, 100. We have now proved mathematically what we previously proved mentally; the ratios are equal, and the proportion is true.

EXAMPLE 2   2 mL : 500 mg = 1 mL : 250 mg

2 : 500 = 1 : 250

$$500 \times 1 = 2 \times 250$$
$$500 = 500$$

The product of the means, 500, equals the product of the extremes, 500. This is a true proportion; the ratios are equal.

EXAMPLE 3   1 mL : 10 U = 2 mL : 20 U

$$10 \times 2 = 20$$
$$20 = 20$$

This is a true proportion.

 It is critical in all mathematics involving proportions that the means and extremes not be mixed up, or an incorrect answer will be obtained.

Here is a memory cue that you can use to prevent confusion. Notice that the **means** are in the **middle** of a proportion. Both of these words begin with an "**m**" (means, middle). The **extremes** are on the **ends** of the proportion. Both of these words begin with an "**e**" (extremes, ends). Use these cues as necessary to prevent mix-ups.

PROBLEM
Determine mathematically if the following are true proportions.

1. 34 mg : 2 mL = 51 mg : 3 mL

2. 15 mg : 4 mL = 45 mg : 12 mL

3. 1.3 mL : 46 mg = 0.65 mL : 23 mg

4. 2.3 mL : 150 U = 1.9 mL : 130 U

5. 40 mg : 1.1 mL = 80 mg : 2.2 mL

6. 0.25 mg : 2 mL = 0.5 mg : 4 mL

ANSWERS 1. True ($2 \times 51 = 102$ and $34 \times 3 = 102$)   2. True ($4 \times 45 = 180$ and $15 \times 12 = 180$)
3. True ($1.3 \times 23 = 29.9$ and $46 \times 0.65 = 29.9$)   4. Not true ($2.3 \times 130 = 299$ and $150 \times 1.9 = 285$)
5. True ($40 \times 2.2 = 88$ and $1.1 \times 80 = 88$)   6. True ($0.25 \times 4 = 1$ and $2 \times 0.5 = 1$)

Dosage Calculation Using R and P Expressed with Colons

Ratio and proportion is important in dosage calculations because it can be used when only **one ratio is known, or complete**, and **the second is incomplete**. Look carefully at the following examples for parenteral dosages, which is where calculations using R and P may frequently be required.

EXAMPLE 1   A solution strength of **8 mg per mL** will be used to prepare a dosage of **10 mg**.

The known ratio is provided by the solution strength available, 8 mg per mL. The incomplete ratio is the dosage to be given, 10 mg, and X is used to represent the mL which will contain 10 mg.

$$8 \text{ mg} : 1 \text{ mL} \quad = \quad 10 \text{ mg} : X \text{ mL}$$

$$\left(\begin{array}{c} \text{complete ratio} \\ \text{drug strength} \end{array} \right) \qquad \left(\begin{array}{c} \text{incomplete ratio} \\ \text{dosage to give} \end{array} \right)$$

 The ratios in a proportion must be written in the same sequence of measurement units.

In the above example they are: mg : mL = mg : mL

Next let's look at the math steps used to determine the value of the unknown, X mL. The math will be familiar because it was covered earlier in the refresher math section.

$8 \text{ mg} : 1 \text{ mL} = 10 \text{ mg} : X \text{ mL}$	check sequence of measurement units; mg : mL = mg : mL
$8 : 1 = 10 : X$	drop the measurement units
$8X = 10$	multiply the means, and the extremes, keeping X on the left of the equation
$X = \dfrac{10}{8}$	divide 10 by the number in front of X
$= \dfrac{10\,^{5}}{8_{4}}$	reduce the numbers by their highest common denominator, 2. Divide the final fraction
$= \mathbf{1.25 \text{ mL}}$	the X in the original proportion was **mL**, so the answer is 1.25 **mL**

The ordered dosage of 10 mg is contained in 1.25 mL

It is routine to check your math twice in dosage calculations. However, it is also necessary to **assess each answer to determine if it seems logical**, and here is where the previous review of relative value of numbers is put to use. Consider the answer just obtained in example 1.

$$8 \text{ mg} : 1 \text{ mL} = 10 \text{ mg} : X \text{ mL}$$

$$X = \mathbf{1.25 \text{ mL}}$$

If **1 mL** contains **8 mg** you will need a **larger** volume than 1 mL to obtain **10 mg**. The answer obtained, 1.25 mL, **is** larger, therefore it is logical. This routine check does not guarantee that your math is correct, but it does indicate that you have not mixed up the means and extremes in your calculations.

Each answer obtained must be assessed to determine if it is logical.

You **can** prove that the proportion is true (and your math correct) by substituting your answer for X in the original proportion.

$$8 \text{ mg} : 1 \text{ mL} = 10 \text{ mg} : \textbf{X mL}$$

$$8 \text{ mg} : 1 \text{ mL} = 10 \text{ mg} : \textbf{1.25 mL}$$

$$10 = 8 \times 1.25$$

$$10 = 10$$

You have now proved mathematically that your answer is correct. **However, in most routine calculations it is neither necessary nor practical to mathematically prove each answer you obtain.** Dosages such as the 1.25 mL in our example are most often rounded to the nearest tenth (1.25 = 1.3 mL). Once this is done, the math proofing the answer may contain small discrepancies which could cause confusion.

| EXAMPLE 2 | The dosage strength available is **25 mg in 1.5 mL**. A dosage of **20 mg** has been ordered. |

$$25 \text{ mg} : 1.5 \text{ mL} = 20 \text{ mg} : \text{X mL}$$ make sure the units are in the same sequence: mg : mL = mg : mL

$$25 : 1.5 = 20 : X$$ drop the measurement units

$$25X = 1.5 \times 20$$ multiply the means, and the extremes; keep X on the left

$$= \frac{30}{25}$$ divide by the number in front of X

$$= \frac{30^{6}}{25_{5}} = 1.2$$ reduce by 5, and divide the final fraction

$$X = \textbf{1.2 mL}$$

The dosage ordered, 20 mg, is a smaller amount of drug than the strength available, 25 mg (in 1.5 mL). So the answer should be smaller than 1.5 mL, and it is, 1.2 mL.

| EXAMPLE 3 | A dosage of **200 mg** must be prepared from a solution strength of **80 mg per mL**. |

$$80 \text{ mg} : 1 \text{ mL} = 200 \text{ mg} : \text{X mL}$$

$$80X = 200$$

$$\frac{200^{5}}{80_{2}} = \frac{5}{2} = \textbf{2.5 mL}$$

The original unknown, X, was mL, so the answer must be mL. The dosage ordered, 200 mg, is larger than the 80 mg per mL strength being used, so it must be contained in more than 1 mL. The answer, 2.5 mL, is larger. Therefore it is logical.

As soon as you are comfortable with the math steps in ratio and proportion you can combine several steps at once, and work even more efficiently. You may already have been doing this, but here are a few examples to demonstrate the short cuts.

EXAMPLE 4   A **300 mg in 1.2 mL** solution will be used to prepare a dosage of **120 mg**.

300 mg : 1.2 mL = 120 mg : X mL   set up the proportion with the known ratios written first

$$X = \frac{1.2 \times 120}{300}$$

multiply the means, and **immediately** divide by the number in front of X

$$\frac{1.2 \times \overset{2}{120}}{\underset{5}{300}} = \frac{2.4}{5} = 0.48 = \textbf{0.5 mL}$$ reduce (by 60). Do final division. Round to nearest tenth.

A dosage of 120 mg will require 0.5 mL

EXAMPLE 5   Prepare a **2 mg** dosage using a **1.5 mg in 0.5 mL** solution.

1.5 mg : 0.5 mL = 2 mg : X mL

$$X = \frac{\overset{1}{0.5} \times 2}{\underset{3}{1.5}} = 0.66 = \textbf{0.7 mL}$$

A dosage of 2 mg will require 0.7 mL

EXAMPLE 6   A **120 mg** dosage is ordered. The solution available is labeled **80 mg/mL**.

80 mg : 1 mL = 120 mg : X mL

$$X = \frac{\overset{3}{120}}{\underset{2}{80}} = \textbf{1.5 mL}$$

A volume of 1.5 mL is necessary to prepare this 120 mg dosage

PROBLEM

Calculate the following dosages. Express answers to the nearest tenth, including the appropriate unit of measure. Assess your answers to determine if they are logical.

1. A dosage of 24 mg has been ordered. The solution strength available is 12.5 mg in 1.5 mL.   _____

2. A 40 mg/2.5 mL solution will be used to prepare a 30 mg dosage.   _____

3. Prepare 0.3 mg from a solution strength of 0.6 mg/0.8 mL.   _____

4. A 36 mg per 2 mL strength solution is used to prepare 24 mg.   _____

5. A dosage of 52 mg is to be prepared from a 78 mg in 0.9 mL solution. _____

6. A dosage of 150 mg has been ordered. The solution strength is 100 mg per mL.   _____

7. A strength of 3 mL containing 750 mcg is available to prepare 600 mcg. _____

8 If the strength available is 1.5 g per cc how many cc will a 4 g dosage require?   _____

9. Prepare a 0.25 mg dosage from a 0.5 mg per 1 mL strength solution.   _____

10. Prepare a 3 g dosage from a 4 g in 2.7 mL strength solution.   _____

ANSWERS   1. 2.9 mL   2. 1.9 mL   3. 0.4 mL   4. 1.3 mL   5. 0.6 mL   6. 1.5 mL   7. 2.4 mL   8. 2.7 cc   9. 0.5 mL   10. 2 mL   If you did not include the units of measure your answers are incorrect.

This completes your introduction to the use of ratio and proportion separated by a colon in solving simple dosage calculation. Turn now to page 139 "Calculations When Drug Weights are in Different Units of Measure" to complete the chapter.

Ratio and Proportion (R & P) Expressed Using Common Fractions

While a ratio is an expression of a significant relationship between two numbers, **a proportion** takes this one step further, and is used **to show the relationship between two ratios**. In a proportion the ratios may be separated by an **equal (=) sign**, or by a **double colon (::)**. For example

$$\frac{1}{50} = \frac{2}{100} \qquad \text{or} \qquad \frac{1}{50} :: \frac{2}{100}$$

The equal (=) sign will be used for all examples of proportion in this text, but you may use the double colon (::) if you prefer this alternate format.

 A true proportion contains two ratios which are equal.

The previous example is a true proportion.

$$\frac{1}{50} = \frac{2}{100}$$

This is a simple comparison, and by using one of our previous drug strength examples we can mentally verify that the ratios are equal, and that the proportion is true.

EXAMPLE 1 $\dfrac{1 \text{ tab}}{50 \text{ mg}} = \dfrac{2 \text{ tab}}{100 \text{ mg}}$

If 1 tablet contains 50 mg, 2 tablets will contain 100 mg.

EXAMPLE 2 $\dfrac{1 \text{ mL}}{50 \text{ mg}} = \dfrac{2 \text{ mL}}{100 \text{ mg}}$

If 1 mL contains 50 mg, 2 mL will contain 100 mg.

You can also prove mathematically that these ratios are equal, and that the proportion is true. Look again at example 1.

$$\frac{1 \text{ tab}}{50 \text{ mg}} = \frac{2 \text{ tab}}{100 \text{ mg}}$$

 In a true proportion the products of cross multiplying will be identical.

To prove a proportion is true cross multiply. The products (answers) you obtain will be identical.

EXAMPLE 1 $\dfrac{1 \text{ tab}}{50 \text{ mg}} = \dfrac{2 \text{ tab}}{100 \text{ mg}}$

$$\frac{1}{50} \diagdown\!\!\!\!\diagup \frac{2}{100 \text{ mg}}$$

$$1 \times 100 = 50 \times 2$$

$$100 = 100$$

The products of cross multiplying in this proportion, 100, are the same. We have now proved mathematically what we previously proved mentally; the ratios are equal, and the proportion is true.

EXAMPLE 2 $$\frac{2\ mL}{500\ mg} \diagdown\!\!\!\diagup \frac{1\ mL}{250\ mg}$$

$$2 \times 250 = 500 \times 1$$

$$500 = 500$$

The products of cross multiplying, 500, are identical. This is a true proportion; the ratios are equal.

EXAMPLE 3 $$\frac{1\ mL}{10\ U} = \frac{2\ mL}{20\ U}$$

$$20 = 20$$

This is a true proportion.

 It is critical in calculations involving proportions that the numbers multiplied not be mixed up.

If necessary make a habit of drawing an X as in the examples just given to make sure you cross multiply correctly.

PROBLEM

Determine mathematically if the following are true proportions.

1. $\dfrac{34\ mg}{2\ mL} = \dfrac{51\ mg}{3\ mL}$ _____

2. $\dfrac{15\ mg}{4\ mL} = \dfrac{45\ mg}{12\ mL}$ _____

3. $\dfrac{1.3\ mL}{46\ mg} = \dfrac{0.65\ mL}{23\ mg}$ _____

4. $\dfrac{2.3\ mL}{150\ U} = \dfrac{1.9\ mL}{130\ U}$ _____

5. $\dfrac{40\ mg}{1.1\ mL} = \dfrac{80\ mg}{2.2\ mL}$ _____

6. $\dfrac{0.25\ mg}{2\ mL} = \dfrac{0.5\ mg}{4\ mL}$ _____

ANSWERS 1. True ($2 \times 51 = 102$ and $34 \times 3 = 102$) 2. True ($4 \times 45 = 180$ and $15 \times 12 = 180$)
3. True ($1.3 \times 23 = 29.9$ and $46 \times 0.65 = 29.9$) 4. Not true ($2.3 \times 130 = 299$ and $150 \times 1.9 = 285$)
5. True ($40 \times 2.2 = 88$ and $1.1 \times 80 = 88$) 6. True ($0.25 \times 4 = 1$ and $2 \times 0.5 = 1$)

Dosage Calculation Using R and P Expressed as Common Fractions

Ratio and proportion is important in dosage calculations because it can be used when only **one ratio is known, or complete,** and **the second is incomplete.** Look carefully at the following examples for parenteral dosages, which is where calculations using R and P may frequently be required.

EXAMPLE 1   A solution strength of **8 mg per mL** will be used to prepare a dosage of **10 mg.**

The known ratio is provided by the solution strength available, 8 mg per mL. The incomplete ratio is the dosage to be given, 10 mg, and X is used to represent the mL which will contain 10 mg.

$$\frac{8\ mg}{1\ mL} \qquad = \qquad \frac{10\ mg}{X\ mL}$$

$$\left(\begin{array}{c}\text{complete ratio}\\ \text{drug strength}\end{array}\right) \qquad \left(\begin{array}{c}\text{incomplete ratio}\\ \text{dosage to give}\end{array}\right)$$

 The ratios in a proportion must be written in the same sequence of measurement units.

In the above example they are.

$$\frac{mg}{mL} = \frac{mg}{mL}$$

Both **numerators** are **mg,** both **denominators** are **mL.**

Next let's review the steps involved in determining the value of the unknown, X mL. The math will be familiar because it was covered earlier in the refresher math section.

$\dfrac{8\ mg}{1\ mL} = \dfrac{10\ mg}{X\ mL}$	set up the proportion to include the measurement units; make sure they are in the same sequence
$\dfrac{8\ mg}{1\ mL} \diagdown\!\!\!\!\diagup\!\!\!\!\diagdown \dfrac{10\ mg}{X\ mL}$	drop the measurement units as you cross multiply
$8X = 10$	keep X on the left of the equation
$X = \dfrac{\overset{5}{10}}{\underset{4}{8}}$	divide 10 by the number in front of X; reduce by highest common denominator (2)
$= 1.25$	divide the final fraction to obtain a decimal fraction
$= 1.25\ \textbf{mL}$	the X in the original proportion was **mL,** so the answer is 1.25 **mL**

The ordered dosage of 10 mg is contained in 1.25 mL

It is routine to check your math twice in dosage calculations. However, it is also necessary to **assess each answer to determine if it seems logical**, and here is where the previous review of relative value of numbers is put to use. Consider the answer you just obtained in example 1.

$$\frac{8 \text{ mg}}{1 \text{ mL}} = \frac{10 \text{ mg}}{X \text{ mL}}$$

$$X = \mathbf{1.25 \text{ mL}}$$

If **1 mL** contains **8 mg** you will need a **larger** volume than 1 mL to obtain **10 mg**. The answer obtained, 1.25 mL, **is** larger, therefore it is logical. This routine check does not guarantee that your math is correct, but it does indicate that you did not mix up the units of measure when you set up the proportion and cross multiplied.

 Each answer obtained must be assessed to determine if it is logical.

You **can** prove that the proportion is true (and your math correct) by substituting your answer for X in the original proportion.

$$\frac{8 \text{ mg}}{1 \text{ mL}} = \frac{10 \text{ mg}}{\mathbf{X \text{ mL}}}$$

$$\frac{8 \text{ mg}}{1 \text{ mL}} = \frac{10 \text{ mg}}{\mathbf{1.25 \text{ mL}}}$$

$$8 \times 1.25 = 10 \times 1$$

$$10 = 10$$

You have now proved mathematically that your answer is correct. **However, in most routine calculations it is neither necessary nor practical to mathematically prove each answer you obtain.** Dosages such as the 1.25 mL in our example are most often rounded to the nearest tenth (1.25 = 1.3 mL). Once this is done, the math of proofing the answer may contain small discrepancies which could cause confusion.

EXAMPLE 2   The strength available is **25 mg in 1.5 mL**. A dosage of **20 mg** has been ordered.

$$\frac{25 \text{ mg}}{1.5 \text{ mL}} = \frac{20 \text{ mg}}{X \text{ mL}}$$
make sure the measurement units are in the correct sequence

$$25X = 1.5 \times 20$$
cross multiply; keep X on left

$$X = \frac{30}{25} \begin{smallmatrix} 6 \\ 5 \end{smallmatrix}$$
reduce by 5, then divide the final fraction

$$= \mathbf{1.2 \text{ mL}}$$
include the measurement unit in your answer

The dosage ordered, 20 mg, is a smaller amount of drug than the strength available, 25 mg (in 1.5 mL). So the answer should be smaller than 1.5 mL, and it is, 1.2 mL.

EXAMPLE 3 A dosage of **200 mg** must be prepared from a solution strength of **80 mg per mL**.

$$\frac{80 \text{ mg}}{1 \text{ mL}} = \frac{200 \text{ mg}}{X \text{ mL}}$$

$$80X = 200$$

$$\frac{200}{\overset{}{\underset{2}{80}}} = 2.5 \text{ mL}$$

The original unknown, X, was mL, so the answer must be mL. The dosage ordered, 200 mg, is larger than the 80 mg per mL strength being used, so it must be contained in more than 1 mL. The answer, 2.5 mL, is larger. Therefore it is logical.

As soon as you are comfortable with the math steps in ratio and proportion you can combine several steps at once, and work even more efficiently. You may already have been doing this, but here are a few examples to demonstrate the short cuts.

EXAMPLE 4 A **300 mg in 1.2 mL** solution will be used to prepare a dosage of **120 mg**.

$$\frac{300 \text{ mg}}{1.2 \text{ mL}} = \frac{120 \text{ mg}}{X \text{ mL}} \qquad \text{set up the proportion with the known ratio written first}$$

$$X = \frac{1.2 \times 120}{300} \qquad \text{cross multiply, and \textbf{immediately} divide by the number in front of X}$$

$$\frac{1.2 \times \overset{2}{120}}{\underset{5}{300}} = \frac{2.4}{5} = 0.48 = \textbf{0.5 mL} \quad \text{reduce (by 60) do final division}$$

A dosage of 120 mg will require 0.5 mL

EXAMPLE 5 Prepare a **2 mg** dosage using **1.5 mg in 0.5 mL** solution.

$$\frac{1.5 \text{ mg}}{0.5 \text{ mL}} = \frac{2 \text{ mg}}{X \text{ mL}}$$

$$X = \frac{0.5 \times \overset{1}{2}}{\underset{3}{1.5}} = 0.66 = \textbf{0.7 mL}$$

A dosage of 2 mg will require 0.7 mL

EXAMPLE 6 A **120 mg** dosage is ordered. The solution available is labeled **80 mg/mL**.

$$\frac{80 \text{ mg}}{1 \text{ mL}} = \frac{120 \text{ mg}}{X \text{ mL}}$$

$$X = \frac{\overset{3}{120}}{\underset{2}{80}} = \textbf{1.5 mL}$$

A volume of 1.5 mL is necessary to prepare this 120 mg dosage

PROBLEM

Calculate the following dosages. Express answers to the nearest tenth, including the appropriate unit of measure. Assess your answers to determine if they are logical.

1. A dosage of 24 mg has been ordered. The solution strength available is 12.5 mg in 1.5 mL. _____

2. A 40 mg/2.5 mL solution will be used to prepare a 30 mg dosage. _____

3. Prepare 0.3 mg from a solution strength of 0.6 mg/0.8 mL. _____

4. A 36 mg per 2 mL strength solution is used to prepare 24 mg _____

5. A dosage of 52 mg is to be prepared from a 78 mg in 0.9 mL solution. _____

6. A dosage of 150 mg has been ordered. The solution strength is 100 mg per mL. _____

7. A strength of 3 mL containing 750 mcg is available to prepare 600 mcg. _____

8 If the strength available is 1.5 g per cc how many cc will a 4 g dosage require? _____

9. Prepare a 0.25 mg dosage from a 0.5 mg per 1 mL strength solution. _____

10. Prepare a 3 g dosage from a 4 g in 2.7 mL strength solution. _____

ANSWERS 1. 2.9 mL   2. 1.9 mL   3. 0.4 mL   4. 1.3 mL   5. 0.6 mL   6. 1.5 mL   7. 2.4 mL   8. 2.7 cc   9. 0.5 mL
10. 2 mL   If you did not include the units of measure your answers are incorrect.

Calculations when Drug Weights are in Different Units of Measure

Consider the following dosage calculations. Follow the examples which use the ratio and proportion method you chose earlier in the chapter.

EXAMPLE 1   The order to give **0.15 g** of medication. The dosage strength available is **200 mg/mL**.

This problem cannot be solved as it is now written because the **drug weights are in different units of measure:** g and mg. In a previous chapter you learned that it may be safer to convert down the scale, higher units to lower, to eliminate or avoid decimals. **Covert the g to mg.**

$$200 \text{ mg} : 1 \text{ mL} = \textbf{0.15 g} : X \text{ mL} \quad \text{or} \quad \frac{200 \text{ mg}}{1 \text{ mL}} = \frac{\textbf{0.15 g}}{X \text{ mL}}$$

$$200 \text{ mg} : 1 \text{ mL} = \textbf{150 mg} : X \text{ mL} \quad \text{or} \quad \frac{200 \text{ mg}}{1 \text{ mL}} = \frac{\textbf{150 mg}}{X \text{ mL}}$$

$$200X = 1 \times 150 \qquad\qquad 200X = 1 \times 150$$

$$X = \frac{150}{200} = 0.75 \qquad\qquad X = \frac{150}{200} = 0.75$$

$$= \textbf{0.8 mL} \qquad\qquad\qquad = \textbf{0.8 mL}$$

150 mg is a smaller dosage than 200 mg so it must be contained in a smaller volume than 1 mL. The answer, 0.8 mL, is logical.

EXAMPLE 2   You have a dosage strength of **200 mcg/mL**. The order is to give **0.5 mg**.

$$200 \text{ mcg} : 1 \text{ mL} = \textbf{0.5 mg} : X \text{ mL} \qquad \text{or} \qquad \frac{200 \text{ mcg}}{1 \text{ mL}} = \frac{\textbf{0.5 mg}}{X \text{ mL}}$$

$$200 \text{ mcg} : 1 \text{ mL} = \textbf{500 mcg} : X \text{ mL} \qquad \text{or} \qquad \frac{200 \text{ mcg}}{1 \text{ mL}} = \frac{\textbf{500 mcg}}{X \text{ mL}}$$

$$200X = 500 \qquad\qquad\qquad\qquad 200X = 500$$

$$X = \textbf{2.5 mL} \qquad\qquad\qquad\qquad X = \textbf{2.5 mL}$$

500 mcg is a larger quantity than 200 mcg so it must be contained in a larger quantity than 1 mL. The answer, 2.5 mL, is logical.

Ratio and proportion is also used to solve dosage calculations for **international units and mEq dosages.**

EXAMPLE 3   The order is to give **1200 U**. The available dosage strength is **1000 U per 1.5 mL**.

$$1000 \text{ U} : 1.5 \text{ mL} = 1200 \text{ U} : X \text{ mL} \qquad \text{or} \qquad \frac{1000 \text{ U}}{1.5 \text{ mL}} = \frac{1200 \text{ U}}{X \text{ mL}}$$

$$1000X = 1.5 \times 1200 \qquad\qquad\qquad 1000X = 1.5 \times 1200$$

$$X = \frac{1.5 \times 1200}{1000} \qquad\qquad\qquad X = \frac{1.5 \times 1200}{1000}$$

$$= \textbf{1.8 mL} \qquad\qquad\qquad\qquad = \textbf{1.8 mL}$$

1200 U is a larger dosage than 1000 U so the answer in mL should be larger, which it is.

EXAMPLE 4   A drug has a dosage strength of **2 mEq/mL**. You are to give **10 mEq**.

$$2 \text{ mEq} : 1 \text{ mL} = 10 \text{ mEq} : X \text{ mL} \qquad \text{or} \qquad \frac{2 \text{ mEq}}{1 \text{ mL}} = \frac{0 \text{ mEq}}{X \text{ mL}}$$

$$2X = 10 \qquad\qquad\qquad\qquad 2X = 10$$

$$X = \textbf{5 mL} \qquad\qquad\qquad\qquad X = \textbf{5 mL}$$

10 mEq is considerably larger than 2 mEq, so the answer should also be significantly larger, and it is.

PROBLEM

Solve the following dosage problems using your preferred R and P method. Express answers to the nearest tenth.

1. The drug label reads 1000 mcg in 2 mL. The order is 0.4 mg.   _____

2. The ordered dosage is 275 mg. The available drug is labeled 0.5 g per 2 mL.   _____

3. A dosage strength of 0.2 mg in 1.5 mL is available. Give 0.15 mg.   _____

4. The strength available is 1 g in 3.6 mL. Prepare a 600 mg dosage.   _____

5. A 10,000 U dosage has been ordered. The dosage strength available is 8,000 U in 1 mL.   _____

6. The dosage available is 20 mEq per 20 mL. You are to prepare 15 mEq.   _____

7. The order is for 200,000 U. The strength available is 150,000 U per 2 mL.   _____

ANSWERS   1. 0.8 mL   2. 1.1 mL   3. 1.1 mL   4. 2.2 mL   5. 1.3 mL   6. 15 mL   7. 2.7 mL

Summary

This concludes the introductory chapter on ratio and proportion and its use in dosage calculations. The important points to remember from this chapter are:

➡ a ratio is composed of two numbers which have a significant relationship to each other

➡ in medication dosages ratios can be used to express the amount of drug contained in a tablet or capsule, or in a certain volume of solution

➡ a true proportion consists of two ratios which are equal to each other

➡ if one number of a proportion is missing it can be determined mathematically by solving an equation to determine the value of X

➡ the available dosage strength provides the complete or known ratio for calculations

➡ the dosage to be given provides the incomplete or unknown ratio

➡ the ratios in a proportion must be set up in the same sequence of measurement units, for example mg : mL = mg : mL

➡ if the measurement units in a calculation are different, for example mg and g, one of these must be converted before the problem can be solved

➡ the math of calculations must always be double checked, and the answer must be assessed logically to determine if X is appropriately larger or smaller than the strength available

➡ if you have any doubt of your accuracy in calculations seek help

Summary Self Test

Page 142

Summary Self Test

Use the ratio and proportion method you have chosen to calculate the following parenteral dosages. Express mL answers to the nearest tenth (or hundredth, where indicated). Use the drug labels provided, and assess each answer you obtain to determine if it is logical. Finally, measure the dosages you calculated on the syringes provided, and have your answers checked by your instructor to be sure you have calculated and measured them correctly.

Dosage Ordered	mL/cc Needed
1. Depo-Provera® 0.25g	_____

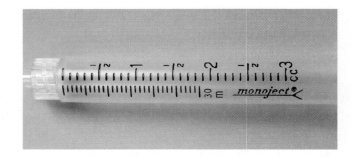

NDC 0009-0248-02
5 ml Vial
Depo-Provera®
Sterile Aqueous Suspension
sterile medroxyprogesterone
acetate suspension, USP
100 mg per ml

For intramuscular use only
See package insert for complete product information.
Shake vigorously immediately before each use.
Store at controlled room temperature 15°-30° C (59°-86° F)
811 851 201
The Upjohn Company
Kalamazoo, Michigan 49001, USA

2. furosemide 15 mg _____

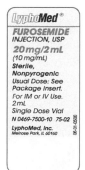

LyphoMed®
FUROSEMIDE
INJECTION, USP
20 mg/2 mL
(10 mg/mL)
Sterile,
Nonpyrogenic
Usual Dose: See
Package Insert.
For IM or IV Use.
2 mL
Single Dose Vial
N 0469-7500-10 75-02
LyphoMed, Inc.
Melrose Park, IL 60160

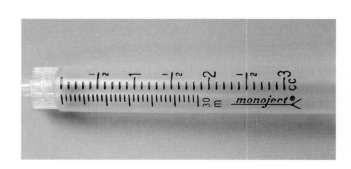

3. heparin 3500 U _____

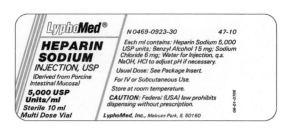

LyphoMed®
HEPARIN SODIUM
INJECTION, USP
(Derived from Porcine Intestinal Mucosa)
5,000 USP Units/ml
Sterile 10 ml
Multi Dose Vial

N 0469-0923-30   47-10
Each ml contains: Heparin Sodium 5,000 USP units; Benzyl Alcohol 15 mg; Sodium Chloride 6 mg; Water for Injection, q.s. NaOH, HCl to adjust pH if necessary.
Usual Dose: See Package Insert.
For IV or Subcutaneous Use.
Store at room temperature.
CAUTION: Federal (USA) law prohibits dispensing without prescription.
LyphoMed, Inc., Melrose Park, IL 60160

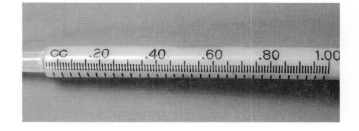

4. Cleocin® 0.75 g   _____
   for an IV additive

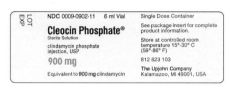

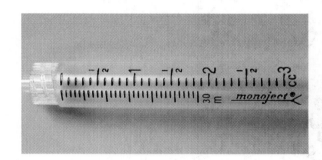

5. atropine 0.35 mg   _____

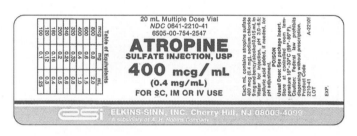

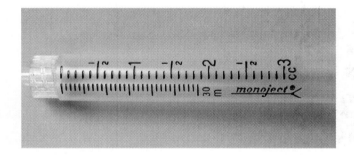

6. hydroxyzine HCl 30 mg   _____

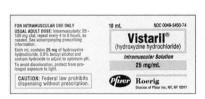

7. Robinul® 150 mcg   _____
   (calculate to the nearest
   hundredth)

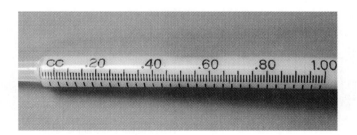

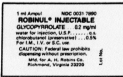

Dosage Ordered   **mL/cc Needed**

8. Tigan® 0.3 g   _____

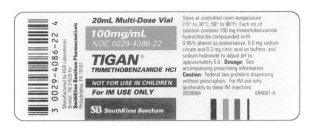

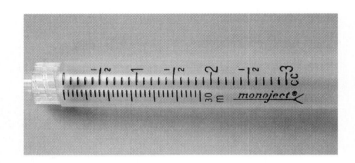

9. aminophylline 0.3 g   _____
    for an IV additive

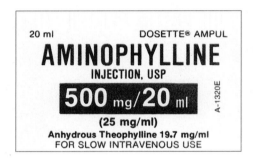

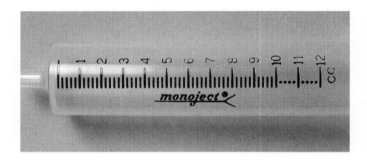

10. cyanocobalamin 800 mcg   _____

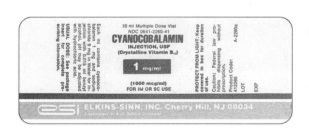

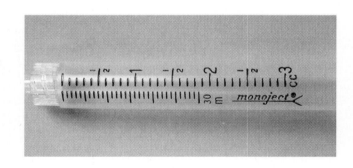

11. tobramycin 30 mg   _____

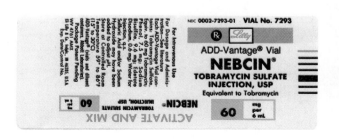

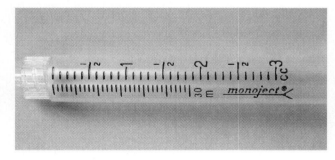

Dosage Ordered **mL/cc Needed**

12. amikacin sulfate 0.12 g _____

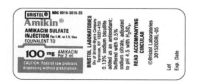

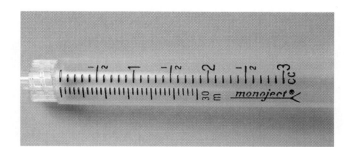

13. Zantac® 70 mg _____

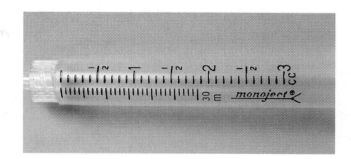

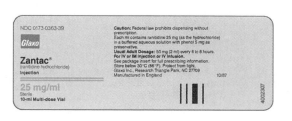

14. calcium gluconate 0.93 mEq _____
    for an IV additive

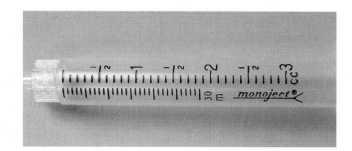

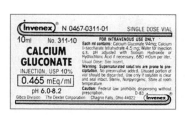

15. diazepam 6 mg _____

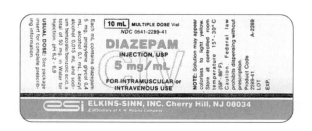

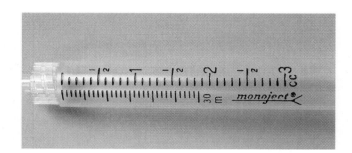

Dosage Ordered	mL/cc Needed

16. heparin 750 U
    (calculate to the nearest
    hundredth)   _____

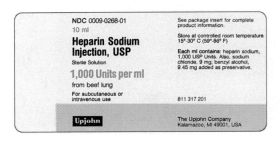

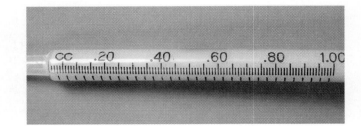

17. perphenazine 3 mg   _____

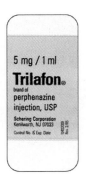

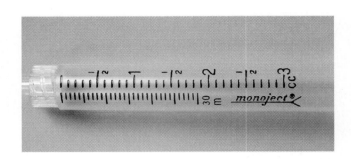

18. phenytoin Na 0.12 g   _____

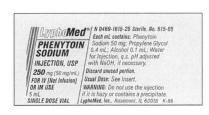

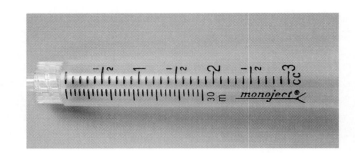

19. medroxyprogesterone 0.9 g _____

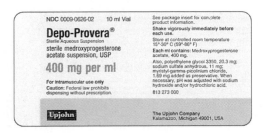

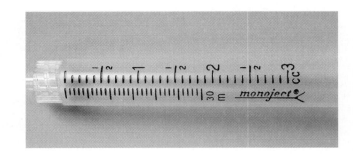

20. gentamicin 70 mg   _____

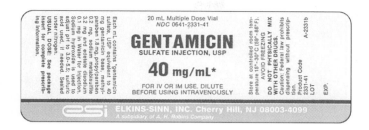

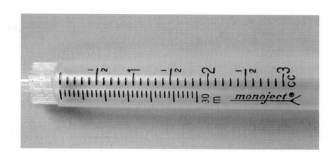

21. lidocaine HCl 60 mg   _____
    for an IV additive

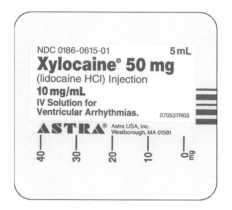

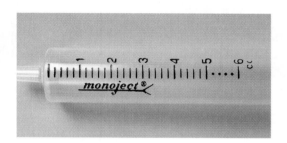

22. sodium chloride 60 mEq   _____
    for an IV additive

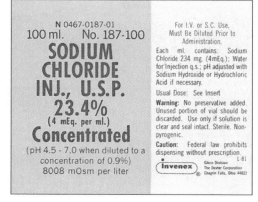

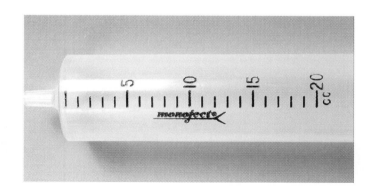

Dosage Ordered   **mL/cc Needed**

23. atropine 500 mcg   _____

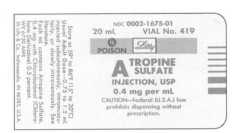

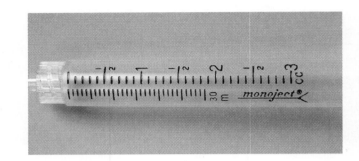

24. meperidine 75 mg   _____

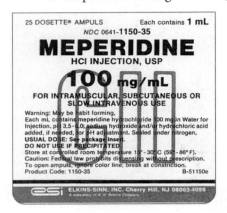

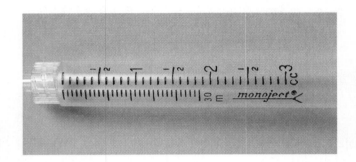

25. cimetidine HCl 0.15 g   _____

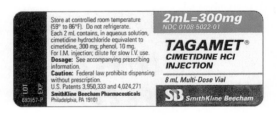

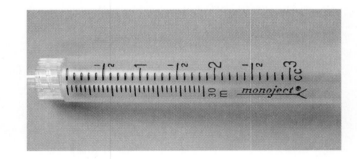

26. clindamycin 0.4 g   _____

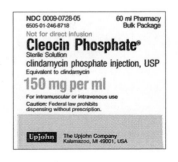

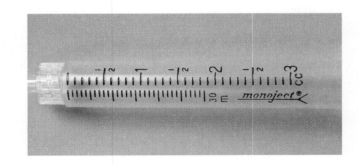

27. morphine sulfate 20 mg _____

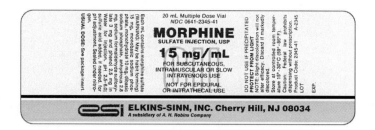

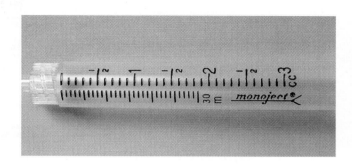

28. Compazine® 12.5 mg _____

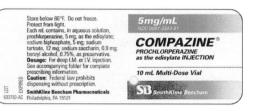

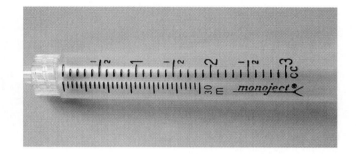

29. nitroglycerin 7.5 mg _____
for an IV additive

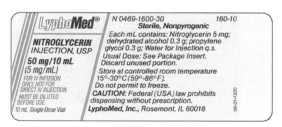

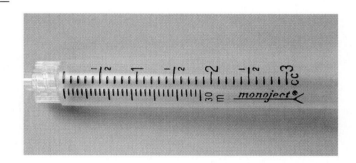

30. doxorubicin HCl 16 mg _____
for an IV additive

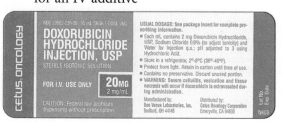

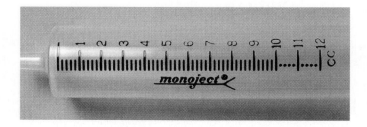

Dosage Ordered   **mL/cc Needed**

31. meperidine HCl 30 mg   _____

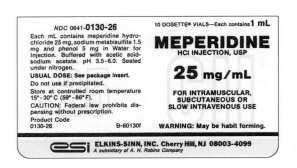   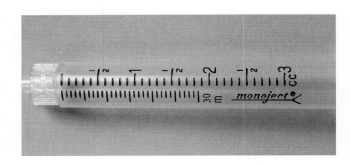

32. methadone HCl 8 mg   _____

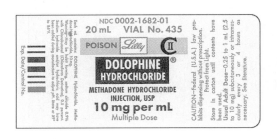   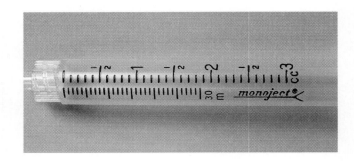

33. Celestone® 12 mg   _____

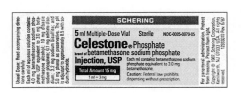   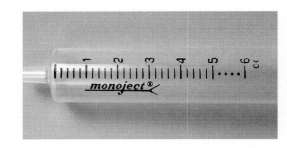

34. naloxone HCl 0.6 mg   _____

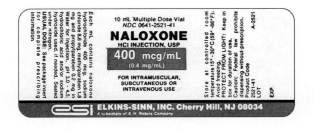   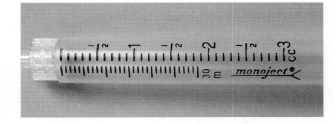

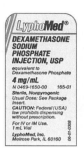
35.　dexamethasone 5 mg　　　_____

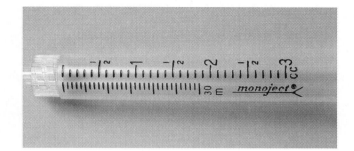

36.　chlorpromazine HCl 40 mg　_____

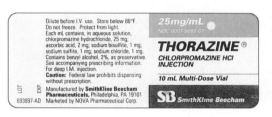

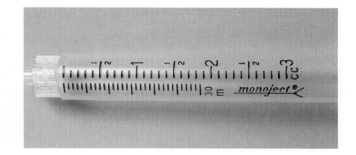

37.　Pronestyl® 0.4 g　　　　_____

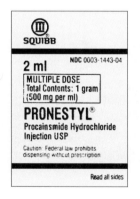

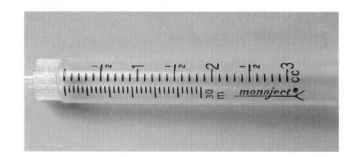

38.　Ergotrate® maleate 100 mcg　_____

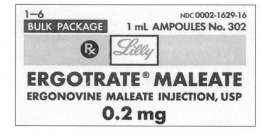

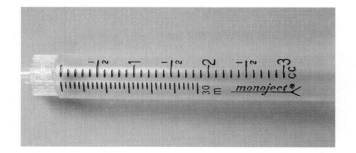

Dosage Ordered   **mL/cc Needed**

39. morphine 15 mg   _____

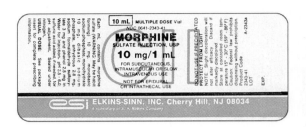

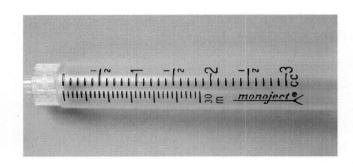

40. Betalin® 0.15 mg   _____

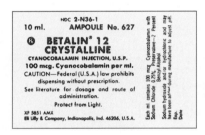

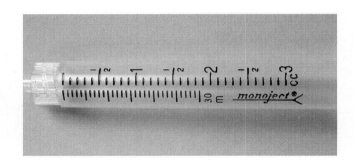

41. tobramycin 70 mg   _____

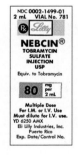

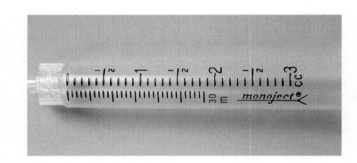

42. aminophylline 0.4 g
    for an IV additive   _____

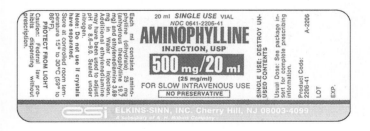

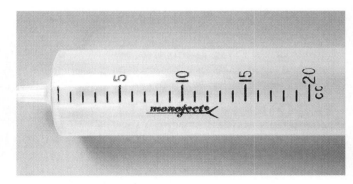

43. Compazine® 12 mg   _____

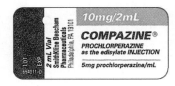

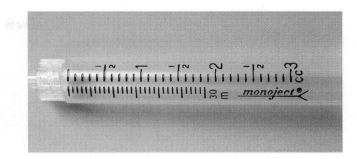

44. Cogentin® 1.5 mg   _____

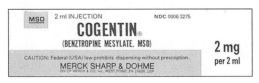

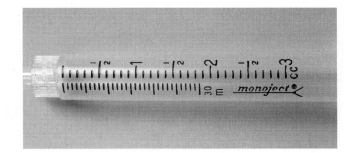

45. chlorpromazine 60 mg   _____

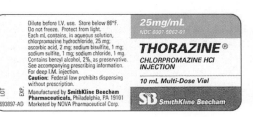

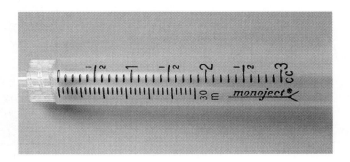

46. gentamicin 0.1 g   _____

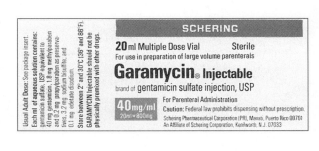

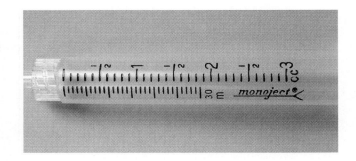

47. Nebcin® 50 mg   _____

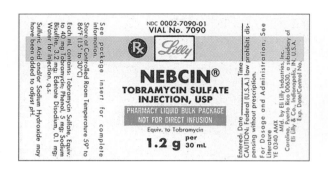

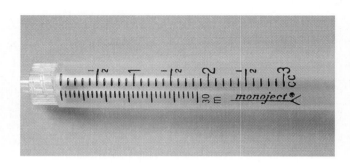

48. Tigan® 0.25 g   _____

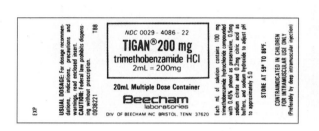

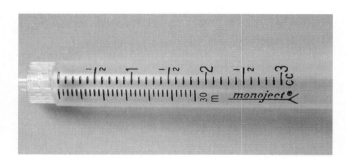

49. penicillin G 400,000 U   _____

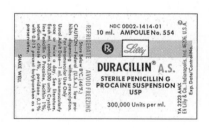

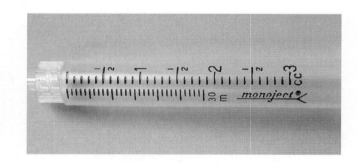

50. Trandate® 8 mg   _____

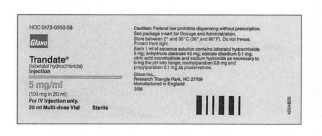

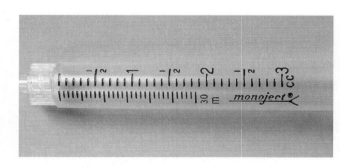

51. potassium chloride 20 mEq _____
    for an IV additive

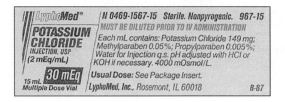

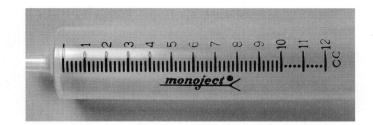

52. oxytocin 25 U　　　　　_____

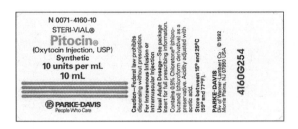

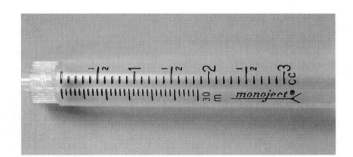

53. betamethasone Na 5 mg　　_____

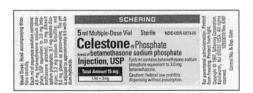

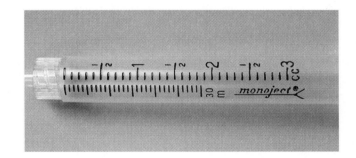

54. Dilantin® 70 mg　　　　_____

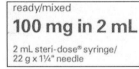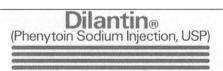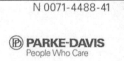

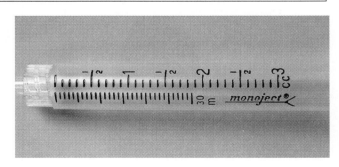

Dosage Ordered   **mL/cc Needed**

55. Depo-Provera® 0.45 g   _____

NDC 0009-0626-01
2.5 ml Vial
Depo-Provera®
Sterile Aqueous Suspension
sterile medroxyprogesterone
acetate suspension, USP
400 mg per ml

For IM use only
See package insert for complete
product information.
Shake vigorously immediately
before each use.
612 224 201
The Upjohn Company
Kalamazoo, Michigan 49001, USA

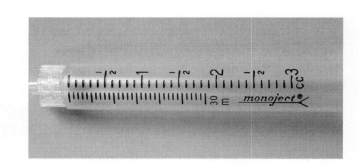

56. prochlorperazine 8 mg   _____

NDC 0007-0C43-01
Keep in a cool place, but avoid freezing
PROTECT FROM LIGHT
Each ml. contains, in aqueous solution, prochlorperazine, 5 mg., as the edisylate; sodium
biphosphate, 5 mg.; sodium tartrate, 12 mg.;
sodium saccharin, 0.9 mg. Contains benzyl
alcohol, 0.75%, as preservative.
See accompanying folder for complete prescribing data.
Patent 2902484

for deep IM or IV injection
Compazine®   10 mL.
brand of
prochlorperazine   Multiple-
dose Vial
Injection   5 mg./mL.
CAUTION—Federal law prohibits
dispensing without prescription.
Smith Kline & French Laboratories
Div. of SmithKline Corp.
Phila., Pa. 19101

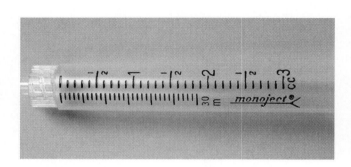

57. furosemide 15 mg   _____

25 DOSETTE® AMPULS   Each contains **2 mL**
NDC 0641-**1425-35**

FUROSEMIDE
INJECTION, USP

20 mg / 2 mL
(10 mg/mL)

**FOR INTRAMUSCULAR OR
SLOW INTRAVENOUS USE**

Each mL contains furosemide 10 mg and sodium chloride 7.5
mg in Water for Injection. pH adjusted to 8.0-9.3 with sodium
hydroxide; hydrochloric acid used, if needed.
PROTECT FROM LIGHT: Store in this box until ready to use.
Do not use if solution is discolored.
Store at controlled room temperature 15°- 30° C (59°- 86° F).
**USUAL DOSE: See package insert for complete prescribing
information.**
Caution: Federal law prohibits dispensing without prescrip-
tion.
To open ampuls, ignore color line; break at constriction.
Product Code: 1425-35   B-51425b

esi ELKINS-SINN, INC. Cherry Hill, NJ 08003-4099
A subsidiary of A. H. Robins Company

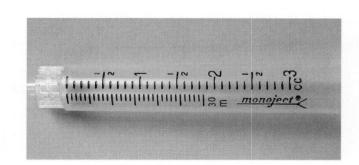

58. atropine 300 mcg   _____

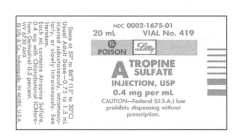
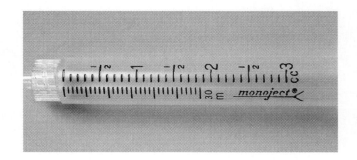

59. phenytoin Na 0.1 g   _____

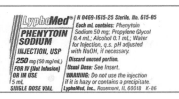
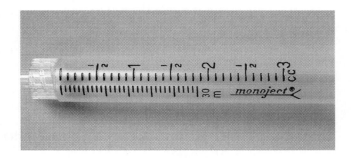

60. methadone 8 mg   _____

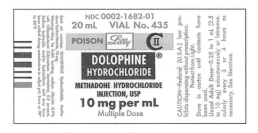
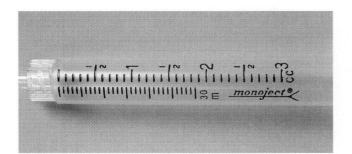

ANSWERS 1. 2.5 mL   2. 1.5 mL   3. 0.7 mL   4. 5 mL   5. 0.9 mL   6. 1.2 mL   7. 0.75 mL   8. 3 mL   9. 12 mL   10. 0.8 mL   11. 3 mL   12. 2.4 mL   13. 2.8 mL   14. 2 mL   15. 1.2 mL   16. 0.75 mL   17. 0.6 mL   18. 2.4 mL   19. 2.3 mL   20. 1.8 mL   21. 6 mL   22. 15 mL   23. 1.3 mL   24. 0.8 mL   25. 1 mL   26. 2.7 mL   27. 1.3 mL   28. 2.5 mL   29. 1.5 mL   30. 8 mL   31. 1.2 mL   32. 0.8 mL   33. 4 mL   34. 1.5 mL   35. 1.3 mL   36. 1.6 mL   37. 0.8 mL   38. 0.5 mL   39. 1.5 mL   40. 1.5 mL   41. 1.8 mL   42. 16 mL   43. 2.4 mL   44. 1.5 mL   45. 2.4 mL   46. 2.5 mL   47. 1.3 mL   48. 2.5 mL   49. 1.3 mL   50. 1.6 mL   51. 10 mL   52. 2.5 mL   53. 1.7 mL   54. 1.4 mL   55. 1.1 mL   56. 1.6 mL   57. 1.5 mL   58. 0.8 mL   59. 2 mL   60. 0.8 mL

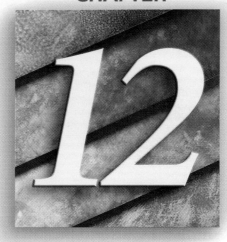
Formula Method

Basic Formula

The formula method may be used for simple one step dosage calculations. It is really just a variation of ratio and proportion, and in other texts has occasionally been presented using different initials. If you are familiar with different initials from those used in this chapter by all means continue to use them. The important thing is the **answer**, not the means of obtaining it.

The initials most commonly used in the formula method are as follows:

$$\frac{D}{H} \times Q = X$$

Here's what these initials means.

D = desired	The dosage **ordered**, in mg, g, etc.
H = have	The dosage strength **available**, in mg, g, etc.
Q = quantity	The **volume** the dosage strength **available** is contained in, mL, cc, etc.
X = the unknown	The **volume** the **desired** dosage will be contained in.

It is necessary to memorize this formula. Stop and do so now. Print the formula several times to help yourself remember it.

The same three precautions which governed calculations using ratio and proportion also apply to the use of the formula: 1. routinely double check all math; 2. assess each answer to determine if it is logical; and, 3. seek help if you have any doubt of your accuracy. Now let's look at some examples of how the formula is used, so you can begin to be comfortable with it.

 The unknown, X, will always be expressed in the same units of measure as Q, the volume the dosage available is contained in.

EXAMPLE 1

A dosage of **80 mg** is ordered. The dosage strength available is **100 mg in 2 mL**. Calculate the mL necessary to administer this dosage.

The desired dosage (D) is 80 mg. You have (H) 100 mg in (Q) 2 mL available. Remember that X will always be expressed in the same units of measure as Q, which in this problem is mL. To ensure accuracy **always set up the formula with the units of measure included.**

$$\frac{(D)\ 80\ mg}{(H)\ 100\ mg} \times (Q)\ 2\ mL = X\ mL$$

$$\frac{80}{100} \times 2 = X = \textbf{1.6 mL}$$

To give a dosage of 80 mg you must administer 1.6 mL

After you have doubled checked your math look at your answer to see if it is logical. The dosage strength available is 100 mg in 2 mL. To prepare 80 mg, which is a smaller dosage, you will need a smaller volume. Your answer, 1.6 mL, is smaller, therefore it is logical.

EXAMPLE 2

The dosage ordered is **0.4 mg**. The strength available is **0.25 mg in 1.2 mL**.

The desired dosage (D) is 0.4 mg. You have (H) 0.25 mg in (Q) 1.2 mL\

$$\frac{0.4\ mg}{0.25\ mg} \times 1.2\ mL = X\ mL$$

$$\frac{0.4}{0.25} \times 1.2 = X = \textbf{1.9 mL}$$

To give a dosage of 0.4 mg you must administer 1.9 mL

0.4 mg is a larger dosage than 0.25 mg and the volume which contains it must be larger, which it is, 1.9 mL.

EXAMPLE 3

A dosage of **750 mcg** has been ordered. The strength available is **1000 mcg per mL**.

$$\frac{750\ mcg}{1000\ mcg} \times 1\ mL = X\ mL$$

$$\frac{750}{1000} \times 1 = X = 0.75 = \textbf{0.8 mL}$$

To give a dosage of 750 mcg you must administer 0.8 mL

The answer should be a smaller quantity than 1 mL, and it is, 0.8 mL.

Determine the volume which will contain the dosage ordered in the following problems. Express answers as decimal fractions to the nearest tenth.

1. A dosage of 0.8 g has been ordered. The strength available is 1 g in 2.5 mL.   _____

2. You have available a dosage strength of 250 mg in 1.5 mL. The order is for 200 mg.   _____

3. The strength available is 1 g in 5 mL. The order is for 0.2 g.   _____

4. A dosage of 300 mcg has been ordered. The strength available is 500 mcg in 1.2 mL.   _____

ANSWERS **1.** 2 mL **2.** 1.2 mL **3.** 1 mL **4.** 0.7 mL

Use with Metric Conversions

Consider the following problem:

A dosage of 200 mcg is ordered. The strength available is 0.3 mg in 1.5 mL.

This problem cannot be solved as it is now written. D and H, the drug strengths, are in different units of measure. One of them must be changed before the problem can be solved.

 D and H, the drug strengths, must be expressed in the same units of measure.

EXAMPLE 1   A dosage of **200 mcg** is ordered. The strength available is **0.3 mg in 1.5 mL**.

• **Convert mg to mcg.**

0.3 mg = 300 mcg

• **Use the formula for the calculation.**

$$\frac{200 \text{ mcg}}{300 \text{ mcg}} \times 1.5 \text{ mL} = X \text{ mL}$$

$$\frac{200}{300} \times 1.5 \text{ mL} = \textbf{1 mL}$$

To give 200 mcg you must administer 1 mL

Your answer must be a smaller quantity, and it is. Therefore it is logical.

EXAMPLE 2   A dosage of **0.7 g** has been ordered. Available is a strength of **1000 mg in 1.5 mL**.

• **Convert g to mg.**

0.7 g = 700 mg

• **Use the formula for the calculation**

$$\frac{700 \text{ mg}}{1000 \text{ mg}} \times 1.5 \text{ mL} = X \text{ mL}$$

$$\frac{700}{1000} \times 1.5 \text{ mL} = \textbf{1.1 mL}$$

To give 0.7 g you must administer 1.1 mL

The answer should be less than 1.5 mL, which it is, 1.1 mL.

PROBLEM

Determine the volume which will be required to prepare the following dosages. Express answers to the nearest tenth.

1. The dosage ordered is 780 mcg. The strength available is 1 mg per mL. _____

2. The available dosage strength is 0.1 g per mL. The dosage ordered is 250 mg. _____

3. Prepare a dosage of 0.6 mg from an available strength of 1000 mcg per 2 mL. _____

4. A dosage of 0.4 g has been ordered. The strength available is 500 mg per 1.3 mL. _____

ANSWERS 1. 0.8 mL 2. 2.5 mL 3. 1.2 mL 4. 1 mL

Use with U and mEq Calculations

Dosages expressed in U or mEq are handled in exactly the same way.

EXAMPLE 1   A dosage of **7500 U** is ordered. The available strength is **10,000 U per mL**.

$$\frac{7500 \text{ U}}{10,000 \text{ U}} \times 1 \text{ mL} = X \text{ mL}$$

$$\frac{7500}{10,000} \times 1 = 0.75 = \textbf{0.8 mL}$$

To give 7500 U administer 0.8 mL

The dosage ordered is less than the strength available, and must be contained in a smaller volume of solution than 1 mL, which it is, 0.8 mL.

EXAMPLE 2   A dosage strength of **40 mEq in 5 mL** is available. You are to prepare **30 mEq**.

$$\frac{30 \text{ mEq}}{40 \text{ mEq}} \times 5 \text{ mL} = X \text{ mL}$$

$$\frac{30}{40} \times 5 = 3.75 = \textbf{3.8 mL}$$

A volume of 3.8 mL is necessary to prepare a 30 mEq dosage

The dosage ordered, 30 mEq, is less than the dosage strength of the solution available. It must be contained in a smaller volume than 5 mL, and the answer, 3.8 mL, indicates that it is.

Determine the volume which will contain the following dosages. Express answers to the nearest tenth.

1. A dosage strength of 1000 U per 1.5 mL is available. Prepare a 1250 U dosage. _____

2. A dosage of 45 U has been ordered. The strength available is 80 U per mL. _____

3. The IV solution available has a strength of 200 mEq per 20 mL. You are to prepare a 50 mEq dosage. _____

4. The strength available is 80 mEq per 5 mL. Prepare 30 mEq. _____

ANSWERS   1. 1.9 mL   2. 0.6 mL   3. 5 mL   4. 1.9 mL

Summary

This concludes the chapter on using the formula method to solve simple dosage calculations. The important points to remember from this chapter are:

➡ the formula method can be used to solve problems expressed in metric, unit, and mEq dosages

➡ when the formula method is used, D and H, the dosage strengths, must be expressed in the same units of measure

➡ the answer obtained, X, will always be in the same unit of measure as Q, the quantity

➡ the math of all calculations is routinely doubled checked

➡ a logical assessment of the answer you obtain is a routine step in calculations

Summary Self Test

Calculate the volume of medication (in mL, cc) necessary to administer the dosages ordered in the following problems. Express your answers as decimal fractions to the nearest tenth.

1. A 50 mg dosage has been ordered. The strength available is 60 mg in 1.5 mL. _____

2. Prepare a 300 mcg dosage. The dosage available is 0.4 mg/mL. _____

3. Prepare 0.45 g. The strength available is 300 mg/mL. _____

4. The medication is labeled 5 mg/mL. An 8 mg dosage has been ordered. _____

5. Prepare a 70 mg dosage from a solution labeled 250 mg in 5 mL. _____

6. The drug is labeled 25 mg per mL; 30 mg has been ordered. _____

7. The label reads 50 mg/mL. Prepare a 60 mg dosage. _____

8. The order is for 12 mg. The vial is labeled 5 mg per mL. _____

9. A dosage of 7 mg has been ordered. The vial labels reads 10 mg per mL. _____

10. The dosage strength is 10mg/1mL; 8 mg has been ordered. _____

11. Prepare a 0.3 g dosage from a medication labeled 900 mg per 6 mL. _____

12. Prepare a 300 mg IV dosage from a vial labeled 0.5 g/20 mL. _____

13. The vial is labeled 0.5 g per 2 mL. A dosage of 750 mg has been ordered. _____

14. Prepare a dosage of 0.2 mg from an available dosage of 250 mcg/5mL. _____

15. The order is for 130 mg and the single use ampule is labeled 0.1 g per 2 mL. _____

16. Draw up a 12 mg dosage from a vial labeled 15 mg in 5 mL. _____

17. The ampule is labeled 20 mg/2 mL. Prepare 14 mg. _____

18. The medication is labeled 1.2 g per 30 mL. Draw up an 800 mg dosage for IV administration. _____

19. Prepare an 80 mg dosage of a medication labeled 100 mg in 2 mL. _____

20. The solution strength is 0.4 mg per mL. A dosage of 300 mcg has been ordered. _____

21. Prepare a 600 mg dosage from an available dosage strength of 0.4 g/mL. _____

22. Draw up a 60 mEq dosage for addition to an IV from a solution labeled 40 mEq per 20 mL. _____

23. The label reads 400 mcg/mL; 0.6 mg has been ordered. _____

24. Prepare a 60 mg dosage from a 75 mg/mL strength. _____

25. Prepare a 0.1 g dosage from a vial labeled 40 mg/mL. _____

26. The drug is labeled 50 mg/10 mL. the order is for 8 mg. _____

27. Measure a 0.8 mg dosage from an available strength of 1000 mcg/cc. _____

28. Prepare 40 mg from a vial labeled 25 mg per mL. _____

29. A dosage of 10 mg has been ordered. You have available a strength of 4000 mcg per mL. _____

30. Prepare 200 mg for IV use of a medication labeled 0.25 g per 25 mL. _____

31. The dosage strength available is 15 mg in 1 mL; 10 mg has been ordered. _____

32. Prepare a 4 mg dosage from a strength available of 5 mg/mL. _____

33. A dosage of 75 U has been ordered from an available strength of 90 U in 1.5 mL. _____

34. You are to prepare 100 mEq for addition to an IV solution. The solution available is labeled 80 mEq per 20 mL. _____

35. Prepare a dosage of 180 mg from a 0.15 g in 1 mL solution. _____

36. Prepare a 750 U dosage from an available strength of 1000 U/mL. _____

37. Draw up a 60 mEq dosage for addition to IV solution from a vial labeled 40 mEq/20 mL. _____

38. 400,000 U has been ordered and you have available 300,000 U in 1 mL. _____

39. A dosage of 0.2 mg per 2 mL is available. Prepare a 250 mcg dosage. _____

40. A dosage of 35 mEq has been ordered for addition to an IV solution. The solution is labeled 50 mEq per 50 mL. _____

ANSWERS   Answers may vary slightly due to rounding.   1. 1.3 mL   2. 0.8 mL   3. 1.5 mL   4. 1.6 mL   5. 1.4 mL   6. 1.2 mL   7. 1.2 mL   8. 2.4 mL   9. 0.7 mL   10. 0.8 mL   11. 2 mL   12. 12 mL   13. 3 mL   14. 4 mL   15. 2.6 mL   16. 4 mL   17. 1.4 mL   18. 20 mL   19. 1.6 mL   20. 0.8 mL   21. 1.5 mL   22. 30 mL   23. 1.5 mL   24. 0.8 mL   25. 2.5 mL   26. 1.6 mL   27. 0.8 cc   28. 1.6 mL   29. 2.5 mL   30. 20 mL   31. 0.7 mL   32. 0.8 mL   33. 1.3 mL   34. 25 mL   35. 1.2 mL   36. 0.8 mL   37. 30 mL   38. 1.3 mL   39. 2.5 mL   40. 35 mL

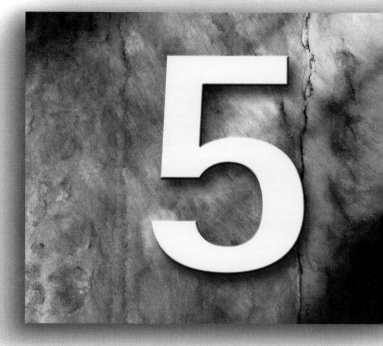

Medication Administration Systems

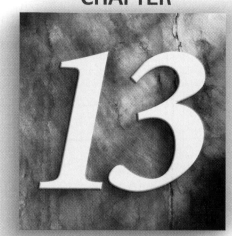

Medication Administration Records

T he system of drug administration most commonly used in hospitals is the medication record system. In this system all the drugs a patient is receiving on a continuing basis are listed on a single record. In some hospitals p.r.n. and IV medications are also listed on this record; in others these are on a separate record, or records. A wide variety of records are in use, and the purpose of this chapter is to provide an introduction to a sufficient number so that you will not be confused by the differences, but rather will recognize and locate essential information which is common to all. The focus will be on identifying the drug, dosage, time, and route of medications being administered on a continuing basis.

Turn to page 169 for a description of the first of the four records you will be introduced to in this chapter.

The student will read medication records to identify
1. drugs ordered on a continuing basis
2. dosage ordered
3. time of administration
4. route of administration

Department of Veterans Affairs — CONTINUING MEDICATION/TREATMENT RECORD

MONTH(S): MAY   YEAR: 20—

ORDER/REORD. DATE	STOP DATE	INITIALS	MEDICATION/TREATMENT DOSE/ROUTE/FREQUENCY	ADMIN. TIMES	3	4	5	6	7	8	9	10	11	12	13	14	15	16
4-28	5-28	AL	Digoxin 0.25 mg p.o. q.d.	0900 JD	JD PM													
5-1	5-15	AL	Furosemide 40 mg p.o. b.i.d.	0900 JD / 1700	JD													
5-1	6-1	AL	Ferrous sulfate 300 mg p.o. q.d.	0900 JD	JD													
5-1	6-1	AL	Allopurinol 300 mg p.o. b.i.d.	0900 JD / 1700	JD													
5-3	5-13	AL	Amoxicillin 250 mg p.o. q.6.h.	0600 JD / 1200 / 1800 / 2400	JD													

ALLERGIES	□ NKA

IMPRINT PATIENT DATA CARD

PATIENT IDENTIFICATION

VA FORM 10-2970C
JUN.1995

IM OR SQ INJECTION SITES

Indicate right (R) or left (L)

1 = abdomen   4 = gluteal area
2 = arm   5 = thigh
3 = iliac crest

OMISSION LEGEND

N = NPO   S = See Progress Notes
R = Refused   P = On Pass
O = Off Ward   H = Held per MD Order
M = Medication Not Available

Medication Record 1

Medication Record 1

On the opposite page is the Continuing Medication/Treatment Record currently being used at Veterans Hospitals in the U.S.A. Notice that from left to right the columns identify the original order/reorder date of the drug; the stop date (expiration date); initials of the nurse who checks for accurate transcription of the order; the drug name, dosage, route, and frequency of administration; the time of administration; and finally, the date columns used by the person administering to initial, indicating that the dosage was given. For example, the initials J.D. have been entered for the 0900 dosages on May 3rd. These initials will be identified on another part of the record. This hospital uses the 24 hour military time clock (0–2400).

Refer back to the drug information. The second drug, furosemide 40 mg, has been ordered p.o. b.i.d., to be given at 0900 and 1700. The administration time column is set up beginning with the earliest administration for the day, and includes all dosages to be given on a continuing basis. The patient identification would be stamped in the lower left corner.

PROBLEM

Read the VA record and identify for each drug listed the name, dosage, route and time of administration.

	Drug	Dosage	Route	Time
1.	_____	_____	_____	_____
2.	_____	_____	_____	_____
3.	_____	_____	_____	_____
4.	_____	_____	_____	_____
5.	_____	_____	_____	_____

6. If it was your responsibility to administer the drugs to this patient at 1700, which ones would you give?   _____

ANSWERS 1. digoxin 0.25 mg p.o. 0900   2. furosemide 40 mg p.o. 0900, 1700   3. ferrous sulfate 300 mg p.o. 0900 4. allopurinal 300 mg p.o. 0900, 1700   5. amoxicillin 250 mg p.o. 0600, 1200, 1800, 2400   6. At 1700 you would give furosemide 40 mg and allopurinal 300 mg

SCHEDULED MEDICATIONS

PHARM USE ONLY		DATE D/M/Y		TIME	1 7/31—	2 8/31—	3 9/31—	4 10/31—	5 11/31—	6 12/31—	7 1/31—
FILL QTY. 1-7	T. FKB R. ✓ BY RN a:tt ✓ BY PHM Anc	**MEDICATION** HUMULIN LENTE **FREQUENCY & DIRECTIONS** QAM **ORDERED DATE** 7/31— **STOP DATE** / /	**DOSE** 22 U **ROUTE** SQ	08	② a:tt	⑥ a:tt	⑱ a:tt				
FILL QTY. 1-7	T. FKB R. ✓ BY RN a:tt ✓ BY PHM Anc	**MEDICATION** DIGOXIN **FREQUENCY & DIRECTIONS** QD **ORDERED DATE** 7/31— **STOP DATE** / /	**DOSE** 0.125 mg **ROUTE** PO	09	a:tt	a:tt	a:tt				
FILL QTY. 1-7	T. FKB R. ✓ BY RN a:tt ✓ BY PHM Anc	**MEDICATION** ENALAPRIL **FREQUENCY & DIRECTIONS** QD **ORDERED DATE** 7/31— **STOP DATE** / /	**DOSE** 2.5 mg **ROUTE** PO	09	a:tt BP 110/90	a:tt BP 145/90	a:tt BP 138/80				
FILL QTY. 1-7	T. FKB R. ✓ BY RN a:tt ✓ BY PHM Ame	**MEDICATION** COLACE **FREQUENCY & DIRECTIONS** BID **ORDERED DATE** 7/31— **STOP DATE** / /	**DOSE** 100 mg **ROUTE** PO	09 21	a:tt JBC	a:tt JBC	a:tt JBC				
FILL QTY. 1-7	T. FKB R. ✓ BY RN a:tt ✓ BY PHM Ame	**MEDICATION** HEPARIN **FREQUENCY & DIRECTIONS** QD **ORDERED DATE** 7/31— **STOP DATE** 10/31—	**DOSE** 5000 U **ROUTE** SQ	09	a:tt ⑪	a:tt ⑤	a:tt ⑯		D/C		
FILL QTY. 1-7	T. FKB R. ✓ BY RN a:tt ✓ BY PHM Anne	**MEDICATION** COUMADIN **FREQUENCY & DIRECTIONS** QD **ORDERED DATE** 7/31— **STOP DATE** / /	**DOSE** 2 mg **ROUTE** PO	18	JBC	JBC	JBC				

LEGEND: T = TRANSCRIBED BY   R = RECOPIED BY

Medication Record 2

Medication Record 2

Take a close look at the medication record on the opposite page, from the University Health Network: Toronto General Hospital, Toronto Western Hospital, Princess Margaret Hospital, Toronto, Canada. You can see that the information it contains is very similar to the VA record, only the arrangement is different. The scheduled (continuing) medications are listed on the left, with the time and date of administration columns to the right. This medical network also uses military time, but omits the hourly zeros (for example 1900 is written as 19). The columns for initials are on this page, but the signature identification is on the reverse of the record, as are the p.r.n. medications.

PROBLEM

Read the University Health Network record and list the drug, dosage, route, and time of all medications ordered.

	Drug	Dosage	Route	Time
1.				
2.				
3.				
4.				
5.				

6. Which drugs were given by JBC on the evening shift on 7-3 (March 7th)? _____

ANSWERS 1. Humulin Lente 22 U s.q. 08 2. Digoxin 0.125 mg p.o. 09 3. Enalapril 2.5 mg p.o. 09 4. Colace 100 mg p.o. 09, 21 5. Heparin 5000 U s.q. 09 6. Colace 100 mg at 21, Coumadin 2 mg at 18

MEDICATION ADMINISTRATION RECORD - 14 DAY

Enter Here
IN PENCIL
Number of
Forms in Use

NAME
ADM. NO.

PATIENT IDENTIFICATION

IMPRINT HERE

DIAGNOSES: _____

ALLERGIC TO: _____
(Record in Red)

DIET: _____

Scheduled Medications

OR. DATE / INITIALS	EXP.DATE / TIME	MEDICATION-DOSAGE-FREQUENCY-RT. OF ADM.	HR.	DATES GIVEN 5/3	5/4	5/5	5/6	5/7	5/8	5/9	5/10	5/11	5/12	5/13	5/14	5/15	5/16
5-3 AMC		Tagamet 300 mg p.o. q.6.h.	6														
			12														
			6														
			12														
5-2 AMC	5-16 59a	Blocadren 10 mg p.o. b.i.d.	9														
			9														
5-3 AMC		Nitro-Bid ung 1" (top) apply to chest q.6.h. while awake	6														
			12														
			6														
			12														
5-3 AMC		Dialose cap ī p.o. t.i.d.	9														
			1														
			9														
5-3 AMC		Bactrim DS ī p.o. b.i.d.	6														
			6														

USE RED ASTERISK *TO INDICATE DOSES
NOT GIVEN - EXPLAIN IN NURSE'S NOTES

Single Orders + Pre-Operatives

OR. DATE / INITIALS	MEDICATION-DOSAGE-RT. OF ADM.	TO BE GIVEN DATE	TIME	NURSE INITIAL	OR. DATE / INITIALS	MEDICATION-DOSAGE-RT. OF ADM.	TO BE GIVEN DATE	TIME	NURSE INITIAL

AGE _____ RELIGION _____ DOCTOR _____ DATE/TIME ADMITTED _____

RM. _____ NAME _____

Lionville Systems, Inc.
© Parke, Davis & Company, 1978
P/N 10104 Rev. H

Medication Record 3

Medication Record 3

Medication Record 3 on the opposite page is produced by Lionville Systems, Inc. Notice that it provides space at the lower left for Single Order and Pre-Operative drugs. The previous records you examined listed these, and p.r.n. drugs, on separate records. IV drugs are also often listed on separate records. The nurse signature identification is not shown, as it is on the back of this particular form.

PROBLEM

Read the Medication Record 3 and list the drug, dosage, and route of each drug that will be administered at 6 p.m.

ANSWERS   Tagamet 300 mg p.o.; Nitro-Bid ung 1" topical to chest; Bactrim DS 1 p.o.

Start / Stop	Medication and Dose	Schedule	Route / Nurse		Date 5-3	Date 5-4	Date 5-5	Date 5-6
5-1	Capoten (captopril) 2.5 mg t.i.d.	08 14 20	p.o. BP	Time / Site / Initials				
				Time / Site / Initials				
				Time / Site / Initials				
				Time / Site / Initials				
				Time / Site / Initials				
				Time / Site / Initials				
				Time / Site / Initials				

Initials	Signature	Initials	Signature	Initials	Signature	Initials	Signature
BP	B.P. Pardis RN						

Physician

Allergies

Room #   Name

Medication Record 4

Medication Record 4

The final record, on the opposite page, is from the University of California Medical Center, San Diego. It also uses military time. Once again you can see the similarities with the previous records, however this record lists both trade and generic drug names in the "Medication and Dose" column.

PROBLEM

Use the drug entry on Medication Record 4 as reference to enter the following drugs, dosages, frequency, and route of administration on the form. Record your initials in the "Nurse" column to indicate you have done the transcribing, and identify your initials appropriately on the record. Have your instructor check your completed record.

1. Coumadin (warfarin Na) 5 mg p.o. q.d. 1800

2. Pronestyl (procainamide) 1000 mg q.6.h. p.o. 0600 1200 1800 2400

3. Mefoxin (cefoxitan Na) 1.5 g q.8.h. IM 0600 1400 2200

4. Ansaid (flurbiprofen) 100 mg p.o. b.i.d. c̄ meals 0800 1800

5. Hismanal (astemizole) 10 mg p.o. q.h.s. 2200

Summary

This concludes your introduction to Medication Administration Records. The important points to remember from this chapter are:

➡ all the drugs the patient is receiving on a continuing basis are entered on a single record

➡ the record contains columns for drug, dosage, route, frequency, and times of administration

➡ dosages are charted and initialed for each calendar day in the appropriate time slots

➡ initials are identified with full signature on each record

➡ p.r.n. and IV medications are frequently recorded on a separate record, or separate section of the continuing medication record

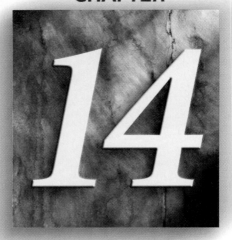

Medication Card Administration

OBJECTIVES

The student will read medication cards to identify

1. drug
2. dosage
3. time of administration
4. route of administration

In the medication card system **a separate card is made for each drug** the patient is to receive. These are usually combined with the medicine cards for all other patients on a unit, and stored in a card rack under **the time of next administration.** If your assignment was to give the 9 a.m. medications you would pull all the cards from the 9 a.m. slot, prepare, administer, and chart them, then sort and return the cards to the time slot of the **next administration**; 1 p.m., 9 p.m., and so on. P.R.N. cards are kept separate.

There are several recognized weaknesses in this system; lost or misplaced cards being one of the more serious. For this reason most hospitals have phased out this system in favor of the medication record system. So, do not do this chapter unless your instructor specifically assigns it.

Reading Medication Cards

Look at the two Medication Cards: A and B. Notice that both cards contain the patient's name, surname first. The room and bed number (frequently written in pencil, so that it can be changed if the patient is moved) is next. Both contain the name of the drug, acetaminophen, the dosage, 600 mg, and the frequency and route of administration, t.i.d. p.o. The time of administration is designated by an X in the appropriate time slot. The shaded areas on these cards identify the evening/night hours. Card B has a built-in weakness in that the time of administration is X'ed in a separate column, leaving open the possibility of misreading the 2100 dosage, for example, as 0900 (this card uses military time).

This information is all you will need to read medication cards. Take the time to read them carefully. Many will be hand printed, as in the examples provided, and not always easy to read. Abbreviations also will vary. The summary self test will provide a representative sampling.

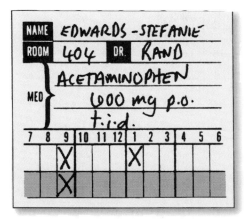

Medication Card A

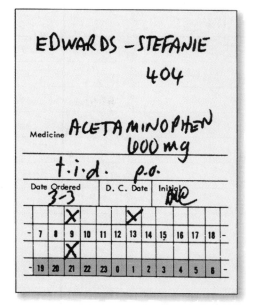

Medication Card B

Summary

The important points to remember about reading medication cards are:

➡ in the medication card system a card is made for each drug the patient is to receive

➡ the patient's name, room number, drug, dosage, frequency and route of administration are all printed on the card

➡ the time of administration is X'ed in the appropriate time space for each dosage to be administered

➡ when the medications for a given time have been administered and charted, the cards are returned to the time slot of the next administration

Summary Self Test

DIRECTIONS

For each of the 12 medication cards shown on the following pages identify the drug, dosage, route, and time of administration. Indicate a.m. or p.m. for dosages given at standard time, but omit these designations if military time is used.

	Drug	Dosage	Route	Time
1.				
2.				
3.				
4.				
5				
6.				
7.				
8.				

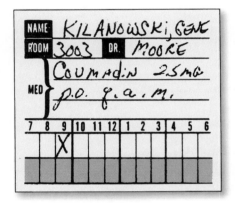

Medication Card 1

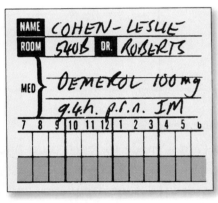

Medication Card 2

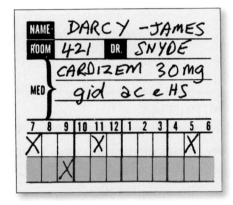

Medication Card 3

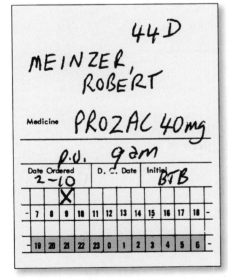

Medication Card 4

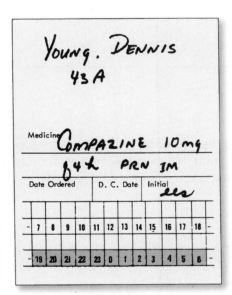

Medication Card 5

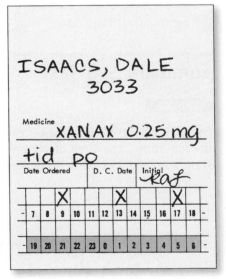

Medication Card 6

	Drug	Dosage	Route	Time
9.	_____	_____	_____	_____
10.	_____	_____	_____	_____
11.	_____	_____	_____	_____
12.	_____	_____	_____	_____

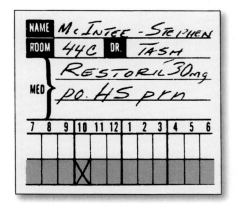

Medication Card 7

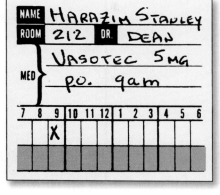

Medication Card 8

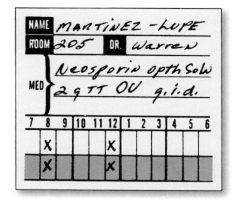

Medication Card 9

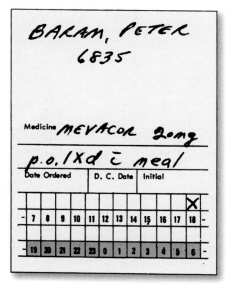

Medication Card 10

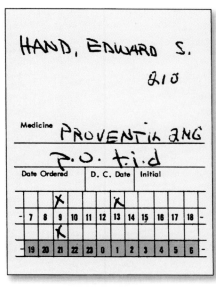

Medication Card 11

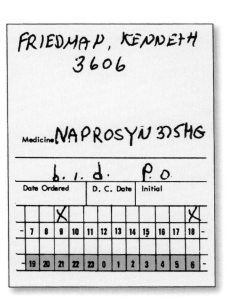

Medication Card 12

ANSWERS					
	1.	Coumadin	2.5 mg	p.o.	9 a.m.
	2.	Demerol	100 mg	IM	q.4.h. p.r.n.
	3.	Cardizem	30 mg	p.o.	7 a.m., 11 a.m., 5 p.m., 9 p.m.
	4.	Prozac	40 mg	p.o.	0900
	5.	Compazine	10 mg	IM	q.4.h. p.r.n.
	6.	Xanax	0.25 mg	p.o.	0900–1300–1700
	7.	Restoril	30 mg	p.o.	h.s. p.r.n. 10 p.m.
	8.	Vasotec	5 mg	p.o.	9 a.m.
	9.	Neosporin opth. soln	2 gtt	OU	8 a.m.–12 p.m.–8 p.m.–12 a.m.
	10.	Mevacor	20 mg	p.o. c̄ meal	1800
	11.	Proventil	2 mg	p.o.	0900–1300–2100
	12.	Naprosyn	375 mg	p.o.	0900–1800

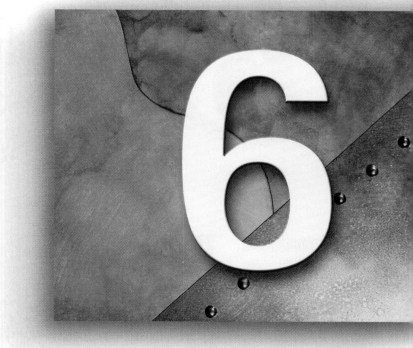

SECTION SIX

Dosage Calculation from Body Weight, and Body Surface Area

CHAPTER

15

Adult and Pediatric Dosages Based on Body Weight

OBJECTIVES

The student will
1. convert body weight from lb to kg
2. convert body weight from kg to lb
3. calculate dosages using mg/kg, mcg/kg, mg/lb
4. determine if dosages ordered are within the normal range

Body weight is a major factor in calculating drug dosages for both adults and children. It is the **most** important determiner of dosages for infants and neonates, whose ability to metabolize drugs is not fully developed. The dosage which will produce optimum therapeutic results for any particular individual, either child or adult, depends not only on dosage but on individual variables, including drug sensitivities and tolerance, age, weight, sex, and metabolic, pathologic, or psychologic conditions.

The doctor will, of course, order the drug and dosage. However it is a nursing responsibility to check each dosage to be sure the order is correct. Each drug label or drug package insert provides specific dosage details, but more complete information is readily available in drug formularies, the PDR, and other nursing and medical references. The hospital pharmacist is an excellent resource person who can also supply additional information.

Individualized dosages may be calculated in terms of mcg per kg, mg per kg, or mg per lb, per day. The total daily dosage may be administered in divided (more than one) doses, for example q.6.h. (4 doses), or t.i.d. (3 doses).

In this chapter you will learn how to calculate dosages based on body weight so that, at any time, you can check an order that appears questionable, or incorrect. However, a preliminary step is necessary to understand conversions between kg and lb, since dosages may be specified in one measure, while body weight is recorded in the other.

Converting lb to kg

Many hospitals still record body weight in lb, but most drug literature states dosages in terms of kg. The most common conversion is therefore from lb to kg. Weights are rounded to the nearest tenth kg.

 There are 2.2 lb in 1 kg

To convert from lb to kg **divide by 2.2**. Since you are dividing, the answer in kg will be **smaller** than the lb you are converting. Answers are expressed to the nearest tenth.

EXAMPLE 1   A child weighs 41 lb. Convert to kg.

$$41 \text{ lb} = 41 \div 2.2 = \textbf{18.6 kg}$$

Your answer should be a smaller number because you are dividing, and it is (41 lb = 18.6 kg).

EXAMPLE 2 Convert the weight of a 144 lb adult to kg.

144 lb = 144 ÷ 2.2 = 65.45 = **65.5 kg**

EXAMPLE 3 Convert the weight of a 27 lb child to kg.

27 lb = 27 ÷ 2.2 = 12.27 = **12.3 kg**

PROBLEM

Convert the following body weights from lb to kg. Round weight to the nearest tenth kg.

1. 14 lb   = _____ kg   6. 134 lb = _____ kg

2. 19 lb   = _____ kg   7. 7 lb   = _____ kg

3. 163 lb = _____ kg   8. 73 lb = _____ kg

4. 31 lb   = _____ kg   9. 121 lb = _____ kg

5. 100 lb = _____ kg   10. 92 lb = _____ kg

ANSWERS 1. 6.4 kg   2. 8.6 kg   3. 74.1 kg   4. 14.1 kg   5. 45.5 kg   6. 60.9 kg   7. 3.2 kg   8. 33.2 kg   9. 55 kg
10. 41.8 kg

Converting kg to lb

To convert in the opposite direction, from kg to lb, always **multiply by 2.2**. Because you are multiplying the answer, in lb, will be **larger** than the kg you started with. Express weight to the nearest lb.

EXAMPLE 1 A child weighs 23.3 kg. Convert to lb.

23.3 kg = 23.3 × 2.2 = 51.2 = **51 lb**

The answer must be larger because you are multiplying, and it is,

23.3 kg = 51 lb.

EXAMPLE 2 Convert an adult weight of 73.4 kg to lb.

73.4 kg = 73.4 × 2.2 = 161.4 = **161 lb**

EXAMPLE 3 Convert the weight of a 14.2 kg child to lb.

14.2 kg = 14.2 × 2.2 = 31.2 = **31 lb**

PROBLEM

Convert the following body weights from kg to lb. Round weights to the nearest lb.

1. 21.3 kg = _____ lb   6. 5.1 kg = _____ lb

2. 99.2 kg = _____ lb   7. 63.8 kg = _____ lb

3. 18.7 kg = _____ lb   8. 57.1 kg = _____ lb

4. 71.4 kg = _____ lb   9. 18.8 kg = _____ lb

5. 10.8 kg = _____ lb   10. 34.9 kg = _____ lb

ANSWERS 1. 47 lb 2. 218 lb 3. 41 lb 4. 157 lb 5. 24 lb 6. 11 lb 7. 140 lb 8. 126 lb 9. 41 lb 10. 77 lb

Calculating Dosages from Drug Label Information

Information you will need to calculate dosages may be on the actual drug label, which is common for pediatric oral liquid medications.

Calculating the dosage is a two step procedure. First the **total daily dosage** is calculated, then it is **divided by the number of doses per day** to obtain the actual dose administered at one time.

Let's start by looking at some pediatric oral antibiotic labels which contain the mg/kg/day dosage guidelines.

EXAMPLE 1

Refer to the information written sideways on the left of the Polymox® label in Figure 67 for children's dosages. Notice that the average dosage range is 20–40 mg/kg/day. This dosage is to be given in divided doses every 8 hours, or a total of 3 doses (24 hr ÷ 8 hr).

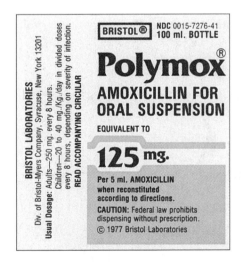

Figure 67

Once you have located the dosage information you can move ahead and calculate the dosage. Let's assume you are checking the dosage ordered for an 18 kg child. Start by calculating the **recommended daily dosage range**.

Lower daily dosage = 20 mg/kg

20 mg × 18 kg (wt of child) = **360 mg/day**

Upper daily dosage = 40 mg/kg

40 mg × 18 kg = **720 mg/day**

The recommended range for this 18 kg child is **360–720 mg/day**.

The drug is to be given in 3 divided doses.

Lower dosage 360 mg ÷ 3 = **120 mg per dose**
Upper dosage 720 mg ÷ 3 = **240 mg per dose**

The dosage range is **120 mg to 240 mg per dose q.8.h.**

Now that you have the dosage range for this child, you are able to assess the accuracy of physician orders. Let's look at some and see how you can use the dosage range you just calculated.

1. **If the order is to give 125 mg q.8.h. is this within the recommended dosage range?**
   Yes, 125 mg q.8.h. is within the average range of 120–240 mg per dose.

2. **If the order is to give 375 mg q.8.h. is this a safe dosage?**
   No, this is an overdosage. The maximum recommended dosage is 240 mg per dose. The 375 mg dose should not be given; the doctor must be called and the order questioned.

3. **If the order is for 75 mg q.8.h. is this an accurate dosage?**
   The recommended lower limit for an 18 kg child is 120 mg. While 75 mg might be safe, it will probably be ineffective. Notify the doctor that the dosage appears to be too low.

4. **If the order is for 250 mg q.8.h. is this accurate?**
   Since 240 mg per dose is the recommended upper limit 250 mg q.8.h. is essentially within normal range. The drug strength is 125 mg per 5 mL and a 250 mg dosage is 10 mL. The doctor has probably ordered this dosage based on available dosage strength, and ease of preparation.

 Discrepancies in dosages are much more significant if the number of mg ordered is small.

For example, the difference between 4 mg and 6 mg is much more critical than the difference between 240 mg and 250 mg, since the drug potency is obviously greater. Additional factors which must be considered are age, weight, and medical condition. While these factors cannot be dealt with at length, keep in mind that **the younger, the older or more compromised by illness the patient is, the more critical a discrepancy is likely to be**.

5. **If the dosage ordered is 125 mg q.4.h. is this an accurate dosage?**
   In this order the frequency of administration, q.4.h., does not fit the recommendations of q.8.h. The total daily dosage of 750 mg (125 mg × 6 doses = 750 mg) is higher than the 720 mg maximum. There may be a reason the doctor ordered this dosage but call to verify the order.

PROBLEM

Refer to the cloxacillin (Tegopen®) label in Figure 68 and answer the following questions.

1. What is the average children's dosage? _____

2. How is this dosage to be administered? _____

3. How many divided doses will this be in 24 hours? _____

4. What will the total daily dose be for a child weighing 10 kg? _____

5. The dosage strength of this oral cloxacillin solution is 125 mg per 5 mL, and the doctor has ordered 125 mg q.6.h. for this 10 kg child. Is there any need to question this order? _____

ANSWERS   1. 50 mg/kg/day   2. equal doses q.6.h.   3. 4 doses in 24 hrs.   4. 500 mg   5. No

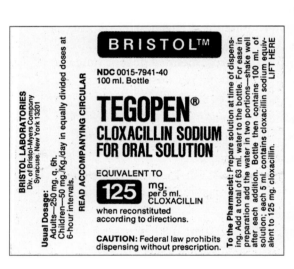

Figure 68

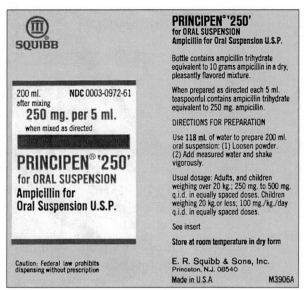

Figure 69

PROBLEM

Refer to the ampicillin (Principen®) label in Figure 69. Answer the following questions for a 12 lb infant.

1. What is the child's body weight in kg to the nearest tenth kg? _____

2. What is the recommended dosage in mg per day for this infant? _____

3. How many doses will this be divided into? _____

4. How many mg will this be per dose? _____

5. The order is to give 125 mg q.6.h. Is this dosage accurate? _____

6. How many mL would you need to administer a 125 mg dosage? _____

ANSWERS   1. 5.5 kg   2. 550 mg   3. 4 doses   4. 137.5 mg   5. Yes   6. 2.5 mL

Calculating Dosages from Drug Literature

The labels you have just been reading were from oral syrups and suspensions, but the same calculation steps are necessary for dosages to be administered by the IV or IM route. Parenteral labels are much smaller in size and usually do not include dosage recommendations. To obtain these, you will have to refer to the drug package inserts, or the PDR, or similar references. These references will contain extensive details about each drug's chemistry, actions, adverse reactions, recommended administration, etc. so it will be necessary for you to search for and select the information you need under the heading "Dosage and Administration." In the following exercises we have done the searching for you, and presented only those excerpts necessary for your calculations.

KEFZOL®, STERILE CEFAZOLIN SODIUM, USP

ADMINISTRATION AND DOSAGE

In children, a total daily dosage of 25 to 50 mg/kg (approximately 10 to 20 mg/lb) of body weight, divided into 3 or 4 equal doses, is effective for most mild to moderately severe infections (Table 5). Total daily dosage may be increased to 100 mg/kg (45 mg/lb) of body weight for severe infections.

TABLE 5. PEDIATRIC DOSAGE GUIDE

Weight		25 mg/kg/Day Divided into 3 Doses		25 mg/kg/Day Divided into 4 Doses	
lb	kg	Approximate Single Dose (mg q8h)	Vol (mL) Needed with Dilution of 125 mg/mL	Approximate Single Dose (mg q6h)	Vol (mL) Needed with Dilution of 125 mg/mL
10	4.5	40 mg	0.35 mL	30 mg	0.25 mL
20	9	75 mg	0.6 mL	55 mg	0.45 mL
30	13.6	115 mg	0.9 mL	85 mg	0.7 mL
40	18.1	150 mg	1.2 mL	115 mg	0.9 mL
50	22.7	190 mg	1.5 mL	140 mg	1.1 mL

Weight		50 mg/kg/Day Divided into 3 Doses		50 mg/kg/Day Divided into 4 Doses	
lb	kg	Approximate Single Dose (mg q8h)	Vol (mL) Needed with Dilution of 225 mg/mL	Approximate Single Dose (mg q6h)	Vol (mL) Needed with Dilution of 225 mg/mL
10	4.5	75 mg	0.35 mL	55 mg	0.25 mL
20	9	150 mg	0.7 mL	110 mg	0.5 mL
30	13.6	225 mg	1 mL	170 mg	0.75 mL
40	18.1	300 mg	1.35 mL	225 mg	1 mL
50	22.7	375 mg	1.7 mL	285 mg	1.25 mL

Figure 70

PROBLEM

Refer to the cefazolin (Kefzol®) insert in Figure 70 and locate the following information for pediatric dosages.

1. What is the dosage range in mg/kg/day for mild to moderate infections? _____

2. What is the dosage range for mild to moderate infections in mg/lb/day? _____

3. The total dosage will be divided into how many doses per day? _____

4. In severe infections, what is the maximum dosage recommended in mg/kg? _____

   mg/lb? _____

ANSWERS 1. 25 mg–50 mg   2. 10 mg–20 mg   3. 3–4 doses per day   4. 100 mg/kg; 45 mg/lb

Notice that in this table, sample dosages are provided for several kg and lb weights, for both the 25 mg and 50 mg dosage, and for both 3 and 4 doses per day. Tables of this sort may be helpful, or harmful. They are helpful if they are easy to understand and the child whose dosage you are calculating fits exactly one of the weights listed; they are harmful if they tend to confuse, which could happen.

The essential information needed to calculate recommended safe dosage ranges is the dosage range in mg/kg/day (or mg/lb/day) and the frequency of administration.

With this information you can quickly calculate what the dosages should be, and determine if the dosages ordered are correct.

PROBLEM

Use the information you just obtained for Kefzol® to calculate the following for a child who weighs 35 lb and has a moderately severe infection.

1. What is the lower daily dosage range? _____

2. What is the upper daily dosage range? _____

3. If the medication is given in 4 divided dosages what will the range be? _____

4. If a dosage of 125 mg q.6.h. is ordered will you need to question it? _____

ANSWERS   1. 350 mg/day   2. 700 mg/day   3. 87.5 mg to 175 mg per dose   4. No; within normal range

PROBLEM

Refer to the dosage information on Mezlin® in Figure 71 and answer the following questions about adult IV dosages.

1. What is the recommended dosage range for serious infections? _____

2. How many divided doses and at what intervals should this dosage be given? _____ _____

3. What is the maximum daily dosage? _____

4. Calculate the dosage range in g for a 176 lb adult. _____

5. If this dosage is to be given q.6.h., what will the individual dosage range be? _____

6. If 2 g per dosage is ordered, what initial assessment would you make? _____

7. If a dosage of 10 g q.6.h. is ordered, what assessment would you make? _____

DOSAGE AND ADMINISTRATION

MEZLIN® (sterile mezlocillin sodium) may be administered intravenously or intramuscularly. For serious infections, the intravenous route of administration should be used. Intramuscular doses should not exceed 2g per injection.

The recommended adult dosage for serious infections is 200-300 mg/kg per day given in 4 to 6 divided doses. The usual dose is 3g given every 4 hours (18g/day) or 4g given every 6 hours (16g/day). For life-threatening infections, up to 350 mg/kg per day may be administered, but the total daily dosage should ordinarily not exceed 24g.

[See table below.]

For patients with life-threatening infections, 4g may be administered every 4 hours (24g/day).

Figure 71

ANSWERS   1. 200 mg/kg to 300 mg/kg   2. 4 to 6 doses; q.6.h. or q.4.h.   3. 24 g   4. 16 g–24 g   5. 4 g–6 g
6. the dosage is too low   7. the dosage is too high

PROBLEM

Refer to the dosage recommendations for Mithracin® in Figure 72 and answer the following questions for treatment of testicular tumors in a patient weighing 240 lbs.

1. What is the recommended dosage range in mcg? _____

2. How often is this dosage to be given, and for how long?

   _____ _____

3. What is the exact dosage range in mg for this patient (calculate to the nearest tenth)? _____

4. If a dosage of 3 mg IV q.a.m. is ordered does this need to be questioned? _____

ANSWERS 1. 25–30 mcg/kg 2. 1 x day; 8–10 days 3. 2.7–3.3 mg 4. No, within normal range

---

MITHRACIN® ℞
(plicamycin)
FOR INTRAVENOUS USE

DOSAGE
The daily dose of Mithracin is based on the patient's body weight. If a patient has abnormal fluid retention such as edema, hydrothorax or ascites, the patient's ideal weight rather than actual body weight should be used to calculate the dose.
Treatment of Testicular Tumors: In the treatment of patients with testicular tumors the recommended daily dose of Mithracin (plicamycin) is 25 to 30 mcg (0.025–0.030 mg) per kilogram of body weight. Therapy should be continued for a period of 8 to 10 days unless significant side effects or toxicity occur during therapy. A course of therapy consisting of more than 10 daily doses is not recommended. Individual daily doses should not exceed 30 mcg (0.030 mg) per kilogram of body weight.

Figure 72

VELOSEF® for INJECTION
Cephradine for Injection USP

DOSAGE AND ADMINISTRATION

Infants and Children
The usual dosage range of VELOSEF is 50 to 100 mg/kg/day (approximately 23 to 45 mg/lb/day) in equally divided doses four times a day and should be regulated by age, weight of the patient and severity of the infection being treated.

PEDIATRIC DOSAGE GUIDE					
		50 mg/kg/day		100 mg/kg/day	
Weight		Approx. single dose	Volume needed @ 208 mg/mL	Approx. single dose	Volume needed @ 227 mg/mL
lbs	kg	mg q6h	dilution	mg q6h	dilution
10	4.5	56 mg	0.27 mL	112 mg	0.5 mL
20	9.1	114 mg	0.55 mL	227 mg	1 mL
30	13.6	170 mg	0.82 mL	340 mg	1.5 mL
40	18.2	227 mg	1.1 mL	455 mg	2 mL
50	22.7	284 mg	1.4 mL	567 mg	2.5 mL

Figure 73

PROBLEM

Refer to the cephradine (Velosef®) literature in Figure 73 and answer the following questions.

1. What is the usual dosage range in mg/kg/day? _____

2. What is the dosage range in mg/lb/day? _____

3. What is the recommended number of dosages per day? _____

4. What will the daily dosage range be for a child weighing 12 kg? _____

5. How many mg will be administered per dose? _____

6. If the order for this child is cephradine 250 mg q.6.h. is this an accurate dosage? _____

7. What is the dosage range for a child weighing 19 lb? _____

8. What amount will be administered per dose? _____

9. If 340 mg q.6.h. is ordered is this an accurate dosage? _____

ANSWERS 1. 50 mg–100 mg/kg/day 2. 23–45 mg/lb/day 3. 4 doses per day 4. 600 mg–1200 mg 5. 150 mg–300 mg 6. Yes 7. 437 mg–855 mg 8. 109–214 mg 9. No, check with the physician

Summary

This concludes the chapter on calculation and assessment of dosages based on body weight. The important points to remember from this chapter are:

→ dosages are frequently ordered on the basis of weight, especially for children

→ dosages may be recommended based on mg/kg/day, mcg/kg/day or mg/lb/day, usually in divided doses

→ body weight may need to be converted from kg to lb, or lb to kg to correlate with dosage recommendations

→ to convert lb to kg divide by 2.2; to convert kg to lb multiply by 2.2

→ calculating dosage is a two step procedure: first calculate the total daily dosage for the weight; then divide this by the number of doses to be administered

→ to check the accuracy of a doctor's order calculate the correct dosage and compare it with the dosage ordered

→ dosage discrepancies are much more critical if the dosage range is low, for example 4–6 mg, as opposed to high, for example 250 mg

→ factors that make discrepancies particularly serious are age, low body weight, and severity of medical condition

→ if the drug label does not contain all the necessary information for safe administration, additional information should be obtained from drug package inserts, the PDR, drug formularies, or the hospital pharmacist

Summary Self Test

DIRECTIONS

Read the dosage labels and literature provided to indicate if dosages are within normal safety limits. If they are not, give the correct range. Express body weight conversions to the nearest tenth, and dosages to the nearest whole number in your calculations.

1. A 45 lb child has an order for Ilosone® (erythromycin) oral susp. 250 mg q.6.h. Read the accompanying label and decide if this is a correct dosage.

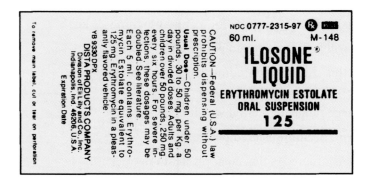

2. Zinacef® (cefuroxime) 375 mg has been ordered IV q.8.h. for a child weighing 44 lb. Determine if this is a safe dosage. _____

3. Zinacef® has also been ordered for a child weighing 84 lb. What would the dosage range be per day, and per dose if the medication is given q.6.h.? _____ _____

4. Oxacillin (Prostaphlin®) 250 mg q.6.h. p.o. has been ordered for a 44 lb child. Determine if this dosage is safe. _____

5. This same oral oxacillin solution has been ordered for a 16 lb infant. The dosage is 125 mg q.6.h. Is this within normal limits? _____

6. A 22 lb child has an order for IV methylprednisolone (Solu-Medrol®) 125 mg q.6.h. for 48 hours. Read the literature and decide if this dosage is within normal range. _____

7. A 7 kg infant has an order for Veetids® 125 mg q.8.h. Comment on this dosage. _____

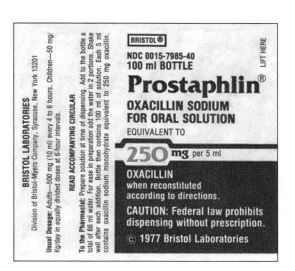

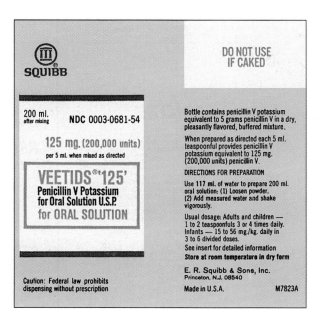

8. A dosage of vancomycin (Vancocin®) 100 mg has been ordered q.6.h. IV for a child weighing 22 lb. Is this a safe dosage? _____

9. Another child weighing 54 lb also has an order for vancomycin IV. Determine what the dosage should be q.6.h. _____

10. Amoxil® oral amoxicillin suspension 125 mg q.8.h. has been ordered for an infant weighing 14 lb. Determine if this is a safe dosage. _____

11. Calculate the dosage range per day and per dose of the amoxicillin oral susp. for a child weighing 41 lb. Given the fact that this child has a severe infection, and that the dosage of the solution is 250 mg per 5 mL, what would you expect the order to be q.8.h?

_____   _____   _____

12. A child weighing 15 kg with a diagnosis of bacterial meningitis has an order for cefuroxime (Kefurox™) 750 mg IV q.6.h. From the available information calculate to determine if this is a correct dosage. _____

VANCOCIN® HCl
[văn 'kō-sĭn ăch 'sē-ĕl]
(vancomycin hydrochloride)
Sterile, USP
IntraVenous

DOSAGE AND ADMINISTRATION

Patients with Normal Renal Function
Adults —The usual daily intravenous dose is 2 g divided either as 500 mg every 6 hours or 1 g every 12 hours. Each dose should be administered over a period of at least 60 minutes. Other patient factors, such as age or obesity, may call for modification of the usual daily dose.
Children —The total daily intravenous dosage of Vancocin® HCl (vancomycin hydrochloride, Lilly), calculated on the basis of 40 mg/kg of body weight, can be divided and incorporated into the child's 24-hour fluid requirement. Each dose should be administered over a period of at least 60 minutes.
Infants and Neonates —In neonates and young infants, the total daily intravenous dosage may be lower. In both neonates and infants, an initial dose of 15 mg/kg is suggested, followed by 10 mg/kg every 12 hours for neonates in the first week of life and every 8 hours thereafter up to the age of 1 month. Close monitoring of serum concentrations of vancomycin may be warranted in these patients.

KEFUROX™
[kĕf 'ŏŏ-rŏcks]
sterile cefuroxime sodium)

DOSAGE AND ADMINISTRATION

Infants and Children Above 3 Months of Age —Administration of 50 to 100 mg/kg/day in equally divided doses every 6 to 8 hours has been successful for most infections susceptible to cefuroxime. The higher dose of 100 mg/kg/day (not to exceed the maximum adult dose) should be used for the more severe or serious infections.
In cases of bacterial meningitis, larger doses of Kefurox are recommended, initially 200 to 240 mg/kg/day intravenously in divided doses every 6 to 8 hours.

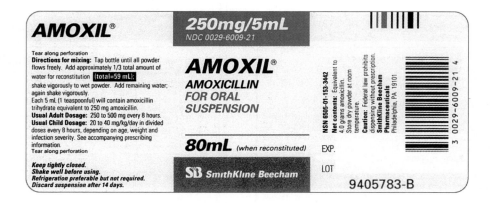

13. An infant suffering from a genitourinary tract infection has an order for IV ampicillin (Omnipen®-N) 125 mg q.6.h. The infant weighs 12 lb. Is this a correct dosage?   _____

14. A 14 lb infant has ampicillin ordered for a respiratory infection. The doctor has ordered 62.5 mg IV q.6.h. Comment on this dosage.   _____

15. A dosage of Ancef® 125 mg q.6.h. has been ordered for a child weighing 16 kg. Calculate the safe dosage range and determine if this dosage is within normal limits.   _____   _____

Wyeth®
Omnipen®-N
(ampicillin sodium)
For Parenteral Administration

Dosage (IM or IV)

Infection	Organisms	Adults	Children*
Respiratory tract	streptococci, pneumococci, nonpenicillinase-producing staphylococci, H. influenzae	250-500 mg q. 6 h.	25-50 mg/kg/day in equal doses q. 6 h.
Gastrointestinal tract	susceptible pathogens	500 mg q. 6 h.	50 mg/kg/day in equal doses q. 6 h.
Genitourinary tract	susceptible gram-negative or gram-positive pathogens	500 mg q. 6 h.	50 mg/kg/day in equal doses q. 6 h.
Urethritis (acute) in adult males	N. gonorrhoeae	500 mg b.i.d. for 1 day (IM)	
	(In complications such as prostatitis and epididymitis, prolonged and intensive therapy is recommended. Gonorrhea cases with suspected primary lesion of syphilis should have dark-field examinations before treatment. In any case suspected of concomitant syphilis, monthly serologic tests for at least 4 months are necessary.)		
Bacterial meningitis	N. meningitidis, H. influenzae	8-14 gram/day	100-200 mg/kg/day
	(Initial treatment is usually by IV drip, followed by frequent [q. 3-4 h.] IM injections.)		
	S. viridans		

*Children's dosage recommendations are intended for those whose weight will not result in a dosage higher than for the adult.

PRESCRIBING INFORMATION

ANCEF®
brand of
sterile cefazolin sodium
and
cefazolin sodium
injection

Pediatric Dosage
In children, a total daily dosage of 25 to 50 mg per kg (approximately 10 to 20 mg per pound) of body weight, divided into three or four equal doses, is effective for most mild to moderately severe infections. Total daily dosage may be increased to 100 mg per kg (45 mg per pound) of body weight for severe infections. Since safety for use in premature infants and in infants under one month has not been established, the use of Ancef (sterile cefazolin sodium) in these patients is not recommended

Pediatric Dosage Guide

Weight		25 mg/kg/Day Divided into 3 Doses		25 mg/kg/Day Divided into 4 Doses	
Lbs	Kg	Approximate Single Dose mg/q8h	Vol. (mL) needed with dilution of 125 mg/mL	Approximate Single Dose mg/q6h	Vol. (mL) needed with dilution of 125 mg/mL
10	4.5	40 mg	0.35 mL	30 mg	0.25 mL
20	9.0	75 mg	0.60 mL	55 mg	0.45 mL
30	13.6	115 mg	0.90 mL	85 mg	0.70 mL
40	18.	150 mg	1.20 mL	115 mg	0.90 mL
50	22.7	190 mg	1.50 mL	140 mg	1.10 mL

Weight		50 mg/kg/Day Divided into 3 Doses		50 mg/kg/Day Divided into 4 Doses	
Lbs	Kg	Approximate Single Dose mg/q8h	Vol. (mL) needed with dilution of 225 mg/mL	Approximate Single Dose mg/q6h	Vol. (mL) needed with dilution of 225 mg/mL
10	4.5	75 mg	0.35 mL	55 mg	0.25 mL
20	9.0	150 mg	0.70 mL	110 mg	0.50 mL
30	13.6	225 mg	1.00 mL	170 mg	0.75 mL
40	18.1	300 mg	1.35 mL	225 mg	1.00 mL
50	22.7	375 mg	1.70 mL	285 mg	1.25 mL

16. Ceftazidime (Tazidime™) 1250 mg IV is ordered q.8.h. for a child weighing 55 lb. How many dosages will the child receive in 24 hr? _____

17. What is this child's weight in kg? _____

18. What is the normal dosage range for IV administration of this drug to this child? _____

19. Is the dosage ordered within the normal range? _____

20. A 198 lb adult is to be treated with IV Ticar® for a respiratory tract infection. What is the daily dosage range in g for this patient? _____

21. If the drug is administered q.4.h. what will the range per dose be? _____

22. Do you need to question a 4 g per dosage order? _____

TAZIDIME™
[tă'zĭ-dĕm]
(ceftazidime)
for injection

DOSAGE AND ADMINISTRATION

The guidelines for dosage of Tazidime™ (ceftazidime, Lilly) are listed in Table 3. The following dosage schedule is recommended:

Table 3: Recommended Dosage Schedule for Ceftazidime

	Dose	Frequency
Adults		
Usual recommended dose	1 g IV or IM	q8 or 12h
Uncomplicated urinary tract infections	250 mg IV or IM	q12h
Bone and joint infections	2 g IV	q12h
Complicated urinary tract infections	500 mg IV or IM	q8 or 12h
Uncomplicated pneumonia; mild skin and skin-structure infections	500 mg–1 g IV or IM	q8h
Serious gynecologic and intra-abdominal infections	2 g IV	q8h
Meningitis	2 g IV	q8h
Very severe life-threatening infections, especially in immunocompromised patients	2 g IV	q8h
Pseudomonal lung infections in patients with cystic fibrosis with normal renal function*	30–50 mg/kg IV to a maximum of 6 g/day	q8h
Neonates (0–4 weeks)	30 mg/kg IV	q12h
Infants and Children (1 month to 12 years)	30–50 mg/kg IV to a maximum of 6 g/day†	q8h

---

TICAR®

brand of
sterile ticarcillin disodium
for Intramuscular or Intravenous Administration

DOSAGE AND ADMINISTRATION

Clinical experience indicates that in serious urinary tract and systemic infections, intravenous therapy in the higher doses should be used. Intramuscular injections should not exceed 2 grams per injection.

Adults:

Bacterial septicemia	200 to 300 mg/kg/day by I.V. infusion in divided doses every 4 or 6 hours.
Respiratory tract infections	(The usual dose is 3 grams given every 4 hours [18 grams/day] or 4 grams given every 6 hours
Skin and soft-tissue infections	[16 grams/day] depending on weight and the severity of the infection.)
Intra-abdominal infections	
Infections of the female pelvis and genital tract	
Urinary tract infections	
Complicated:	150 to 200 mg/kg/day by I.V. infusion in divided doses every 4 or 6 hours.
	(Usual recommended dosage for average [70 kg] adults: 3 grams q.i.d.)
Uncomplicated:	1 gram I.M. or direct I.V. every 6 hours.

23. An adult weighing 77.3 kg with good cardio-renal function who tolerated a test dose of Fungizone® is to receive this drug IV. What will the dosage be to the nearest tenth mg? _____

24. Another patient who weighs 67.4 kg is to receive Fungizone® for a severe infection. What will this dosage be to the nearest tenth mg? _____

25. Dosages can be increased to a maximum of how much? What would this be to the nearest tenth mg for a patient weighing 63.6 kg? _____

FUNGIZONE® INTRAVENOUS ℞
Amphotericin B For Injection USP

WARNING

This drug should be used *primarily* for treatment of patients with progressive and potentially life-threatening fungal infections; it should not be used to treat noninvasive forms of fungal disease such as oral thrush, vaginal candidasis and esophegeal candidiasis in patients with normal neutrophil counts.

DOSAGE AND ADMINISTRATION

CAUTION: Under no circumstances should a total daily dose of 1.5 mg/kg be exceeded. Amphotericin B overdoses can result in cardio-respiratory arrest (see OVERDOSAGE).
FUNGIZONE Intravenous should be administered by *slow* intravenous infusion. Intravenous infusion should be given over a period of approximately 2 to 6 hours (depending on the dose) observing the usual precautions for intravenous therapy (see PRECAUTIONS, General). The recommended concentration for intravenous infusion is 0.1 mg/mL (1 mg/10 mL).
Since patient tolerance varies greatly, the dosage of amphotericin B must be individualized and adjusted according to the patient's clinical status (e.g., site and severity of infection, etiologic agent, cardio-renal function, etc.).
A single intravenous **test dose** (1 mg in 20 mL of 5% dextrose solution) administered over 20–30 minutes may be preferred. The patient's temperature, pulse, respiration, and blood pressure should be recorded every 30 minutes for 2 to 4 hours.
In patients with **good cardi-renal function and a well tolerated test dose**, therapy is usually initiated with a daily dose of 0.25 mg/kg of body weight. However, in those patients having **severe and rapidly progressive fungal infection**, therapy may be initiated with a daily dose of 0.3 mg/kg of body weight. In patients with **impaired cardio-renal function** or a **severe reaction to the test dose**, therapy should be initiated with smaller daily doses (i.e., 5 to 10 mg).
Depending on the patient's cardio-renal status (see PRECAUTIONS, Laboratory Tests), doses may gradually be increased by 5 to 10 mg per day to final daily dosage of 0.5 to 0.7 mg/kg.

16

Adult and Pediatric Dosages Based on Body Surface Area

OBJECTIVES

The student will
1. calculate BSA using formulas for weight and height
2. use BSA to calculate dosages
3. assess the accuracy of dosages prescribed on the basis of BSA
4. recognize the West nomogram as an alternative for determining BSA

Body surface area (BSA or SA) is a major factor in calculating dosages for some drugs, because many of the body's physiologic processes are more closely related to body surface than they are to weight. One of the major drug categories for which body surface is used to calculate dosages is antineoplastic agents, for cancer chemotherapy. However, an increasing number of other drugs are also calculated using BSA. The nursing responsibility for checking dosages based on BSA varies widely among hospitals, therefore this chapter will cover all three essentials: calculation of BSA, calculation of dosages based on BSA, and assessment of physician orders based on BSA.

Body surface is calculated in **square meters (m²)** using the patient's **weight and height**. The safest way to calculate BSA is by using a calculator which has square root ($\sqrt{}$) capabilities (fortunately most do) and a simple formula. Two formulas are available, one for kg and cm measurements, and another for lb and in (inch) measurements.* We'll look at these separately.

Calculating BSA from kg and cm

The formula used to calculate BSA from kg and cm measurements is very easy to remember.

FORMULA

$$BSA = \sqrt{\frac{\text{wt (kg) x ht (cm)}}{3600}}$$

EXAMPLE 1 Calculate the BSA of a man who weighs 104 kg and whose height is 191 cm. Express BSA to the nearest hundredth.

$$\sqrt{\frac{104 \text{ (kg)} \ x \ 191 \text{ (cm)}}{3600}}$$

$$= \sqrt{5.517}$$

$$= 2.348 = \mathbf{2.35 \ m^2}$$

---

*Taketomo, Carol K. *Pediatric Dosage Handbook.* Hudson/Cleveland/Akron: Lexi-Comp, Inc., 1998-1999.

Calculators may vary in the way square root must be obtained, but here's how this BSA was calculated:

$$104. \times 191. \div 3600. = 5.517, \text{ then immediately enter } \sqrt{}$$

Only the final m² BSA is rounded to hundredths. Your answers may vary slightly depending on how your calculator is set. Consider answers within 2–3 hundredths correct. Fractional weights and heights are also simple to calculate.

EXAMPLE 2 Calculate the BSA of an adolescent who weighs 59.1 kg and is 157.5 cm in height. Express BSA to the nearest hundredth.

$$\sqrt{\frac{59.1 \text{ (kg)} \times 157.5 \text{ (cm)}}{3600}}$$

$$= \sqrt{2.585}$$

$$= 1.607 = \mathbf{1.61 \text{ m}^2}$$

EXAMPLE 3 A child who is 96.2 cm tall weighs 15.7 kg. What is his BSA in m² to the nearest hundredth?

$$\sqrt{\frac{15.17 \text{ (kg)} \times 96.2 \text{ (cm)}}{3600}}$$

$$= \sqrt{0.4195}$$

$$= 0.647 = \mathbf{0.65 \text{ m}^2}$$

PROBLEM

Calculate the BSA in m² for the following patients. Express to the nearest hundredth.

1. An adult weighing 59 kg whose height is 160 cm. _____

2. A child whose weight is 35.9 kg and height 63.5 cm. _____

3. A child whose weight is 7.7 kg and height 40 cm. _____

4. An adult whose weight is 92 kg and height 178 cm. _____

5. A child whose weight is 46 kg and height 102 cm. _____

ANSWERS 1. 1.62 m²   2. 0.8 m²   3. 0.29 m²   4. 2.13 m²   5. 1.14 m²

Calculating BSA from lb and in

The formula for calculating BSA from lb and in measurements is equally as easy to use. **The only difference is the denominator, which is 3131.**

FORMULA

$$BSA = \sqrt{\frac{wt\ (lb) \times ht\ (in)}{3131}}$$

EXAMPLE 1   Calculate BSA to the nearest hundredth of a child who is 24 in tall weighing 34 lb.

$$\sqrt{\frac{34\ (lb)\ x\ 24\ (in)}{3131}}$$

$$= \sqrt{0.260}$$

$$= 0.510 = \mathbf{0.51\ m^2}$$

EXAMPLE 2   Calculate BSA to the nearest hundredth of an adult who is 61.3 in tall and weighs 142.7 lb.

$$\sqrt{\frac{142.7\ (lb)\ x\ 61.3\ (in)}{3131}}$$

$$= \sqrt{2.793}$$

$$= 1.671 = \mathbf{1.67\ m^2}$$

EXAMPLE 3   A child weighs 105 lb and is 51 in tall. Calculate BSA to the nearest hundredth.

$$\sqrt{\frac{105\ (lb)\ x\ 51\ (in)}{3131}}$$

$$= \sqrt{1.71}$$

$$= 1.307 = \mathbf{1.31\ m^2}$$

PROBLEM

Determine the BSA for the following patients. Express to the nearest hundredth.

1. A child weighing 92 lb who measures 35 in. _____
2. An adult of 175 lb who is 67 in tall. _____
3. An adult who is 70 in tall and weighs 194 lb. _____
4. A child who is 72.4 lb and 40.5 in tall. _____
5. A child who measures 26 in and weighs 36 lb. _____

ANSWERS   1. $1.01\ m^2$ 2. $1.94\ m^2$ 3. $2.08\ m^2$ 4. $0.97\ m^2$ 5. $0.55\ m^2$

Dosage Calculation Based on BSA

Once you know the BSA, dosage calculation is simple multiplication.

EXAMPLE 1 Dosage recommended is 5 mg per m^2. The child has a BSA of 1.1 m^2.

$$1.1 \ (m^2) \ x \ 5 \ mg \ = \ \textbf{5.5 mg}$$

EXAMPLE 2 The recommended child's dosage is 25–50 mg per m^2. The child has a BSA of 0.76 m^2.

Lower dosage $0.76 \ (m^2) \ x \ 25 \ mg = \ 19 \ mg$

Upper dosage $0.76 \ (m^2) \ x \ 50 \ mg = \ 38 \ mg$

The dosage range is **19–38 mg**.

PROBLEM

Determine the child's dosage for the following drugs. Express answers to the nearest whole number.

1. The recommended child's dosage is 5–10 mg/m^2.
   The BSA is 0.43 m^2.   _____

2. A child with a BSA of 0.81 m^2 is to receive a drug with
   a recommended dosage of 40 mg/m^2.   _____

3. Calculate the dosage of a drug with a recommended child's
   dosage of 20 mg/m^2 for a child with a BSA of 0.50 m^2. _____

4. An adult is to receive a drug with a recommended dosage of
   20–40 U per m^2. The BSA is 1.93 m^2.   _____

5. The adult recommended dosage is 3–5 mg per m^2.
   Calculate dosage for 2.08 m^2.   _____

ANSWERS   1. 2–4 mg   2. 32 mg   3. 10 mg   4. 39–77 U   5. 6–10 mg

Assessing Orders Based on BSA

In most situations where you will have to check a dosage against m^2 recommendations you will be referring to drug package inserts, medication protocols, or the PDR to determine what the dosage should be.

EXAMPLE 1 Refer to the vinblastine information insert in Figure 74 on page 200 and calculate the first dose for an adult whose BSA is 1.66 m^2. Calculations are to the nearest whole number.

Recommended first dose $= \ 3.7 \ mg/m^2$

$$1.66 \ (m^2) \ x \ 3.7 \ mg \ = \ 6.14 \ = \ \textbf{6 mg}$$

EXAMPLE 2 A child with a BSA of 0.96 m^2 is to receive her fourth dose of vinblastine.

Recommended fourth dose $=$ 6.25 mg/m^2

0.96 (m^2) x 6.25 mg $=$ **6 mg**

cetus oncology

STERILE VINBLASTINE SULFATE, USP

DOSAGE AND ADMINISTRATION

Caution: It is extremely important that the needle be properly positioned in the vein before this product is injected.

If leakage into surrounding tissue should occur during intravenous administration of vinblastine sulfate, it may cause considerable irritation. The injection should be discontinued immediately, and any remaining portion of the dose should then be introduced into another vein. Local injection of hyaluronidase and the application of moderate heat to the area of leakage help disperse the drug and are thought to minimize discomfort and the possibility of cellulitis.

There are variations in the depth of the leukopenic response which follows therapy with vinblastine sulfate. For this reason, it is recommended that the drug be given no more frequently than *once every 7 days.* It is wise to initiate therapy for adults by administering a single intravenous dose of 3.7 mg/M^2 of body surface area (bsa); the initial dose for children should be 2.5 mg/M^2. Thereafter, white-blood-cell counts should be made to determine the patient's sensitivity to vinblastine sulfate. A reduction of 50% in the dose of vinblastine is recommended for patients having a direct serum bilirubin value above 3 mg/100 mL. Since metabolism and excretion are primarily hepatic, no modification is recommended for patients with impaired renal function.

A simplified and conservative incremental approach to dosage *at weekly intervals* may be outlined as follows:

	Adults	Children
First dose	3.7 mg/M^2 bsa	2.5 mg/M^2 bsa
Second dose	5.5 mg/M^2 bsa	3.75 mg/M^2 bsa
Third dose	7.4 mg/M^2 bsa	5 mg/M^2 bsa
Forth dose	9.25 mg/M^2 bsa	6.25 mg/M^2 bsa
Fifth dose	11.1 mg/M^2 bsa	7.5 mg/M^2 bsa

The above-mentioned increases may be used until a maximum dose (not exceeding 18.5 mg/M^2 bsa for adults and 12.5 mg/M^2 bsa for children) is reached. The dose should not be increased after that dose which reduces the white-cell count to approximately 3000 cells/mm^3. In some adults, 3.7 mg/M^2 bsa may produce this leukopenia; other adults may require more than 11.1mg/M^2 bsa; and, very rarely, as much as 18.5 mg/M^2 bsa may be necessary. For most adult patients, however, the weekly dosage will prove to be 5.5 to 7.4 mg/M^2 bsa.

Figure 74

PROBLEM

Calculate the following dosages of vinblastine from the information available in Figure 74. Calculate dosages to the nearest whole number.

1. Calculate the dosage for an adult's third dose. The patient's BSA is 1.91 m^2. ____________
2. Calculate the first child's dosage for a patient with a BSA of 1.2 m^2. ____________
3. Calculate the fifth adult dosage. BSA is 1.53 m^2. ____________
4. Calculate the second child's dosage for a BSA of 1.01 m^2. ____________
5. Calculate the second adult dose for a BSA of 2.12 m^2. ____________

ANSWERS 1. 14 mg 2. 3 mg 3. 17 mg 4. 4 mg 5. 12 mg

BICNU®
[bĭk'nū]
(sterile carmustine [BCNU])
℞

DOSAGE AND ADMINISTRATION
The recommended dose of BiCNU as a single agent in previously untreated patients is 150 to 200 mg/m² intravenously every 6 weeks. This may be given as a single dose or divided into daily injections such as 75 to 100 mg/m² on 2 successive days. When BiCNU is used in combination with other myelo-suppressive drugs or in patients in whom bone marrow reserve is depleted, the doses should be adjusted accordingly.

Figure 75

PROBLEM

Refer to Figure 75 for BiCNU® and locate the following information. Express all dosages to the nearest whole number.

1. What is the dosage per m² if the drug is to be given in a single dose? _____

2. If the patient has a BSA of 1.91 m² what will the dosage range be? _____

3. If the order for this patient is a single dosage of 325 mg is there any need to question it? _____

4. If the dosage ordered is 450 mg is there any need to question it? _____

ANSWERS   1. 150–200 mg/m²   2. 287–382 mg   3. No   4. Yes, too high

Calculation of BSA Using a Nomogram

A nomogram is a **chart of average or normal values**. In the case of nomograms used to calculate BSA, these averages are based on height and weight. A variety of BSA nomograms are in use, the best known perhaps, and the one we will explain, is the West nomogram. Nomograms are not easy to use. They contain columns of heights, weights, and BSA's which are transected with a straightedge to locate the BSA. **If the ruler is even slightly off either height or weight, the BSA will be incorrect.**

Until the advent of calculators, which simplified square root calculations, the nomogram was the best tool available for determining BSA. Nomograms are still in use in some hospitals, and your instructor may wish you to do some practice calculations to understand them. However, check before you commit time and effort to this instruction. If you are omitting this section turn now to the summary on page 203.

Use of the West Nomogram

Refer to Figure 76 of the West nomogram, which can be used to calculate BSA for individuals weighing up to 180 lb (80 kg).

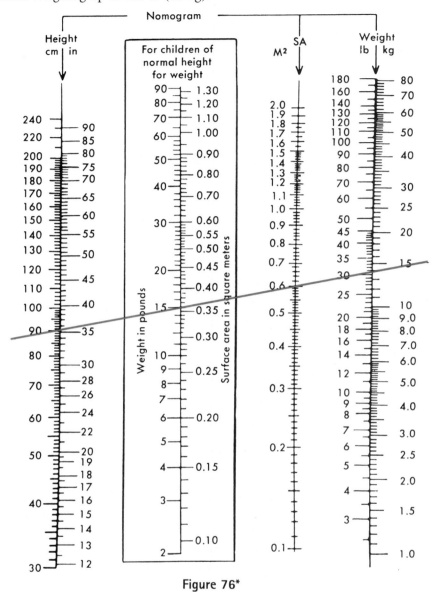

Figure 76*

If the patient is a child of roughly normal height and weight for his or her age, the BSA can be determined from weight alone. If you refer to the enclosed column second from the left on the nomogram you can see, for example, that a child weighing 30 lb has a BSA of 0.60 m².

Before you move on to determining BSA's on your own, you must be aware of a peculiarity of nomograms that could cause confusion. Notice that neither the calibrations nor the numbers identifying them rise consistently from the bottom to the top of the graph. **To identify the correct values you must first read the numbers, then determine what the calibrations between them are measuring.** Refer to the column second from the left again, and notice that there is a very large space between 2 and 3 lb at the bottom, while at the top of the scale there is a very narrow space between 80 and 90 lb. Between 15 and 20 lb there are 1 lb increments in calibration representing 16, 17, 18, and 19 lb, but between 80 and 90 lb only one calibration, which represents 85 lb. Similarly, on the bottom of the m² scale there are four calibrations between 0.10 and 0.15, which represent 0.11,

*West Nomogram. From Behman, R. E. and Vaughan, V. C. *Nelson Textbook of Pediatrics*, Philadelphia, W. B. Saunders Co.

0.12, 0.13, and 0.14 m². On the top of the m² scale there is only one calibration between 1.20 and 1.30 which represents 1.25 m². So once again look at the numbers and calibrations very carefully to determine what the measurements are.

PROBLEM

Read the nomogram provided and indicate the BSA in m² for the following children of normal height and weight.

1. A child weighing 24 lb. _____
2. A child weighing 42 lb. _____
3. A child weighing 11 lb. _____
4. A child weighing 52 lb. _____
5. A child weighing 75 lb. _____

ANSWERS 1. 0.50 m² 2. 0.78 m² 3. 0.29 m² 4. 0.90 m² 5. 1.15 m²

The BSA can also be calculated from the nomogram using both weight and height. The extreme left column for height (in cm and inches), and the extreme right column for weight (in lb and kg) are used for this determination. A ruler is placed on the graph from the height column on the left to the weight column on the right, and the surface area (SA) in m² is indicated where this line intersects the SA column second from the right. For example the line already on the nomogram identifies a BSA of 0.59 m² for a child weighing 30 lb and measuring 35 inches.

PROBLEM

Use the nomogram provided to calculate the following BSA's.

1. The child is 100 cm long and weighs 55 lb. _____
2. A child whose length is 120 cm and weight 40 kg. _____
3. A child whose height and weight are 65 cm and 13 kg. _____
4. A child whose height is 58 in and weight 12 kg. _____
5. A child whose length is 45 in and weight 18 lb. _____

ANSWERS 1. 0.86 m² 2. 1.2 m² 3. 0.51 m² 4. 0.66 m² 5. 0.49 m²

Summary

This concludes dosage calculation based on BSA. The important points to remember from this chapter are:

➡ BSA is calculated from a patient's weight and height

➡ BSA is more important than weight alone in calculating some drug dosages because many physiologic processes are more closely related to surface area than they are to weight

➡ BSA is calculated in square meters (m2) using a formula

➡ the formulas for calculation of BSA are:

$$\sqrt{\frac{wt\ (kg)\ x\ ht\ (cm)}{3600}} \quad and \quad \sqrt{\frac{wt\ (lb)\ x\ ht\ (in)}{3131}}$$

➡ once the BSA has been obtained it can be used to calculate specific drug dosages, and assess accuracy of physician orders

➡ nomograms can be used to determine BSA but they are not as accurate as the formula method

Summary Self Test

Use the formula method to calculate the following BSA's. Express BSA to the nearest hundredth.

1. The weight is 58 lb, height is 36 in. _____

2. An adult weighing 74 kg and measuring 160 cm. _____

3. A child who is 14.2 kg and measures 64 cm. _____

4. An adult weighing 69 kg whose height is 170 cm. _____

5. An adolescent who is 55 in and 103 lb. _____

6. A child who is 112 cm and weighs 25.3 kg. _____

7. An adult who weighs 55 kg and measures 157.5 cm. _____

8. An adult who weighs 65.4 kg and is 132 cm in height. _____

9. A child whose height is 58 in and weight 26.5 lb. _____

10. A child whose height and weight are 60 cm and 13.6 kg. _____

Read the drug insert information provided on pages 204–206 and answer the following questions pertaining to it. Calculate dosages to the nearest whole number.

11. Read the information on children's dosage for Periactin® syrup and calculate the dosage for a child whose BSA is 0.78 m². _____

12. If a dosage of 4 mg is ordered for this patient would you question it? _____

13. What would the daily dosage be for a child whose BSA is 0.29 m²? _____

14. What would the daily dosage be for a child with a BSA of 0.51 m²? _____

15. A patient is to receive the antineoplastic drug Mutamycin® IV. The patient's BSA is 1.46 m². _____

16. Another patient with a BSA of 2.12 m² is also to receive Mutamycin®. What will the dosage be? _____

PERIACTIN® Syrup ℞
(Cyproheptadine HCl, MSD), U.S.P.

DOSAGE AND ADMINISTRATION

DOSAGE SHOULD BE INDIVIDUALIZED ACCORDING TO THE NEEDS AND THE RESPONSE OF THE PATIENT. Each PERIACTIN tablet contains 4 mg of cyproheptadine hydrochloride. Each 5 mL of PERIACTIN syrup contains 2 mg of cyproheptadine hydrochloride.
Although intended primarily for administration to children, the syrup is also useful for administration to adults who cannot swallow tablets.
Children
The total daily dosage for children may be calculated on the basis of body weight or body area using approximately 0.25 mg/kg/day (0.11 mg/lb/day) or 8 mg per square meter of body surface (8 mg/M²). In small children for whom the calculation of dosage based upon body size is most important, it may be necessary to use PERIACTIN syrup to permit accurate dosage.

MUTAMYCIN® ℞
[*mū"-tĕ-mī'-sĭn*]
(mitomycin for injection) USP

DOSAGE AND ADMINISTRATION
Mutamycin should be given intravenously only, using care to avoid extravasation of the compound. If extravasation occurs, cellulitis, ulceration, and slough may result.
Each vial contains either mitomycin 5 mg and mannitol 10 mg, mitomycin 20 mg and mannitol 40 mg, or mitomycin 40 mg and mannitol 80 mg. To administer, add Sterile Water for Injection, 10 mL, 40 mL or 80 mL, respectively. Shake to dissolve. If product does not dissolve immediately, allow to stand at room temperature until solution is obtained.
After full hematological recovery (see guide to dosage adjustment) from any previous chemotherapy, the following dosage schedule may be used at 6- to 8-week intervals:
  20 mg/m² intravenously as a single dose via a functioning intravenous catheter.
Because of cumulative myelosuppression, patients should be fully reevaluated after each course of Mutamycin, and the dose reduced if the patient has experienced any toxicities. Doses greater than 20 mg/m² have not been shown to be more effective, and are more toxic than lower doses.
The following schedule is suggested as a guide to dosage adjustment:

PARAPLATIN® ℞
[păr-a-plătin]
(carboplatin for injection)

DOSAGE AND ADMINISTRATION
NOTE: Aluminum reacts with carboplatin causing precipitate formation and loss of potency, therefore, needles or intravenous sets containing aluminum parts that may come in contact with the drug must not be used for the preparation or administration of PARAPLATIN.
PARAPLATIN, as a single agent, has been shown to be effective in patients with recurrent ovarian carcinoma at a dosage of 360 mg/m² IV on day 1 every 4 weeks. In general, however, single intermittent courses of PARAPLATIN should not be repeated until the neutrophil count is at least 2,000 and the platelet count is at least 100,000.
The dose adjustments shown in the table below are modified from a controlled trial in previously treated patients with ovarian carcinoma. Blood counts were done weekly, and the recommendations are based on the lowest posttreatment platelet or neutrophil value.

BLENOXANE® ℞
[blĕ-nŏk'sān]
(sterile bleomycin sulfate, USP)
vial, 15 units NSN 6505-01-060-4278(m)

DOSAGE
Because of the possibility of an anaphylactoid reaction, lymphoma patients should be treated with two units or less for the first two doses. If no acute reaction occurs, then the regular dosage schedule may be followed.
The following dose schedule is recommended: Squamous cell carcinoma, lymphosarcoma, reticulum cell sarcoma, testicular carcinoma—0.25 to 0.50 units/kg (10 to 20 units/m²) given intravenously, intramuscularly, or subcutaneously weekly or twice weekly.
Hodgkin's Disease—0.25 to 0.50 units/kg (10 to 20 units/m²) given intravenously, intramuscularly, or subcutaneously weekly or twice weekly. After a 50% response, a maintenance dose of one unit daily or five units weekly intravenously or intramuscularly should be given.
Pulmonary toxicity of Blenoxane appears to be dose related with a striking increase when the total dose is over 400 units. Total doses over 400 units should be given with great caution.

---

17. A patient is to be treated with the drug Paraplatin® for ovarian carcinoma. Her BSA is 1.61 m². What will the dosage be? _____

18. Another patient, who weighs 130 lb and measures 62 in, is to receive Paraplatin®. What will her dosage be? _____

19. A third patient receiving Paraplatin® has a dosage of 637 mg IV ordered. She is 161 cm tall and weighs 70 kg. Assess this dosage. _____

20. A patient with Hodgkins disease who weighs 60 kg and is 142 cm tall is to receive Blenoxane® IV. What is her BSA? _____

    What will her dosage range be? _____

    If a dosage of 20 U is ordered must you question it? _____

21. Another patient receiving Blenoxane® weighs 91 kg and measures 190 cm. What will his dosage range be? _____

22. A patient receiving Novantrone® is to have an induction dosage. The BSA is 1.97 m². _____

PLATINOL® ℞
[plă'tĭ-nŏl'']
(cisplatin for injection, USP)

DOSAGE AND ADMINISTRATION
Note: Needles or intravenous sets containing aluminum parts that may come in contact with PLATINOL® (cisplatin for injection, USP) should not be used for preparation or administration. Aluminum reacts with PLATINOL, causing precipitate formation and a loss of potency.
Metastatic Testicular Tumors—The usual PLATINOL dose for the treatment of testicular cancer in combination with other approved chemotherapeutic agents is 20 mg/m² IV daily for 5 days.
Metastatic Ovarian Tumors—The usual PLATINOL dose for the treatment of metastatic ovarian tumors in combination with Cytoxan or other approved chemotherapeutic agents is 75–100 mg/m² IV once every 4 weeks, (Day 1).[1,2]
The dose of Cytoxan when used in combination with PLATINOL is 600 mg/m² IV once every 4 weeks, (Day 1).[1,2]
For directions for the administration of Cytoxan refer to the Cytoxan package insert.
In combination therapy, PLATINOL and Cytoxan are administered sequentially.
As a single agent, PLATINOL should be administered at a dose of 100 mg/m² IV once every 4 weeks.

NOVANTRONE® ℞
[nŏ-văn-trōne]
Mitoxantrone for Injection Concentrate

DOSAGE AND ADMINISTRATION
(See WARNINGS.)
NOVANTRONE SOLUTION MUST BE DILUTED PRIOR TO USE.
Combination Initial Therapy for ANLL in Adults: For induction, the recommended dosage is 12 mg/m² of NOVANTRONE daily on days 1 to 3 given as an intravenous infusion, and 100 mg/m² cytosine arabinoside for 7 days given as a continuous 24-hour infusion on days 1 to 7.
Most complete remissions will occur following the initial course of induction therapy. In the event of an incomplete antileukemic response, a second induction course may be given. NOVANTRONE mitoxantrone for Injection Concentrate should be given for 2 days and cytosine arabinoside for 5 days using the same daily dosage levels.
If severe or life-threatening nonhematologic toxicity is observed during the first induction course, the second induction course should be withheld until toxicity clears.
Consolidation therapy which was used in two large, randomized, multicenter trials consisted of NOVANTRONE 12 mg/m² given by intravenous infusion daily for days 1 and 2 and cytosine arabinoside 100 mg/m² for 5 days given as a continuous 24-hour infusion on days 1 to 5. The first course was given approximately 6 weeks after the final induction course; the second was generally administered 4 weeks after the first. Severe myelosuppression occurred. (See CLINICAL PHARMACOLOGY.)

---

23. Cytosine arabinoside is to be given at the same time as the Novantrone®.What dosage does the Novantrone® literature specify for cytosine?

    _____

    What will the dosage be for this patient?

    _____

24. A second patient receiving these drugs has a BSA of 1.84 m². What will the dosage of Novantrone® be?

    _____

    What will the dosage of cytosine be?

    _____

25. Platinol® is being given for metastatic ovarian carcinoma. What is the dosage range of this drug for a patient with a BSA of 1.29 m²?

    _____

26. Another patient with metastatic testicular carcinoma is to receive Platinol®. He weighs 173 lb and is 65 in tall. What is his BSA?

    _____

    What will his dosage be?

    _____

27. Zovirax® is to be given IV to a child with herpes simplex encephalitis. This patient weighs 34 lb and is 24 in tall. What is the BSA?

    _____

    What will the dosage be?

    _____

28. An immunocompromised 10 year old child with a herpes simplex infection is to be medicated with Zovirax®. Her weight is 72 lb and height 40 in. What is her BSA?

    _____

    What will the hourly dosage be?

    _____

29. Another immunosuppressed child is to receive Zovirax® for a varicella zoster infection. His weight is 43 lb and height 28 in. What is his BSA?

    _____

30. What will the dosage be for this patient?

    _____

ZOVIRAX® Sterile Powder ℞
[zō"vĭ'răx]
(Acyclovir Sodium)
FOR INTRAVENOUS INFUSION ONLY

DOSAGE AND ADMINISTRATION
CAUTION— RAPID OR BOLUS INTRAVENOUS AND IN-TRAMUSCULAR OR SUBCUTANEOUS INJECTION MUST BE AVOIDED. Therapy should be initiated as early as possible following onset of signs and symptoms. For diagnosis—see INDICATIONS.
Dosage:
HERPES SIMPLEX INFECTIONS
MUCOSAL AND CUTANEOUS HERPES SIMPLEX (HSV-1 and HSV-2) INFECTIONS IN IMMUNOCOMPROMISED PATIENTS —5 mg/kg infused at a constant rate over 1 hour, every 8 hours (15 mg/kg/day) for 7 days in adult patients with normal renal function. In children under 12 years of age, more accurate dosing can be attained by infusing 250 mg/m² at a constant rate over 1 hour, every 8 hours (750 mg/m²/day) for 7 days.

SEVERE INITIAL CLINICAL EPISODES OF HERPES GENITALIS —The same dose given above—administered for 5 days.
HERPES SIMPLEX ENCEPHALITIS —10 mg/kg infused at a constant rate over at least 1 hour, every 8 hours for 10 days. In children between 6 months and 12 years of age, more accurate dosing is achieved by infusing 500 mg/m², at a constant rate over at least one hour, every 8 hours for 10 days.
VARICELLA ZOSTER INFECTIONS
ZOSTER IN IMMUNOCOMPROMISED PATIENTS —10 mg/kg infused at a constant rate over 1 hour, every 8 hours for 7 days in adult patients with normal renal function. In children under 12 years of age, equivalent plasma concentrations are attained by infusing 500 mg/m² at a constant rate over at least 1 hour, every 8 hours for 7 days. Obese patients should be dosed at 10 mg/kg (Ideal Body Weight). A maximum dose equivalent to 500 mg/m² every 8 hours should not be exceeded for any patient.

ANSWERS 1. 0.82 m² 2. 1.81 m² 3. 0.50 m² 4. 1.81 m² 5. 1.35 m² 6. 0.89 m² 7. 1.55 m² 8. 1.55 m²
9. 0.70 m² 10. 0.48 m² 11. 6 mg per day 12. Yes; too low 13. 2 mg per day 14. 4 mg 15. 29 mg 16. 42 mg
17. 580 mg 18. 576 mg 19. Accurate 20. 1.54 m²; 15-31 U; No 21. 22-44 U 22. 24 mg 23. 100 mg/m²;
197 mg 24. 22 mg; 184 mg 25. 97-129 mg 26. 1.90 m²; 38 mg 27. 0.51 m²; 255 mg 28. 0.96 m²; 240 mg
29. 0.62 m² 30. 310 mg

SECTION SEVEN

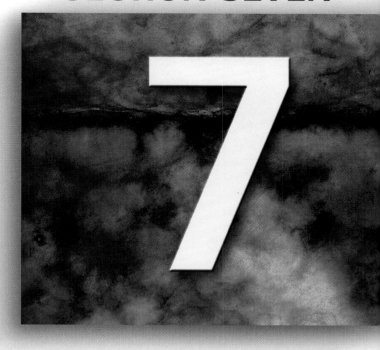

Intravenous Calculations

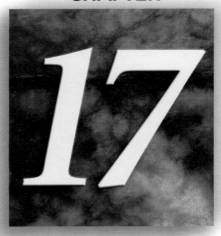

CHAPTER 17

Introduction to IV Therapy

The calculations associated with IV's will be easier to understand if you have some general understanding of IV therapy. IV fluid and medication administration is one of the most challenging of all nursing responsibilities. There are currently estimated to be over 200 different IV fluids being manufactured, and at least as many additives used with IV fluids, including medications, electrolytes, and nutrients. In addition there are hundreds of different types of IV administration sets and components, and dozens of different models of electronic devices used to infuse and monitor IV fluids. This would appear to make the entire subject of IV therapy overwhelming, but it is not. This chapter will present the essentials in understandable segments, and give you an excellent base of instruction on which to build. Let's begin by looking at a basic sterile IV setup, which is referred to as a primary line.

Primary Line

Refer to Figure 77, which shows a typical primary line connecting the IV fluid bag or bottle to the needle or cannula in a vein.

As the photo illustrates, the IV tubing is connected to the IV solution bag (using sterile technique), and the bag is hung on an IV stand.

 Close all roller clamps on the tubing before connecting to solution bag. This step prevents air bubbles forming in the tubing.

The **drip chamber**, A, is then squeezed to **half fill** it with fluid. This level is very important because **IV flow rates are set and monitored by counting the drops falling in this chamber.** If the chamber is too full the drops cannot be counted. On the other hand if the outlet at the bottom of the chamber is not completely covered air can enter the tubing during infusions, and subsequently the vein and circulatory system. So the half full fluid level is very important.

Next notice B, the **roller clamp**. This is adjusted while the drops falling in the drip chamber are counted to set the flow rate. It provides an extremely accurate control of rate. A second type of clamp, C, called a **slide clamp**, is present on tubings. The slide clamp can be used to temporarily stop an IV without disturbing the rate set on the roller clamp.

Next notice D, the **injection ports**. Rubber ports are located in several locations on the tubing, typically near the cannula end, drip chamber and middle of the line, and on most IV solution bags. Ports allow injection of medication directly into the line or bag, or the attachment of secondary IV lines containing compatible IV fluids or medications to the primary line.

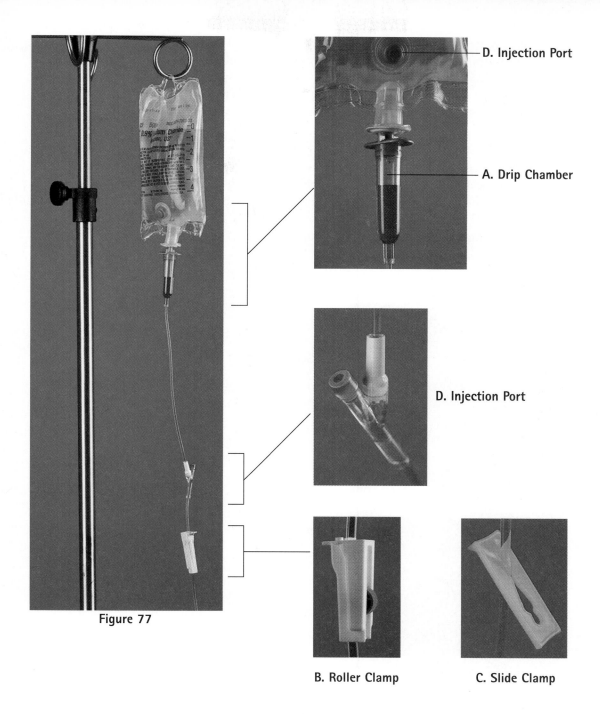

D. Injection Port

A. Drip Chamber

D. Injection Port

Figure 77

B. Roller Clamp

C. Slide Clamp

Intravenous fluids run by gravity flow. This necessitates that the IV solution bag be hung **above the patient's heart level** to exert sufficient pressure to infuse. Three feet is the average height.

 The higher an IV bag is hung, the greater the pressure, and the faster the IV will infuse.

This pressure differential also means that if the flow rate is adjusted while the patient is lying in bed it will slow down if she/he sits or stands, and in fact changes slightly with each turn from side to side. For this reason **monitoring IV flow rate is on-going**, officially done every hour, but routinely checked after each major position change.

There are two additional terms relating to primary lines that you must know. If an arm (or less commonly leg) vein is used for an infusion it is referred to as a **peripheral line**. This is to distinguish it from a **central line**, which uses a special catheter whose tip is located centrally in a deep chest vein. Central lines may access the chest vein either directly through the chest wall, or via a neck vein, or a peripheral vein in the arm or leg.

Secondary Line

Secondary lines attach to the primary line at an injection port. They are used primarily to infuse medications, frequently on an intermittent basis, for example every 6-8 hours. They may also be used to infuse other compatible IV fluids. Secondary lines are commonly referred to as **IV piggybacks**. They are abbreviated **IVPB**. Refer to Figure 78, which illustrates a primary and secondary line setup.

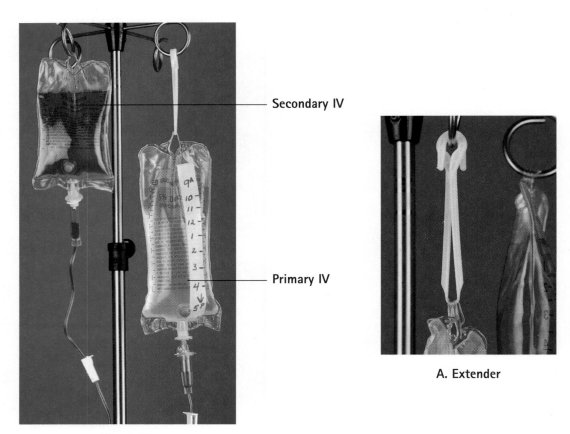

Secondary IV

Primary IV

A. Extender

Figure 78

The IVPB is connected to a port located below the drip chamber on the primary line. Notice that **the IVPB bag is hanging higher than the primary**. This gives it greater pressure, and causes it to **infuse first**. Each IVPB set includes a metal or plastic **extender**, A, which is used to lower the primary solution bag to obtain this pressure differential. The flow rate for the IVPB is set by a separate roller clamp located on the secondary line. When the IVPB bag has emptied the primary line will automatically resume its flow. Secondary medication bags are usually much smaller than primary bags. Fifty, 100 and 150 cc bags are frequently used. An example is the Cefotan® medication bag in Figure 79, which as you can see is completely labeled with the drug name and dosage.

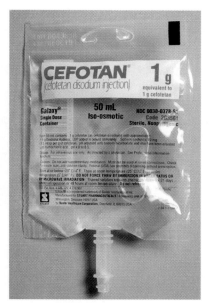

Figure 79

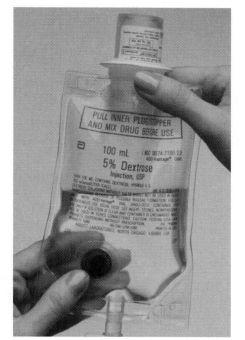

Figure 80

Another type of secondary medication setup is provided by Abbott Laboratories **ADD-Vantage®system** (Figure 80). In this system a specially designed IV fluid bag which contains a **medication vial port** is used. The medication vial containing the ordered drug and dosage is inserted into the port, and the drug (frequently in powdered form) is mixed using IV fluid as the diluent, as illustrated in Figure 81. The vial contents are then displaced back into the solution bag and thoroughly mixed in the total solution prior to infusion. The vial remains in the solution bag port throughout the infusion, making it possible to cross check the vial label for drug and dosage at any time.

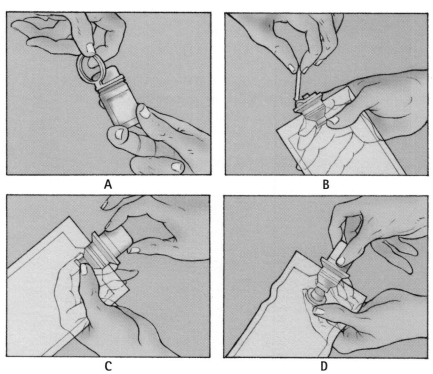

Figure 81 Abbott Laboratories ADD-Vantage® IV medication system **A.** The ADD-Vantage® Medication vial is opened first. **B.** The medication vial port on the IV bag is opened. **C.** The vial top is inserted into the IV bag port and twisted to lock tightly in place. **D.** The vial stopper is removed "inside" the IV bag and the medication and solution thoroughly mixed prior to infusion.

If a drug is not available in either of these pre-packaged or ADD-Vantage® formats it is often totally prepared and labeled by the hospital pharmacy. And finally, an IV medication may be prepared, added to the appropriate IV fluid, thoroughly mixed, labeled and initialed, and administered by the nurse who initiates the infusion.

Volume Controlled Burettes

For greater accuracy in the measurement of **small volume** IV medications and fluids, a **calibrated burette chamber** such as the one in Figure 82 may be used. The total capacity of burettes varies from 100 to 150 mL, calibrated in 1 mL increments. Many burettes are calibrated to deliver very small drops (microdrops), which also contributes to their accuracy. Burettes are most often referred to by their trade names, for example Buretrols®, Solusets®, or Volutrols®. Burette chambers are often connected to a secondary solution bag and used as a secondary line, but they can also be primary lines. When medication is ordered, it is injected into the burette through its injection port. The exact amount of IV fluid is then added as diluent. After thorough mixing the flow rate is set using a separate clamp on the burette line. Burettes are extensively used in pediatric and intensive care units, where both medication dosages and fluid volumes are critical.

Indwelling Infusion Ports/Intermittent Locks

When a continuous IV is not necessary, but intermittent IV medication administration is, an **infusion port adapter** (Figure 83) can be attached to an indwelling cannula in a vein. Infusion ports are frequently referred to as **heplocks** or **saline locks (or ports)**. This terminology evolved because the ports must be irrigated with 1-2 cc of sterile saline every 6-8 hours, or a heparin lock flush solution (100 U/mL) to prevent clotting and blockage. To infuse medication, the protective cap is removed from the port, its latex top is cleansed, and the medication line is attached. When the infusion is complete, the line is disconnected until the next dosage is due. Ports are also used for **direct injection of medication using a syringe**, which is called an **IV push, or bolus**.

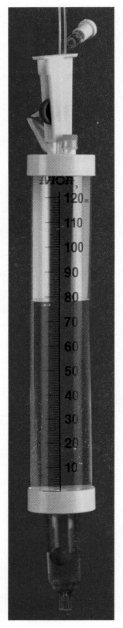

Figure 82

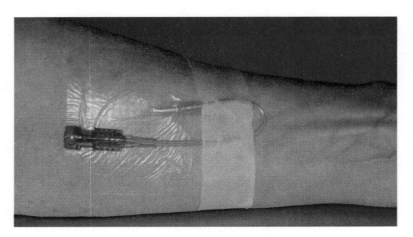

Figure 83

PROBLEM

Answer the following questions about IV administration sets as briefly as possible.

1. What is the correct fluid level for an IV drip chamber? _____

2. Which clamp is used to regulate IV flow rate? _____

3. When might a slide clamp be used? _____

4. What is a peripheral line? _____

5. What is a central line? _____

6. What is the common abbreviation for an intravenous piggyback? _____

7. Is this a primary or secondary line? _____

8. What must the height of a primary solution bag be when a secondary bag is infusing? _____

9. When is a saline lock used? _____

ANSWERS 1. middle of chamber   2. roller clamp   3. stop the IV temporarily without disturbing the rate set on the roller clamp   4. arm or leg vein   5. IV catheter inserted into a large chest vein   6. IVPB   7. secondary 8. lower than secondary bag   9. intermittent infusions when a continuous IV is not necessary

Electronic Infusion Devices (EID's)

Because the flow rate of IV's can easily be altered or obstructed by a patient's positional changes, electronic infusion devices are widely used for fluid and medication infusions. There are four major categories of devices: Rate Controllers, Volumetric Pumps, Syringe Pumps, and PCA's (Patient Controlled Analgesia devices). Many different models of these devices are available, and it is only possible to talk about them in terms of their general function, rather than specific operation. How to use them must await hands-on experience. The function of these devices will be discussed separately.

Electronic Rate Controllers

Controllers work on the same principle of gravity as a regular IV, with the rate of flow being maintained by rapid compression/decompression of the IV tubing by a pincher mechanism inside the controller. Refer to the controller in Figure 84 on page 214.

Notice first that the IV tubing is inserted in the controller at A, where the pincher mechanism is located. A **drop sensor**, B, is clipped to the tubing's drip chamber. This sensor monitors the flow rate, and causes the controller to adjust and compensate for flow rate changes. The desired **flow rate in mL/hr** is set on the controller at the flow rate panel, C (some models may be set in **gtt/min**).

Here is an example of how the controller would function. An IV is started, and the controller is set to deliver a rate of 125 mL/hr. Inadvertently the patient rolls on to and partially obstructs the IV tubing. The drip sensor immediately senses the slowed rate and causes the controller to adjust its compression/decompression cycle to re-establish the pre-set flow rate. **If the controller cannot maintain this rate it will alarm.**

Remember that a controller works on the principle of gravity; its control is not unlike a roller clamp, in that it adjusts the flow rate by changing the pressure on the IV tubing. The advantage of the controller is that the adjustment is instant, and continuous.

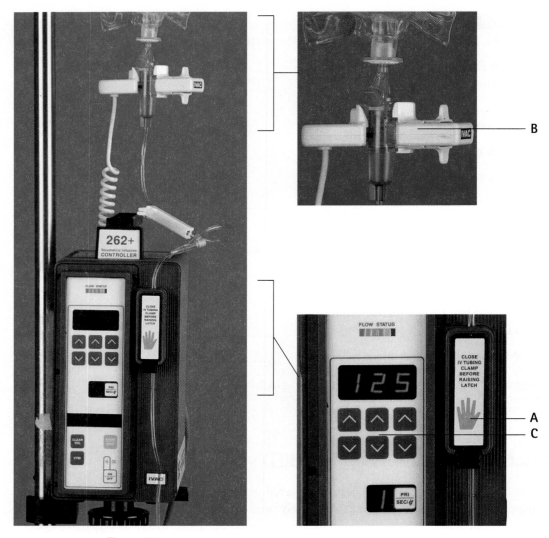

Figure 84

 Because controllers work by gravity the height of the solution bag is critical, and must be maintained at a minimum of 36 inches (3 feet) above the controller.

Volumetric Pumps

Volumetric pumps look very much like controllers (see Figure 85), but their function is quite different.

 A volumetric pump forces fluids into the vein under pressure, and against resistance.

Pumps are **always used for infusion of drugs whose dosage must be carefully regulated (titrated).** Some examples are dopamine, heparin, and pitocin. The flow rate is set in mL/hr to be infused. A sensor may be used on the drip chamber with a pump, however its function is not to monitor and adjust the flow rate, but to alarm when the drip chamber (and solution bag) is empty. Gravity is not a factor in the use of a pump, and the height of the IV solution bag is not a critical factor. As with controllers, when the pre-set rate cannot be maintained the pump will alarm.

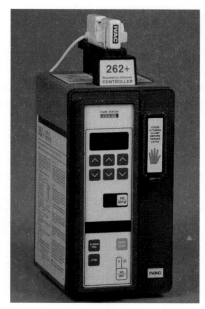
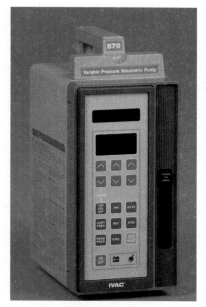
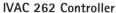

IVAC 262 Controller   IVAC 570 Volumetric Pump

Figure 85

 A pump will continue to force IV fluids even if the cannula becomes dislodged and is no longer in the vein.

This can not only be very painful but, depending on the type of solution infusing, can be very damaging to the tissues. For this reason when pumps are used on peripheral lines the IV site must be checked frequently for swelling, coolness, or discomfort, which could indicate infiltration.

Horizon Nxt™ Pump

One of the most sophisticated IV pumps available is the B. Braun/McGaw Horizon Nxt™ illustrated in Figure 86. Infusions can be set on this pump not only by flow rate but by drug dosage to be administered. Notice the display panel at the upper right which identifies the drug and dosage being infused (Dopamine 8.83 mcg/kg/min), the time of infusion left, the amount of solution infused, and the occlusion limit (pressure at the infusion site). The flow rate and volume to be delivered is displayed in red near the top left (25 mL/hr, 250 mL).

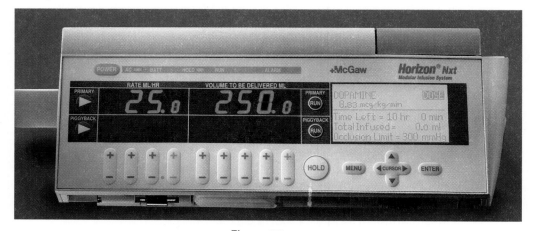

Figure 86

If a flow rate change is entered the display will instantly reflect the new dosage infusing; similarly if a dosage change is entered the flow rate necessary to infuse it will display instantly. Some additional features of the pump include the capability to deliver intermittent drug infusions; a built in safety feature which compares drug dosages entered with normal ranges; and sophisticated IV site monitoring features. The importance of this pump in the infusion of critical physiological altering drugs has led to its use becoming standard in many critical care units.

Syringe Pumps

Syringe pumps, as their name implies, are devices which use a syringe to administer medications or fluids (Figure 87).

Syringe pumps are particularly valuable when **drugs which cannot be mixed with other IV solutions or medications** must be administered at a controlled rate over a short period of time, for example 5, 10, or 20 minutes. The drug is measured in the syringe, which is inserted into the device, and the medication is infused at the rate set.

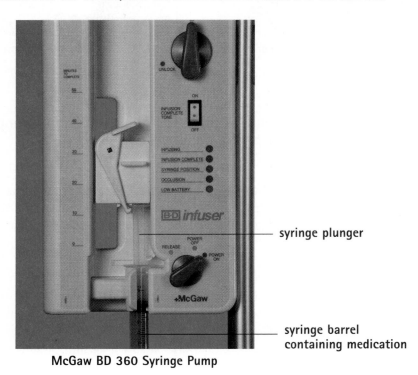

McGaw BD 360 Syringe Pump

Figure 87

Patient Controlled Analgesia (PCA) Devices

PCA's allow a patient to **self administer medication to control pain**. A pre-filled syringe or medication bag containing pain medication is inserted into the device (Figure 88) and the **dosage and frequency of administration ordered by the doctor is set**. The patient presses the control button, A, as medication is needed, and it is administered and recorded by the PCA.

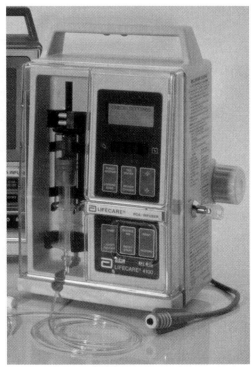

Abbott LIFECARE® PCA 4100 INFUSER

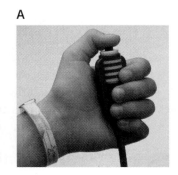

A

Figure 88

The device also keeps a record of the number of times a patient **attempts** to use it, and thus provides a record of the effectiveness of the dosage prescribed. If a patient's pain is not being relieved new orders must be obtained, and the PCA reset to administer the new dosage.

 All electronic devices must be monitored to be sure they are functioning properly.

Is the IV infusing at the rate which was set? Is the patient who activates a PCA getting relief of pain? If not, is it possible the PCA itself is malfunctioning? Electronic devices have been in use for many years and are relatively trouble free, but if the desired goal is not being obtained, in the absence of other obvious reasons, the possibility of malfunction must always be considered.

PROBLEM

Answer the following questions about EID's as briefly as possible.

1. What do electronic controllers control? ______________________
2. What is the optimum height of the solution bag in relation to a controller? ______________________
3. Why? ______________________
4. What is the function of a volumetric pump? ______________________
5. When might a syringe pump be used? ______________________
6. What is a PCA? ______________________

ANSWERS **1.** IV flow rate **2.** 36 inches **3.** IV runs by gravity flow and needs pressure to infuse **4.** forces fluids against resistance at a controlled rate **5.** to infuse drugs which are not compatible with other drugs and fluids **6.** patient controlled analgesia device

Introduction to IV Fluids

IV fluids are prepared in plastic solution bags or glass bottles in volumes ranging from 50 cc (bags only) to 1000 cc. The 500 and 1000 cc sizes are the most commonly used. IV bags and bottles are labeled with the **complete name** of the fluid they contain, and fine print under the solution name identifies the exact amount of each component of the fluid. IV **orders and charting**, however, are most often done **using abbreviations**. Some examples of frequently used fluids are: 5% Dextrose in Water, which may be abbreviated D5W; and 5% Dextrose in Normal Saline, which may be abbreviated D5NS.

In IV fluid abbreviations D always identifies dextrose; W always identifies water; S identifies saline, NS normal saline; and numbers identify percentage (%) strengths.

Solutions may be abbreviated in different ways; for example in addition to D5W you may see 5%D/W, D5%W, or other combinations. But the initials and percentage have the identical meaning regardless of the way they are abbreviated. Normal saline solutions are frequently written with the .9 or % sign included, for example D5 .9NS, or D5 0.9%S. IV fluids with different percentages of saline are also available: 0.45%, often written as 1/2 (0.45% is half of 0.9%), and 0.225%, sometimes written as 1/4 (1/4 of 0.9) are examples. Some typical orders might be abbreviated D5 1/2S, or D5 1/4NS.

Another commonly used solution is **Ringers Lactate**, a balanced electrolyte solution, which is also called Lactated Ringers Solution. As you would now expect, this solution is abbreviated **RL** or **LR**, and possibly RLS. Electrolytes may also be added to the basic fluids (DW and DS) just discussed. One electrolyte so commonly added that it must be mentioned is potassium chloride, which is abbreviated KCl. It is measured in milliequivalents (mEq).

PROBLEM

List as briefly as possible the components and percentage strengths of the following IV solutions.

1. D10 NS _____

2. D5 NS _____

3. D2.5 1/2S _____

4. D5 1/4S _____

5. D20W _____

6. D5NS _____

7. D5NS 20 mEq KCl _____

8. D5RL _____

ANSWERS 1. 10% Dextrose in 0.9% Saline 2. 5% Dextrose in Normal (0.9%) Saline 3. 2.5% Dextrose in 0.45% Saline 4. 5% Dextrose in 0.225% Saline 5. 20% Dextrose in Water 6. 5% Dextrose in Normal (0.9%) Saline 7. 5% Dextrose in 0.9% Saline with 20 mEq potassium chloride 8. 5% Dextrose in Ringers Lactate solution

Determining Percentages in IV Fluids

You may recall that **percent means grams of drug per 100 mL of fluid**. This means that a 5% dextrose solution will have 5 g of dextrose in each 100 mL. A 500 mL bag of a 5% solution will contain 5 g $\times$ 5, or 25 g of dextrose. The fine print on IV labels always lists the name and amount of all ingredients, but this can also be calculated using R&P.

EXAMPLE 1   **Calculate the amount of dextrose in 1000 mL 10% DW.**

% = g per 100 mL therefore 10% = 10 g per 100 mL

10 g : 100 mL = X g : 1000 mL
        X = 100 g

1000 mL 10% DW contains 100 g of dextrose

EXAMPLE 2   **Determine the amount of dextrose and NaCl in 500 mL 5% DNS.**

Dextrose   5 g : 100 mL = X g : 500 mL
            X = **25 g dextrose**

NaCl   0.9 g : 100 mL = X g : 500 mL
            X = **4.5 g NaCl**

500 mL 5% DNS contains 25 g of dextrose and 4.5 g NaCl

EXAMPLE 3   Determine the amount of dextrose and NaCl in 250 mL D5 1/2S.

Dextrose   5 g : 100 mL = X g : 250 mL
X = **12.5 g dextrose**

NaCl   0.45 g : 100 mL = X g : 250 mL
X = **1.13 g NaCl**

250 mL D5 1/2S contains 12.5 g dextrose and 1.13 g NaCl

PROBLEM

Calculate the amount of dextrose and NaCl in the following IV solutions.

1. 500 mL D5 1/2S   dextrose = _____   NaCl = _____

2. 750 mL D5NS   dextrose = _____   NaCl = _____

ANSWERS   1. 25 g dextrose; 2.25 g NaCl   2. 37.5 g dextrose; 6.75 g NaCl

The point illustrated by these calculations is that IV fluids contain significant quantities of dextrose, salts, and electrolytes. This highlights the importance of IV flow rates, and the considerations necessary when IV's are discovered to have infused ahead of or behind schedule.

Parenteral Nutrition

One of the options available for providing nutrition when a patient is unable to eat is to administer a nutrient solution via a peripheral or central vein. This is referred to as parenteral nutrition. The solutions infused are generally high caloric, and contain varying percentages of glucose, amino acids, and/or fat emulsions. A number of abbreviations/ descriptions are used for parenteral nutrients, two of the more common being TPN (total parenteral nutrition), PPN (partial parenteral nutrition), and hyperalimentation (nutrition in excess of maintenance needs). There is a noticeable difference in fluids which contain lipids (fat, intralipids) in that they are opaque-white in appearance, not unlike non-fat milk. These fluids are normally infused slowly, but not usually in excess of 24 hours, because they can spoil and support bacterial growth. All precautions applicable to IV's in general apply equally to parenteral nutrients, with more care necessary for the IV site to prevent infection. Flow rate and infusion time calculations covered in subsequent chapters are also applicable for parenteral nutrition solutions.

IV Medication Guidelines/Protocols

IV drugs far outnumber those given by any other parenteral route. The number of IV drugs has become so large, and the specifics of their administration so varied, that hospitals are increasingly compiling IV **Medication Guidelines or Protocols** to cover all the pertinent details of their administration. This information is compiled from pharmaceutical manufacturers specifications, which in turn are based on clinical testing of a drug. The information contained in protocols may include usual dosage, dilution for IV administration, infusion rates and time, compatibility with other drugs and IV fluids, and patient observations specific for drug action, for example pulse or blood pressure.

Refer to the sample guidelines for adult medications in Figure 89, and notice that this particular protocol has columns for Drug Name (with trade name in parenthesis); Administration (IVPB or Push); Dosage, Rate, and Recommended Dilution; and Comments (precautions in use and administration).

GUIDELINES FOR THE ADMINISTRATION OF IV DRUGS

DRUG	ADMINISTRATION	DOSAGE, RATE, RECOMMENDED DILUTION	COMMENTS
Theophylline (Aminophyllin)	IV Drip **IVAC	500 mg/1000 cc 35–50 mg/hr (75–100 cc/hr)	1. Do not mix with any other drug
	IVPB	250 mg/50 cc (30 min) 500 mg/100 cc (50 min)	2. Do not exceed 25 mg/min 3. Assess: P for tachycardia, arrhythmias; BP for hypotension
Vancomycin (Vanocin)	IVPB	0–500 mg/100 cc (30 min) 0.5–1 g/250 cc (30 min)	
Penicillin G	IVPB	0–2 M units/50 cc (45 min) 2–6 M units/100 cc (60 min) 10–20 M units/250–1000 cc (6-8 hrs)	1. Note: Allergies
Pipracillin (Pipracil)	IVPB	< 3 g/50 mL (30 min) > 3 g/100 mL (30 min)	
	IV Push	5 cc diluent/g (3–5 min)	
Oxacillin (Prostaphlin)	IVPB	< 1 g/50 mL NS (30 min) > 1 g/100 mL NS (30 min) > 2 g/250 mL NS (60 min)	
	IV Push	1 g/10 cc in sterile water (20 min)	

Figure 89

Courtesy Scripps Memorial Hospital, La Jolla, CA.

This sample protocol provides a very simplified introduction to IV medications, but it will give you an idea of the kinds of information they may contain, and what information you will be expected to locate and understand.

PROBLEM

Examine the information contained on the IV Drug Guidelines in Figure 89, and answer the following questions.

1. If Vanocin 400 mg is to be given IVPB, how much solution must it be diluted in? _____

   What time is specified for its administration? _____

2. When aminophyllin is administered IVPB, what observations are required to monitor the patient's reaction to the drug? _____

3. If Pipracil 2.5 g is to be administered IVPB, what amount of diluent is specified for its dilution? _____

4. What time is specified for the administration of a 4 g dosage of pipracillin IVPB? _____

5. What type of diluent must be used to dilute oxacillin for IVPB administration? _____

   For IV Push administration? _____

6. How much diluent must be used for a 6 M (million) U penicillin dosage IVPB? _____

   What time is specified for the infusion? _____

ANSWERS   1. 100 cc; 30 min   2. P, BP   3. 50 mL   4. 30 min   5. NS; Sterile Water   6. 100 cc; 60 min

Summary

This concludes your introduction to IV therapy. The important points to remember from this chapter are:

→ sterile technique is used to set up all IV solutions, tubings and devices

→ the correct fluid level for an IV drip chamber is half full

→ injection ports on an IV line are used to connect secondary lines, and infuse medications

→ a peripheral line refers to an IV infusing in a hand, arm or leg vein

→ a central line refers to an IV infusing into a deep chest vein

→ IV's flow by gravity pressure, and the higher the solution bag the faster the IV will infuse

→ the average height for an IV solution bag above the patient's heart level is 3 feet

→ secondary solution bags must hang higher than the primary bag to infuse first

→ volume controlled burettes are used for very exact measurement of IV medications and fluids

→ intermittent infusion locks or ports are used to infuse IV medications or fluids on an intermittent basis when a continuous IV is not necessary

→ controllers are electronic devices which regulate gravity flow IV rates

→ volumetric pumps are electronic devices which force fluids into a vein under pressure

→ syringe pumps are used to infuse medications which cannot be mixed with other fluids or medications

→ patient controlled analgesia (PCA) devices allow a patient to self administer pain medication

→ in IV fluid abbreviations D identifies Dextrose, W identifies Water, S identifies Saline, NS identifies Normal Saline, RL and LR identify Lactated Ringers Solution, and numbers identify percentage (%) strengths

→ IV Medication Guidelines/Protocols have been developed to clarify hospital policy on the specific details of IV medication administration

Summary Self Test

You are to assist with some IV procedures. Answer the following situational questions concerning these.

1. A patient is admitted and an IV of 1000 cc D5RL is started. These initials identify what type of solution? _____

   This is referred to as what type of line? _____

2. All roller clamps on the IV tubing are closed before connection to the solution bag. Why? _____

3. The IV is started in the back of the patient's left hand. This makes it what type of line? _____

4. You are asked to check the fluid level in the drip chamber, and you observe that it is correct, which is _____

5. You are then asked to adjust the flow rate. You will use what type of clamp to do this? _____

6. It is decided to use an electronic infusion control device to monitor this gravity flow IV. The device used is a _____

7. An IV antibiotic is ordered for the patient. This is sent from the pharmacy already prepared in a small volume IV solution bag. The setup used to infuse this medication is referred to as an IV _____

   This is abbreviated how? _____

8. In order for the antibiotic to infuse first, it must be hung how in relation to the original solution bag? _____

9. When you assisted with the IV antibiotic infusion, you noticed that the staff nurse referred to a printed sheet of instructions pertaining to IV medication administration. What terminology is used to identify these instructions? _____ or _____

10. Some days later the patient's IV is to be discontinued, but he is to continue to receive IV antibiotics. The device used for this intermittent administration is called what? _____

11. The patient had a PCA in use for one day. What do these initials mean? _____

    What does this device control? _____

Answer the following questions as briefly as possible.

12. A small volume IV medication is to be diluted in 20 mL and infused. This can be most accurately measured using a _____ _____ .

13. These devices are calibrated in _____ mL increments.

14. When an IV medication is injected directly into the vein via a port it is called an IV _____ or _____ .

15. Ports may be irrigated with _____ cc of _____ to prevent blockage every _____ hr.

16. A volumetric pump differs from a controller in that it _____ fluids into a vein.

17. What happens if an IV infiltrates while a pump is being used?

_____

18. What is the function of the sensor on the drip chamber when a controller is being used? _____

19. In IV fluid abbreviations D5RL identifies what IV fluid? _____

20. How many grams of NaCl are in 500 mL of D5 0.9NS? _____

21. How many grams of dextrose does 1000 mL D10W contain? _____

ANSWERS 1. 5% Dextrose in Ringers Lactate; primary 2. to prevent air entering the tubing 3. peripheral 4. half full 5. roller 6. controller 7. piggyback; IVPB 8. higher 9. Guidelines or Protocols 10. intermittent infusion port; saline or heparin lock 11. patient controlled analgesia; pain 12. calibrated burette 13. 1 mL 14. Push or bolus 15. 1-2; Normal Saline; 6-8 16. forces 17. fluid continues to be forced into the tissues 18. counts the drops to regulate the flow 19. 5% Dextrose in Ringers Lactate 20. 4.5 g 21. 100 g

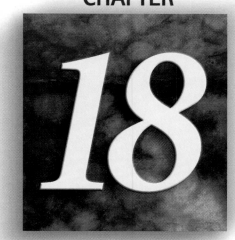

IV FLOW RATE CALCULATION

T There are a number of ways to calculate IV flow rates, and this chapter will present three, using ratio and proportion, the formula method, and the division factor method. Large volumes of intravenous fluids are most often ordered on the basis of **mL/hr** to be administered, for example 125 mL/hr. With the widespread use of electronic infusion devices which can be set to deliver a mL/hr rate, simply setting the rate ordered on the device and making sure it is working properly is all that is required for most infusions. Some infusion devices can also be set at a **gtt/min** (drop per minute) rate, which is much less frequently ordered than the mL/hr rate.

The most common calculation, which is necessary **when an infusion device is not being used**, involves **converting an IV order to the gtt/min rate necessary to infuse it**. This calculation may be required for **large volume orders** written designating a **mL/hr** rate, for example 1000 mL to infuse at **125 mL/hr**, for infusions of **mL per multiple hours**, for example 3000 mL/24 hr, or for **small volume orders**, usually involving medication administration, for example 100 mL/40 min.

OBJECTIVES
The student will
1. identify the calibrations in gtt/mL on IV administration sets
2. calculate flow rates using ratio and proportion
3. calculate flow rates using the formula method
4. calculate flow rates by the division factor method
5. recalculate flow rates to correct off–schedule infusions

IV Tubing Calibration

The size of IV drops is regulated by the type of IV set being used, which is **calibrated in number of gtt/mL**. Unfortunately all sets (and their drop size) are not the same. Each hospital uses at least two sizes of infusion sets, the standard or **macrodrip set**, **calibrated at 10, 15 or 20 gtt/mL**, which is used for routine adult IV administrations; and a **mini or microdrip set calibrated at 60 gtt/mL**. These are used when more exact measurements are needed, for example to infuse medications, or in critical care and pediatric units where they are often routinely used.

 IV administration sets are calibrated in gtt/mL.

The gtt/mL calibration of each IV set is clearly printed on each package, and the first step in calculating flow rates is to identify the gtt/mL calibration of the set to be used for infusion.

PROBLEM

Refer to the IV set packages provided and identify the calibration in gtt/mL of each.

1. _____

2. _____

3. _____

4. _____

5. _____

PRIMARY I.V. SET
No. 8083

Nonvented, 100 Inch
BACKCHECK VALVE AND 3 Y-INJECTION SITES.
Piggyback MICRODRIP® with OPTION-LOK™

60 DROPS/mL

Package 1

2C5419 s
Baxter-Travenol
Vented Basic Set
10 drops/mL
10

Package 2

Twin-Site® Venoset®
with CAIR™ Clamp
 ABBOTT
No. 8957
15 drops/ml.

100 inch I.V. Set (254 cm.), with CAIR* (constant accurate infusion rate) clamp,
drip chamber providing approximately 15 drops per ml., bacterial retentive air filter,
and two Y injection sites 6 and 39 inches (15 and 99 cm.) from male adapter.
Dimensions are nominal.

*Precision roller clamp mfd. for Abbott by Adelberg R&D Laboratories. U.S. Pat. No. 3,685,787; Canadian Pat. No. 926,371.

Package 3

code 880-02
**60" (152 cm)
I.V. Set**
20 ga x 11/2" (3.8 cm) needle
screw clamp
20 Drops=1ml (approx.)

Package 4

Catalog Number: *IV3DO6*
*Non-Vented Burette Set With Microbore Tubing
And Luer-Lock*   *Macrodrop Set: Approx. 20 drops/ml*

IVION CORPORATION
A wholly-owned subsidiary of Medex, Inc.

Package 5

ANSWERS   **1.** 60 gtt/mL   **2.** 10 gtt/mL   **3.** 15 gtt/mL   **4.** 20 gtt/mL   **5.** 20 gtt/mL

Calculating Large Volume gtt/min Rates from mL/hr Ordered

Since only one **macrodrip** calibrated set of either **10, 15 or 20 gtt/mL** is used in most hospital or clinical settings, a **mL/hr to gtt/min conversion chart** may be available. If one is not available the following method is one of the safest and most logical ways to **convert the mL/hr ordered to a gtt/min flow rate**. It can be used if the rate ordered is mL/hr, for example 125 mL/hr, or mL per multiple hr, for example 3000 mL/24 hr. Let's now look at some calculations which involve both of these types of orders.

EXAMPLE 1   An IV is ordered to infuse at a rate of **125 mL/hr** using a set calibrated at **10 gtt/mL**. Calculate the **gtt/min** flow rate.

You are calculating **gtt/min** so start by determining how many **mL/min** this order represents. This is done by **dividing the 125 mL/hr rate by 60 min**.

- **Change the mL/hr ordered to mL/min.**

    125 mL ÷ 60 min = **2 mL/min**

- **Calculate the gtt/min rate for the 2 mL/min obtained.** To establish consistency you may wish to **enter the set calibration first.**

    10 gtt : 1 mL = X gtt : 2 mL   or $\dfrac{10\ gtt}{1\ mL} : \dfrac{X\ gtt}{2\ mL}$ = **20 gtt**
    X = **20 gtt**

    To infuse an IV at 125 mL/hr using a set calibrated at 10 gtt/mL set the manual drip rate at 20 gtt/min.

EXAMPLE 2   An IV of **150 mL** is to infuse in **1 hr** using a set calibrated at **15 gtt/mL**. Calculate the **gtt/min** flow rate.

- **Change the mL/hr ordered to mL/min.**

    150 mL ÷ 60 min = **2.5 mL/min**

- **Calculate the gtt/min rate.**

    15 gtt : 1 mL = X gtt : 2.5 mL   or $\dfrac{15\ gtt}{1\ mL} : \dfrac{X\ gtt}{2.5\ mL}$ = 37.5 = **38 gtt**
    X = 37.5 = **38 gtt**

    To infuse 150 mL/hr using a set calibrated at 15 gtt/mL set the manual drip rate at 38 gtt/min.

 Flow rates are routinely rounded to the nearest whole number.

Let's now look at some IV's ordered to infuse in more than one hour.

EXAMPLE 3   An IV of **2500 mL** is to infuse in **24 hr** using a **20 gtt/mL** calibrated set. Calculate the **gtt/min** flow rate.

- **Calculate the mL/hr to infuse.**

    2500 mL ÷ 24 hr = 104.1 = **104 mL/hr**

- **Calculate the mL/min to infuse.**

    104 mL ÷ 60 min = **1.7 mL/min**

• **Calculate the gtt/min rate.**

$$20 \text{ gtt} : 1 \text{ mL} = X \text{ gtt} : 1.7 \text{ mL} \quad \text{ or } \quad \frac{20 \text{ gtt}}{1 \text{ mL}} : \frac{X \text{ gtt}}{1.7 \text{ mL}} = \textbf{34 gtt}$$
$$X = \textbf{34 gtt}$$

To infuse an IV of 2500 mL in 24 hr using an IV set calibrated at 20 gtt/mL set the manual flow rate at 34 gtt/min.

EXAMPLE 4   An IV of **1000 mL** is ordered to infuse in **5 hr** using a set calibrated at **15 gtt/mL**.

• **Calculate the mL/hr to infuse.**

$$1000 \text{ mL} \div 5 \text{ hr} = \textbf{200 mL/hr}$$

• **Calculate the mL/min to infuse.**

$$200 \text{ mL} \div 60 \text{ min} = \textbf{3.3 mL/min}$$

• **Calculate the gtt/min rate.**

$$15 \text{ gtt} : 1 \text{ mL} = X \text{ gtt} : 3.3 \text{ mL} \quad \text{ or } \quad \frac{15 \text{ gtt}}{1 \text{ mL}} : \frac{X \text{ gtt}}{3.3 \text{ mL}} = \textbf{50 gtt}$$
$$X = 49.5 = \textbf{50 gtt}$$

To infuse 1000 mL in 5 hr using a set calibrated at 15 gtt/mL set the rate at 50 gtt/min.

Flow rate answers may vary by 1–2 gtt/min depending on how the numbers are rounded in calculations, or calculator setting if one is used.

A 1-2 gtt/min variation is considered insignificant for most infusions, because flow rates fluctuate as the patient bends the infusion arm, changes position in bed, or ambulates. Thus manually set rates are always approximate.

PROBLEM

Calculate the gtt/min manual IV flow rates for the following infusions. Round rates to the nearest whole number.

1. An IV of 2000 mL is to infuse over 12 hr using a 10 gtt/mL set.   _____

2. 3500 mL are ordered to infuse in 24 hr using a set calibrated at 20 gtt/mL.   _____

3. Infuse 500 mL in 3 hr using a 15 gtt/mL set.   _____

4. A volume of 1500 mL is to infuse in 5 hr using a 15 gtt/mL set.   _____

5. 1750 mL are ordered to infuse in 9 hr using a 20 gtt/mL set.   _____

6. An IV of 2500 mL is to infuse in 18 hr on a set calibrated at 10 gtt/mL.   _____

7. A 3000 mL volume is to infuse in 24 hr on a set calibrated at 20 gtt/mL.   _____

8. A volume of 2750 mL is to infuse in 22 hr on a 15 gtt/mL set.   _____

9. An IV of 750 mL is ordered to infuse in 8 hr on a 10 gtt/mL set.   _____

10. A volume of 1250 mL is to infuse in 12 hr using a 15 gtt/mL set.   _____

ANSWERS   Note: Answers which vary by 1-2 gtt/min may be considered correct.   **1.** 27 gtt/min   **2.** 48 gtt/min   **3.** 41 gtt/min   **4.** 75 gtt/min   **5.** 64 gtt/min   **6.** 23 gtt/min   **7.** 40 gtt/min   **8.** 30 gtt/min   **9.** 16 gtt/min   **10.** 26 gtt/min

Calculating Small Volume gtt/min Rates from mL/min Ordered

Small volume IV solutions are most frequently ordered to administer medications. Because of the immediacy of IV medication action each dosage is routinely double checked for accuracy before administration. A small volume flush of IV solution is usually ordered to follow the medication to ensure that all the medication has cleared the line. The flush volume may vary from 2–15 mL depending on the length of the IV tubing between the medication source and the injection site.

There are three common administrative techniques used for small volume infusions. **Very small volumes** are most often administered by **syringe**, either **manually** or **via syringe pump**. If a syringe pump (see chapter 17, page 216) is used the primary responsibilities are to make sure the rate is set correctly on the device, **and** that it is working properly.

The two other methods of small volume administration are via **burettes** calibrated in 1–2 mL increments, with a capacity of 100–150 mL (chapter 17, page 212); or via **commercial or pharmacy prepared IV bags containing medication** with a volume of 50–250 mL (chapter 17, page 211).

It is when a **burette** or **small volume IV solution bag** is to be infused **without the use of an electronic device** that a gtt/min flow rate will need to be calculated. With regard to burettes one precaution must be particularly stressed: **while most are calibrated in 60 gtt/mL microdrips, this calibration cannot be taken for granted.** Some burettes are specifically manufactured for use with electronic infusion devices (pumps most commonly) and may have, for example, a 20 gtt/mL calibration. When pumps are used with their companion tubings their setting accommodates for the gtt size, and the main administrative precaution becomes **matching the correct tubing to its pump**, setting the rate correctly, and as always, making sure the device is working properly.

Let's now look at calculation of small volume flow rates when no infusion device is used.

EXAMPLE 1 An IV medication of **100 mL** is to be infused in **40 min** using a set calibrated at **15 gtt/mL**. Calculate the **gtt/min** flow rate.

- **Calculate the mL/min to be administered.**

$$100 \text{ mL} : 40 \text{ min} = X \text{ mL} : 1 \text{ min} \quad \text{or} \quad \frac{100 \text{ mL}}{40 \text{ min}} : \frac{X \text{ mL}}{1 \text{ min}} = \textbf{2.5 mL}$$
$$X = \textbf{2.5 mL}$$

- **Calculate the gtt/min rate.**

$$15 \text{ gtt} : 1 \text{ mL} = X \text{ gtt} : 2.5 \text{ mL} \quad \text{or} \quad \frac{15 \text{ gtt}}{1 \text{ mL}} : \frac{X \text{ gtt}}{2.5 \text{ mL}} = 37.5 = \textbf{38 gtt}$$
$$X = 37.5 \text{ gtt} = \textbf{38 gtt}$$

To administer an infusion of 100 mL in 40 min using a 15 gtt/mL calibrated set the flow rate must be 38 gtt/min.

EXAMPLE 2 An IV medication with a volume of **60 mL** is ordered to infuse in **30 min**. The set calibration is **20 gtt/mL**. Calculate the **gtt/min** flow rate.

- **Calculate the mL/min to be administered.**

$$60 \text{ mL} : 30 \text{ min} = X \text{ mL} : 1 \text{ min} \quad \text{or} \quad \frac{60 \text{ mL}}{3 \text{ min}} : \frac{X \text{ mL}}{1 \text{ min}} = \textbf{2 mL/min}$$
$$X = \textbf{2 mL/min}$$

- **Calculate the gtt/min rate.**

$$20 \text{ gtt} : 1 \text{ mL} = X \text{ gtt} : 2 \text{ mL} \quad \text{or} \quad \frac{20 \text{ gtt}}{1 \text{ mL}} : \frac{X \text{ gtt}}{2 \text{ mL}} = \textbf{40 gtt/min}$$
$$X = \textbf{40 gtt}$$

To infuse a volume of 60 mL in 30 min using a set calibrated at 20 gtt/mL set the flow rate at 40 gtt/min.

EXAMPLE 3 A volume of **50 mL** is ordered to infuse in **20 min** using a **10 gtt/mL** calibrated set. Calculate the **gtt/min** flow rate.

• Calculate the mL/min to be administered.

$$50 \text{ mL} : 20 \text{ min} = X \text{ mL} : 1 \text{ min} \quad \text{or} \quad \frac{50 \text{ mL}}{20 \text{ min}} : \frac{X \text{ mL}}{1 \text{ min}} = \textbf{25 gtt/min}$$
$$X = \textbf{2.5 mL/min}$$

• Calculate the gtt/min rate.

$$10 \text{ gtt} : 1 \text{ mL} = X \text{ gtt} : 2.5 \text{ mL} \quad \text{or} \quad \frac{10 \text{ gtt}}{1 \text{ mL}} : \frac{X \text{ gtt}}{2.5 \text{ mL}} = \textbf{25 gtt}$$
$$X = \textbf{25 gtt}$$

To infuse a volume of 50 mL in 20 min using a set calibrated at 10 gtt/mL set the flow rate at 25 gtt/min.

PROBLEM

Calculate the flow rates in gtt/min for the following small volume infusions. Round rates to the nearest whole gtt.

1. A medication of 75 mL is to be administered in 50 min using a set calibrated at 10 gtt/mL. _____

2. A set calibrated at 15 gtt/mL is to be used to infuse 80 mL in 50 min. _____

3. A volume of 40 mL is to be infused in 20 min using a set calibrated at 20 gtt/mL. _____

4. A 10 gtt/mL set is being used to administer 20 mL in 20 min. _____

5. A 70 mL volume is to infuse in 40 min using a 15 gtt/mL set. _____

ANSWERS Note: Answers which vary by 1-2 gtt/min may be considered correct. **1.** 15 gtt/min **2.** 24 gtt/min **3.** 40 gtt/min **4.** 10 gtt/min **5.** 27 gtt/min

Formula Method of Flow Rate Calculation

The flow rate can also be determined by using the following formula, which is useful when the rate can be expressed as **mL/60 min or less**.

$$\textbf{Flow Rate} = \frac{\textbf{Volume} \times \textbf{Set Calibration}}{\textbf{Time (in min)}}$$

EXAMPLE 1 An IV is ordered to infuse at **125 mL/hr**. Calculate the **gtt/min** rate for a set calibrated at **10 gtt/mL**.

• Convert the hr to min

$$\frac{125 \text{ (mL)} \times 10 \text{ (gtt/mL)}}{60 \text{ (min)}}$$

• Calculate the gtt/min rate

$$\frac{125 \times 10}{60} = 20.8 = \textbf{21 gtt/min}$$

EXAMPLE 2 Administer an IV medication of **100 mL** in **40 min** using a set calibrated at **15 gtt/mL**.

$$\frac{100 \times 15}{40} = 37.5 = \textbf{38 gtt/min}$$

EXAMPLE 3   A **75 mL** volume of IV medication is ordered to infuse in **45 min**. The set is calibrated at **20 gtt/mL**.

$$\frac{75 \times 20}{45} = 33.3 = \textbf{33 gtt/min}$$

PROBLEM

Calculate the flow rate in gtt/min for the following infusions using the formula method.

1. Administer an IV of 110 mL/hr using a set calibrated at 20 gtt/mL. _____

2. An IV solution is ordered at 200 mL/hr using a set calibrated at 15 gtt/mL. _____

3. A volume of 80 mL is to be infused in 20 min using a 10 gtt/mL set. _____

4. An IV is ordered to infuse at 150 mL/hr using a 10 gtt/mL calibrated set. _____

5. An IV rate of 90 mL/hr is ordered using a 15 gtt/mL calibrated set. _____

ANSWERS Note: Consider answers within 1 gtt/min correct. **1.** 37 gtt/min **2.** 50 gtt/min **3.** 40 gtt/min **4.** 25 gtt/min **5.** 23 gtt/min

When an IV is ordered to infuse in **more than one hour** the formula method can still be used. However, to keep the numbers you are working with as small as possible it is best to add a preliminary step, and determine the **mL/hr** the ordered volume will represent.

EXAMPLE 1   Calculate the gtt/min flow rate for an IV of **1000 mL** to infuse in **8 hr** on a set calibrated at **20 gtt/mL**.

• **Calculate the mL/hr.**

  1000 mL/8 hr = 1000 ÷ 8 = **125 mL/hr**

• **Calculate the gtt/min flow rate.**

$$\frac{125 \text{ (mL)} \times 20 \text{ (gtt/mL)}}{60 \text{ (min)}} = 41.6 = \textbf{42 gtt/min}$$

EXAMPLE 2   Calculate the gtt/min flow rate for a volume of **2500 mL** to infuse in **24 hr** on a set calibrated at **10 gtt/mL**.

• **Calculate the mL/hr.**

  2500 mL/24 hr = 2500 ÷ 24 = **104 mL/hr**

• **Calculate the gtt/min flow rate.**

$$\frac{104 \times 15}{60} = 17.3 = \textbf{17 gtt/min}$$

EXAMPLE 3   An IV of **1200 mL** is to infuse in **16 hr** on a set calibrated at **15 gtt/mL**.

1200 mL/16 hr = 1200 ÷ 16 = **75 mL/hr**

$$\frac{75 \times 15}{60} = 18.7 = \textbf{19 gtt/min}$$

PROBLEM

Calculate the gtt/min flow rate for the following infusions using the formula method.

1. A volume of 2000 mL to infuse in 24 hr on a set calibrated at 15 gtt/mL. _____

2. A volume of 300 mL to infuse in 6 hr on a 60 gtt/mL micro-drip set. _____

3. A volume of 500 mL to infuse in 4 hr on a 15 gtt/mL calibrated set. _____

4. A 10 hr infusion of 1200 mL using a 20 gtt/mL set. _____

5. An infusion of 500 mL in 5 hr on a set calibrated at 10 gtt/mL. _____

ANSWERS Note: Answers which vary by 1-2 gtt/min may be considered correct. **1.** 21 gtt/min **2.** 50 gtt/min **3.** 31 gtt/min **4.** 40 gtt/min **5.** 17 gtt/min

Division Factor Method of Calculation

In a clinical setting where all the macrodrip IV sets have the same calibration, either 10, 15 or 20 gtt/mL, an alternate "division factor" method can be used to calculate flow rates. However, **this method can only be used if the rate is expressed in mL/hr (mL/60 min)**. Let's start by looking at how the division factor is obtained.

EXAMPLE Administer an IV at **125 mL/hr**. The set calibration is **10 gtt/mL**. Calculate the gtt/min rate. Express the hr rate as 60 min.

$$\frac{125 \text{ (mL)} \times \overset{1}{10} \text{ (gtt/mL)}}{\underset{6}{60} \text{ (min)}} = 20.8 = \textbf{21 gtt/min}$$

Look at the completed equation, and notice that because you are restricting the time to 60 min, the set calibration (10) will be divided into 60 (min) to obtain a constant number (6). This constant, (6), is the division factor for a 10 gtt/mL calibrated set.

 The division factor can be obtained for any IV set by dividing 60 by the calibration of the set.

PROBLEM

Determine the division factor for the following IV sets.

1. 20 gtt/mL _____

2. 15 gtt/mL _____

3. 60 gtt/mL _____

4. 10 gtt/mL _____

ANSWERS **1.** 3 **2.** 4 **3.** 1 **4.** 6

Once the division factor is known, the gtt/min rate can be calculated in one step, by dividing the mL/hr rate by the division factor. Look again at the example.

$$\frac{125 \text{ (mL)} \times \overset{1}{10} \text{ (gtt/mL)}}{\underset{6}{60} \text{ (min)}} = 20.8 = \textbf{21 gtt/min}$$

$$\text{or } 125 \text{ (mL/hr)} \div 6 = 20.8 = \textbf{21 gtt/min}$$

The 125 mL/hr flow rate divided by the division factor 6 gives the same 21 gtt/min rate.

 The gtt/min flow rate can be calculated for mL/hr IV orders in one step by dividing the mL/hr to be infused by the division factor of the set.

EXAMPLE 1   Infuse an IV at **100 mL/hr** using a set calibrated at **10 gtt/mL.**

Determine the division factor: 60 ÷ 10 = **6**

Calculate the flow rate: 100 mL ÷ 6 = 16.6 = **17 gtt/min**

EXAMPLE 2   Infuse an IV at **125 mL/hr** using a set calibrated at **15 gtt/mL.**

60 ÷ 15 = **4**   125 mL ÷ 4 = 31.2 = **31 gtt/min**

EXAMPLE 3   A set calibrated at **20 gtt/mL** is used to infuse **90 mL per hr.**

60 ÷ 20 = **3**   90 mL ÷ 3 = **30 gtt/min**

PROBLEM

Calculate the flow rates in gtt/min for the following infusions using the division factor method.

1. A rate of 110 mL/hr via a set calibrated at 20 gtt/mL.   _____
2. A set is calibrated at 15 gtt/mL. Infuse at 130 mL/hr.   _____
3. Infuse 150 mL/hr using a 10 gtt/mL set.   _____
4. A set calibrated at 20 gtt/mL is used to infuse 45 mL/hr.   _____
5. Infusion is ordered at 75 mL/hr with a set calibrated at 15 gtt/mL.   _____

ANSWERS Note: Answers which vary by 1-2 gtt/min may be considered correct. **1.** 37 gtt/min **2.** 33 gtt/min **3.** 25 gtt/min **4.** 15 gtt/min **5.** 19 gtt/min

All of the above examples and problems using the division factor method were for **macrodrip** sets. Let's now look what happens when a **microdrip** set calibrated at **60 gtt/mL** is used.

EXAMPLE   Infuse at **50 mL/hr** using a **60 gtt/mL** microdrip.

60 ÷ 60 = **1**   50 mL ÷ 1 = **50 gtt/min**

Because the set calibration is 60, and the division factor is based on a 60 min (hr) time, the division factor is 1. So, for microdrip sets the gtt/min flow rate will be identical to the mL/hr ordered.

> When a 60 gtt/mL microdrip set is used the flow rate in gtt/min is identical to the volume in mL/hr.

PROBLEM

What is the drip rate in gtt/min for the following infusions if a microdrip is used?

1. 120 mL/hr   _____

2. 90 mL/hr   _____

3. 100 mL/hr   _____

4. 75 mL/hr   _____

5. 80 mL/hr   _____

ANSWERS 1. 120 gtt/min 2. 90 gtt/min 3. 100 gtt/min 4. 75 gtt/min 5. 80 gtt/min

The division factor method can be used to calculate the flow rate of **any volume that can be expressed in mL/hr.** Larger volumes can be divided, and smaller volumes multiplied and expressed in mL/hr. This does require an extra step, and if you find it confusing you may elect not to use it.

EXAMPLE 1   2400 mL/24 hr = 2400 ÷ 24 = **100 mL/hr**

EXAMPLE 2   1800 mL/8 hr = 1800 ÷ 8 = **225 mL/hr**

EXAMPLE 3   10 mL/30 min = 10 × 2 (2 × 30 min) = **20 mL/hr**

EXAMPLE 4   15 mL/20 min = 15 × 3 (3 × 20 min) = **45 mL/hr**

Regulating Flow Rate

The flow rate is regulated by **counting the number of drops falling in the drip chamber.** The standard procedure for doing this is to hold a watch next to the drip chamber and actually **count the drops for 15-60 seconds** (sec count may vary depending on agency or state regulations), while using the roller clamp to adjust the flow rate to the desired gtt/min. For example, if the required rate is 41 gtt/min you would adjust the flow rate to 10 gtt in 15 seconds (41 ÷ 4 = 10; 10/sec is as close as you can get for a 15 sec count).

PROBLEM

Answer the following questions about 15 second drip rates.

1. The 15 second count of an IV flow rate is 7 gtt. A 29 gtt/min rate is required. Is this rate correct?   _____

2. You are to regulate a newly started IV to deliver 67 gtt/min. Using a 15 second count, how would you set the flow rate?   _____

3. An IV is to run at 48 gtt/min. What must the 15 second drip rate be?   _____

4. How many gtt will you count in 15 seconds if the rate is 55 gtt/min?   _____

5. An IV is to run at 84 gtt/min. What will the 15 second rate be?   _____

ANSWERS Note: Answers which vary by 1 gtt/min may be considered correct. 1. yes 2. 17 gtt/15 sec
3. 12 gtt/15 sec 4. 14 gtt/15 sec 5. 21 gtt/15 sec

Correcting Off-Schedule Rates

Because a patient's positional changes can alter the rate slightly, IV's occasionally infuse ahead of or behind schedule. When this occurs the usual procedure is to recalculate the flow rate using the volume and time remaining, and adjust the rate accordingly. However, each situation must be individually evaluated, especially if the discrepancy is large. If too much fluid has infused, immediately assess the patient's response to the increased intake, and take appropriate action. If too little fluid has infused it will first be necessary to assess the patient's ability to tolerate an increased rate, and secondly to consider the type of fluid/medication involved. Some medications in particular have restrictions on rate of administration. Both of these factors must be considered before rates can be increased to "catch up." In addition, many hospitals will have specific policies to cover over or under infusion due to altered flow rates, and you will be responsible for knowing these.

The following are some examples of how the rate can be recalculated. Because IV's are usually checked hourly, we will focus first on recalculation using exact hours. Some recalculations have also been included using fractions of hours, rounded to the nearest quarter hour (15 min): 15 min = 0.25 hr, 30 min = 0.5 hr, and 45 min = 0.75 hr. These equivalents are close enough for uncomplicated infusions, since the exact time of completion is not totally predictable. IV's needing exact infusion would hopefully be monitored by electronic infusion devices.

EXAMPLE 1 An IV of **1000 mL** was ordered to infuse over **10 hr** at a rate of **25 gtt/min**. The set calibration is **15 gtt/mL**. After **5 hr** a total of **650 mL** have infused, instead of the **500 mL** ordered. Recalculate the new gtt/min flow rate to complete the infusion on schedule.

Time remaining 10 hr – 5 hr = **5 hr**

Volume remaining 1000 mL – 650 mL = **350 mL**

350 mL ÷ 5 hr = **70 mL/hr**

Set calibration is **15 gtt/mL.**

70 ÷ 4 (division factor) = 17.5 = **18 gtt/min**

Slow the rate from 25 gtt/min to 18 gtt/min

EXAMPLE 2 An IV of **800 mL** was to infuse over **8 hr** at **20 gtt/min**. After **4 hr 15 min** only **300 mL** have infused. Recalculate the **gtt/min** rate to complete on schedule. The set calibration is **15 gtt/mL.**

Time remaining 8 hr – 4.25 hr = **3.75 hr**

Volume remaining 800 mL – 300 mL = **500 mL**

500 mL ÷ 3.75 hr = 133.3 = **133 mL/hr**

Set calibration is **15 gtt/mL.**

133 ÷ 4 (division factor) = 33.2 = **33 gtt/min**

Increase the rate to 33 gtt/min

EXAMPLE 3

An IV of **500 mL** is infusing at **28 gtt/min**. It was to complete in **3 hr**, but after **1 1/2 hr** only **175 mL** have infused. Recalculate the **gtt/min** rate to complete the infusion on schedule. Set calibration is **10 gtt/mL**.

Time remaining 3 hr – 1.5 hr = **1.5 hr**

Volume remaining 500 mL – 175 mL = **325 mL**

325 mL ÷ 1.5 hr = 216.6 = **217 mL/hr**

Set calibration is **10 gtt/mL**.

217 ÷ 6 (division factor) = 36.1 = **36 gtt/min**

Increase the rate to 36 gtt/min

EXAMPLE 4

A volume of **250 mL** was to infuse **56 gtt/min** in **1 1/2 hr** using a set calibrated at **20 gtt/mL**. After **30 min 175 mL** have infused. Recalculate the flow rate.

Time remaining 1.5 hr – 30 min = **1 hr**

Volume remaining 250 mL – 175 mL = **75 mL**

Set calibration is **20 gtt/mL**.

75 ÷ 3 (division factor) = **25 gtt/min**

Decrease the rate to 25 gtt/min

PROBLEM

Recalculate the following IV rates so that the infusions will complete on schedule.

1. An IV of 500 mL was ordered to infuse in 3 hours using a 15 gtt/mL set. With 1 1/2 hours remaining you discover only 150 mL is left in the bag. At what rate will you need to reset the flow? _____

2. An IV of 1000 mL was scheduled to run in 12 hours. After 4 hours only 220 mL have infused. The set calibration is 20 gtt/mL. Recalculate the rate for the remaining solution. _____

3. An IV of 1000 mL was ordered to infuse in 8 hours. With 3 hours of infusion time left you discover that 600 mL have infused. The set delivers 20 gtt/mL. Recalculate the drip rate and indicate how many drops you will count in 15 seconds to set the new rate.

   _____ _____

4. An IV of 750 mL was ordered to run over 6 hours with a set calibrated at 10 gtt/mL. After 2 hours you notice that 300 mL have infused. Recalculate the flow rate, and indicate how many drops you will count in 15 seconds to reset the rate. _____ _____

5. An IV of 800 mL was started at 9 a.m. to infuse in 4 hours. At 10 a.m. 150 mL have infused. The set is calibrated at 15 gtt/mL. Recalculate the flow rate in gtt/min. _____

ANSWERS Note: Answers which vary by 1-2 gtt/min may be considered correct. **1.** 25 gtt/min **2.** 33 gtt/min **3.** 44 gtt/min; 11 gtt/15 sec **4.** 19 gtt/min; 4–5 gtt/15 sec **5.** 54 gtt/min

Summary

This concludes the chapter on IV flow rate calculation and monitoring. The important points to remember from this chapter are:

➡ IV's are ordered as mL/hr or mL/min to be administered

➡ manual flow rates are counted in gtt/min

➡ IV tubings are calibrated in gtt/mL

➡ macrodrip IV sets will have a calibration of 10, 15, or 20 gtt/mL

➡ mini or microdrip sets have a calibration of 60 gtt/mL

➡ the formula for calculating flow rates is

$$\frac{\text{Volume} \times \text{set calibration}}{\text{time (min)}}$$

➡ the division factor method can only be used to calculate flow rates if the volume to be administered is specified in mL/hr (60 min)

➡ the division factor is obtained by dividing 60 by the set calibration

➡ flow rate by the division factor method is determined by dividing the mL/hr to be administered by the division factor

➡ because micro and minidrips have a calibration of 60 gtt/mL, their division factor is 1, and the flow rate in gtt/min is the same as the mL/hr ordered

➡ if an IV runs ahead of or behind schedule a standard procedure is to use the time and mL remaining and calculate a new flow rate

➡ if a rate must be increased to compensate for running behind schedule, the type of fluid being infused and the patient's ability to tolerate an increased rate must be assessed

Summary Self Test

DIRECTIONS

Answer the following questions as briefly as possible.

1. Determine the division factor for the following IV sets.

   a) 60 gtt/mL   _____

   b) 15 gtt/mL   _____

   c) 20 gtt/mL   _____

   d) 10 gtt/mL   _____

2. How is the flow rate determined in the division factor method?   _____

3. The division factor method can only be used if the volume to be administered is expressed in   _____

4. An IV is to infuse at 50 gtt/min. How will you set it using a 15 second count?   _____

5. You are to adjust an IV at a rate of 60 gtt/min. What will the 15 second count be?   _____

Calculate the flow rate in gtt/min for each of the following IV solutions and medications. Don't let the types of solutions confuse you. Concentrate on locating the information you need for your calculations.

6. D5W 2000 mL has been ordered to run 16 hr. Set calibration is 10 gtt/mL. _____

7. The order is for 500 mL Normal Saline in 8 hr. The set is calibrated at 15 gtt/mL. _____

8. Administer 150 mL of Sodium Chloride 0.45% over 3 hr. A microdrip is used. _____

9. 1500 mL D5W with 40 mEq KCl/L has been ordered to run over 12 hr. Set calibration is 20 gtt/mL. _____

10. An IV medication of 30 mL is to be administered over 30 min using a 15 gtt/mL set. _____

11. Administer 100 mL 0.9% NaCl in 1 hour using a 15 gtt/mL set. _____

12. Infuse 500 mL intralipids IV in 6 hours. Set calibration is 10 gtt/mL. _____

13. The doctor orders a liter of D5W to infuse over 10 hours. At the end of 8 hours you notice that there is 500 mL left in the bag. What would the new flow rate be if the set calibration is 10 gtt/mL? _____

14. An IV was started at 9 a.m. with orders to infuse 500 mL over 6 hrs. At 12 noon the IV infiltrated with 350 mL left in the bag. At 1 p.m. the IV was restarted. The set calibration is 20 gtt/mL. Calculate the new flow rate to deliver the fluid on time. _____

15. A 50 mL piggyback IV is to infuse over 15 min. The set calibration is 15 gtt/mL. After 5 minutes the IV contains 40 mL. Calculate the flow rate to deliver the volume on time. _____

16. An IV of 1000 cc D5 1/4 NaCl with 20 mEq KCl is ordered to run at 25 mL/hr using a microdrip set. _____

17. Ringers Lactate 800 mL has been ordered to run in over 5 hours. Set calibration is 10 gtt/mL. _____

18. Administer 1500 mL D5 Lactated Ringers solution over 8 hours using a set calibrated at 20 gtt/mL. _____

19. The order is for D5 1/2 NaCl 750 mL over 6 hours. Set calibration is 15 gtt/mL. _____

20. An IV of 1000 mL was ordered to run over 8 hours. After 4 hours only 250 mL have infused. The set calibration is 20 gtt/mL. Recalculate the rate for the remaining solution. _____

21. The order is to infuse 50 mL of a piggyback antibiotic over 1 hour. The set calibration is a microdrip. _____

22. An IV of 500 mL D5W is to infuse over 6 hours. You will be using a set calibration of 10 gtt/mL. _____

23. Infuse 120 mL gentamicin via IVPB over 1 hour. Set calibration is 10 gtt/mL. _____

24. Administer 12 mL of an IV medication in 22 min using a
    microdrip set.   _____

25. A patient is to receive 3000 mL of D5W over 20 hours.
    Set is calibrated at 20 gtt/mL.   _____

26. Infuse 1 liter of D5W over 5 hours using a set calibration of
    15 gtt/mL.   _____

27. A hyperalimentation solution of 1180 mL is to infuse over
    12 hours using a set calibration of 20 gtt/mL.   _____

28. 150 mL of an antibiotic solution is to infuse over 30 minutes.
    At the end of 20 minutes you discover that 100 mL has infused.
    The set calibration is 10 gtt/mL. Should the flow rate be adjusted?
    If so, what is the new rate?   _____   _____

29. Two 500 mL units of whole blood are ordered. Both units are
    to be completed in 5 hours. The set calibration is 20 gtt/mL. _____

30. Infuse 15 mL of IV medication over the next 14 minutes using
    a 20 gtt/mL set.   _____

31. The patient is to receive 1000 mL 0.9% NaCl in 10 hours
    using a 20 gtt/mL calibration.   _____

32. A minidrip is used to administer 12 mL in 17 minutes.   _____

33. Infuse 2750 mL over 20 hours using a 10 gtt/mL set.   _____

34. D5W 1800 mL is to infuse in the next 15 hours with a
    15 gtt/mL set.   _____

35. Infuse 600 mL intralipids IV in 6 hours with a 10 gtt/mL set. _____

36. Administer 22 mL of an IV antibiotic solution in 18 minutes
    using a minidrip set.   _____

37. 1800 mL of D5W with 30 mEq of KCl per liter has been
    ordered to infuse in 10 hours. Set calibration is 20 gtt/mL. _____

38. Infuse 8 mL in 9 minutes using a minidrip.   _____

39. A patient is to receive 4000 mL D5W IV in the next 20 hours.
    A 20 gtt/mL set is used.   _____

40. An IV of 500 mL D5W which was to infuse in 2 hr is discovered
    to have only 150 mL left after 30 min. Recalculate the flow rate.
    Set calibration is 15 gtt/mL.   _____

ANSWERS   Note: Consider answers which vary by 1-2 gtt/min accurate.   1. a) 1 b) 4 c) 3 d) 6
2. mL/hr ÷ division factor   3. mL/hr (mL/60 min)   4. 13 gtt/15 sec   5. 15 gtt/15 sec   6. 21 gtt/min   7. 16 gtt/min
8. 50 gtt/min   9. 42 gtt/min   10. 15 gtt/min   11. 25 gtt/min   12. 14 gtt/min   13. 42 gtt/min   14. 58 gtt/min
15. 60 gtt/min   16. 25 gtt/min   17. 27 gtt/min   18. 63 gtt/min   19. 31 gtt/min   20. 63 gtt/min   21. 50 gtt/min
22. 14 gtt/min   23. 20 gtt/min   24. 33 gtt/min   25. 50 gtt/min   26. 50 gtt/min   27. 33 gtt/min   28. No, rate is
correct at 50 gtt/min   29. 67 gtt/min   30. 21 gtt/min   31. 33 gtt/min   32. 42 gtt/min   33. 23 gtt/min
34. 30 gtt/min   35. 17 gtt/min   36. 73 gtt/min   37. 60 gtt/min   38. 53 gtt/min   39. 67 gtt/min   40. 25 gtt/min

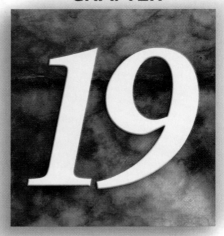

Calculating IV Infusion and Completion Times

The student will calculate IV infusion times using
1. volume and hourly rate of infusion
2. volume, gtt/min rate of infusion and set calibration
3. start time and infusion time to determine completion times
4. an IV solution bag tape to label the start, progress and completion times

T he three main reasons for calculating IV infusion times are: 1) to know when a particular solution bag or bottle will be completed, so that any additional solutions ordered can be prepared in advance and ready to hang; 2) to discontinue an IV when it has completed; and 3) to label an IV bag or bottle with start, progress, and completion times so that the infusion can be monitored and adjusted as necessary to keep it on schedule. Knowing the infusion time is also important because laboratory studies are sometimes made before, during, or after specified amounts of IV solutions have infused. The infusion time may be calculated in hours and/or minutes, depending on the amount and type of solution, and individual patient needs.

Calculating from Volume and Hourly Rate Ordered

Most IV orders are written specifying the total volume to be infused and hourly rate of administration, for example 2000 mL at 100 mL per hr. The largest IV solution bag/bottle is 1000 mL, so this 2000 mL volume (or any volume) may require a combination of several 1000 mL, 500 mL, or 250 mL bags or bottles.

Since most large volume IV's take several hours to infuse the unit of time being calculated is most often hours (hr). An easy one step calculation is used to obtain the infusion time. To use it you will divide the **total volume to be infused** by the **mL/hr rate** of infusion.

 The infusion time is calculated by dividing the total volume to be infused by the mL/hr flow rate.

| EXAMPLE 1 | Calculate the infusion time for an IV of **500 mL** D5W ordered to infuse at **50 mL/hr.** |

> **Infusion Time = total volume ÷ mL/hr rate**
>
> = 500 mL ÷ 50 mL/hr = **10 hr**

The infusion time for an IV of 500 mL infusing at 50 mL/hr is 10 hr

| EXAMPLE 2 | The order is to infuse **1000 mL** of D5NS at **75 mL/hr.** Calculate the infusion time. |

> 1000 mL ÷ 75 mL/hr = **13.33 hr**

In this example the 13 represents 13 hr, while the **.33 represents the fraction of an additional hr.**

Fractional hr are converted to min by multiplying 60 min by the fraction obtained.

Calculate the min by multiplying 60 min by the fractional hr

60 min × .33 = 19.8 = **20 min**

The total infusion time is 13 hr 20 min

EXAMPLE 3   An IV of **1000 mL** D5W is infusing at **90 mL/hr**. How long will it take to complete?

1000 mL ÷ 90 mL/hr = **11.11 hr**

Remember that .11 represents the fraction of an additional hr. Convert this to minutes by multiplying 60 min by .11.

60 min × .11 = 6.6 = **7 min**

The total infusion time is 11 hr 7 min

EXAMPLE 4   Calculate the infusion time for an IV of **750 mL** RL ordered at a rate of **80 mL/hr**.

750 mL ÷ 80 mL/hr = **9.38 hr**

60 min × .38 = 22.8 = **23 min**

The infusion time is 9 hr 23 min

EXAMPLE 5   A rate of **75 mL/hr** is ordered for a total volume of **500 mL** D5W. Calculate the infusion time.

500 mL ÷ 75 mL/hr = **6.67 hr**

60 min × .67 = 40.2 = **40 min**

The infusion time is 6 hr 40 min

PROBLEM

1. What is the infusion time for an IV of 900 mL RL ordered to infuse at 80 mL/hr?   _____

2. A volume of 250 mL is to be infused at 30 mL/hr. Calculate the infusion time.   _____

3. Calculate the infusion time if a 25 mL/hr rate is ordered for an infusion of 180 mL of NS.   _____

4. What is the infusion time for a volume of 1000 mL D5W ordered at a rate of 60 mL/hr?   _____

5. Calculate the infusion time for 150 mL ordered to infuse at 80 mL/hr.   _____

ANSWERS   Note: Answers may vary by 1-2 min due to rounding, or calculator setting if one is used. These may be considered correct. 1. 11 hr 15 min   2. 8 hr 20 min   3. 7 hr 12 min   4. 16 hr 40 min   5. 1 hr 53 min

Calculating Infusion Time from gtt/min Rate and Set Calibration

In some instances the only information you may have to calculate the infusion time is the the gtt/min rate at which the IV is infusing, the set calibration, and the total volume to be infused. The first step is to use the gtt/min flow rate and gtt/mL set calibration to calculate the mL/min, then the mL/hr rate.

EXAMPLE 1   Calculate the infusion time for an IV of **1000 mL** of D5W running at **25 gtt/min** on a set calibrated at **10 gtt/mL**.

- **Convert gtt/min to mL/min**

  10 gtt : 1 mL = 25 gtt : X mL   or $\dfrac{10 \text{ gtt}}{1 \text{ mL}} : \dfrac{25 \text{ gtt}}{X \text{ mL}} = $ **2.5 mL/min**
  X = **2.5 mL/min**

- **Convert mL/min to mL/hr**

  60 min × 2.5 mL/min = **150 mL/hr**

- **Calculate the infusion time by dividing the total volume to be infused by the mL/hr rate you have just obtained**

  1000 mL ÷ 150 mL/hr = **6.67 hr**

- **Multiply 60 min by the .67 hr fraction to obtain the min of infusion**

  60 min × .67 = 40.2 = **40 min**

The total infusion time is 6 hr 40 min

EXAMPLE 2   A volume of **750 mL** D5RL is running at **12 gtt/min** on a set calibrated at **10 gtt/mL**. Calculate the infusion time.

- **Convert gtt/min to mL/min**

  10 gtt : 1 mL = 12 gtt : X mL   or $\dfrac{10 \text{ gtt}}{1 \text{ mL}} : \dfrac{12 \text{ gtt}}{X \text{ mL}} = $ **1.2 mL/min**
  X = **1.2 mL/min**

- **Convert mL/min to mL/hr**

  60 min × 1.2 mL/min = **72 mL/hr**

- **Calculate the infusion time in hr and min**

  750 mL ÷ 72 mL/hr = **10.42 hr**

  60 min × .42 = 25.2 = **25 min**

The infusion time is 10 hr 25 min

EXAMPLE 3

Determine the infusion time for **100 mL** D5NS infusing at a rate of **40 gtt/min** using a **microdrip set.**

• **Convert gtt/min to mL/min**

$$60 \text{ gtt} : 1 \text{ mL} = 40 \text{ gtt} : \text{X mL} \qquad \text{or} \qquad \frac{60 \text{ gtt}}{1 \text{ mL}} : \frac{40 \text{ gtt}}{\text{X mL}} = \textbf{0.67 mL/min}$$
$$\text{X} = \textbf{0.67 mL/min}$$

• **Convert mL/min to mL/hr**

60 min × .67 mL/min = 40.2 = **40 mL/hr**

• **Calculate the infusion time in hr and min**

100 mL ÷ 40 mL/hr = **2.5 hr**

60 min × .5 = **30 min**

The infusion time is 2 hr 30 min

EXAMPLE 4

Calculate the infusion time for a volume of **150 mL** infusing at a rate of **20 gtt/min** on a **15 gtt/mL** calibrated set.

• **Convert gtt/min to mL/min**

$$15 \text{ gtt} : 1 \text{ mL} = 20 \text{ gtt} : \text{X mL} \qquad \text{or} \qquad \frac{15 \text{ gtt}}{1 \text{ mL}} : \frac{20 \text{ gtt}}{\text{X mL}} = \textbf{1.3 mL/min}$$
$$\text{X} = 1.33 = \textbf{1.3 mL/min}$$

• **Convert mL/min to mL/hr**

60 min × 1.3 mL/min = **78 mL/hr**

• **Calculate the infusion time in hr and min**

150 mL ÷ 78 mL/hr = **1.92 hr**

60 min × .92 = 55.2 = **55 min**

The infusion time is 1 hr 55 min

EXAMPLE 5

A volume of **1100 mL** hyperalimentation solution is infusing at a flow rate of **10 gtt/min** on a set calibrated at **10 gtt/mL.** Calculate the infusion time.

• **Convert gtt/min to mL/min**

$$10 \text{ gtt} : 1 \text{ mL} = 10 \text{ gtt} : \text{X mL} \qquad \text{or} \qquad \frac{10 \text{ gtt}}{1 \text{ mL}} : \frac{10 \text{ gtt}}{\text{X mL}} = \textbf{1 mL/min}$$
$$\text{X} = \textbf{1 mL/min}$$

• **Convert mL/min to mL/hr**

60 min × 1 mL/min = **60 mL/hr**

• **Calculate the infusion time in hr and min**

1100 mL ÷ 60 mL/hr = **18.33 hr**

60 min × .33 = 19.8 = **20 min**

The infusion time is 18 hr 20 min

PROBLEM

1. Determine the infusion time for 1 L D5W at a flow rate of 33 gtt/min using a set calibrated at 15 gtt/mL. _____

2. What is the infusion time for 250 mL D5RL infusing at 25 gtt/min using a 10 gtt/mL calibrated set? _____

3. A volume of 100 mL is to infuse at 10 gtt/min using a 10 gtt/mL set. Calculate the infusion time. _____

4. Calculate the infusion time for a volume of 900 mL running at a rate of 30 gtt/min using a 20 gtt/mL calibrated set. _____

5. What is the infusion time for an IV of 200 mL infusing at 18 gtt/min on a set calibrated at 15 gtt/mL? _____

ANSWERS   Note: Consider answers which vary by 1-2 min correct. **1.** 7 hr 35 min   **2.** 1 hr 40 min   **3.** 1 hr 40 min   **4.** 10 hr   **5.** 2 hr 47 min

Calculating Small Volume Infusion Times of Less Than 1 hr

Many small volume infusions will complete in less than 1 hr. Since the infusion time being calculated is **min**, the calculation will be shorter. Calculate the **mL/min** rate first, then **divide** the **total volume** by the **mL/min** rate.

EXAMPLE 1   An IV medication with a volume of **40 mL** is ordered to infuse at **45 gtt/min**. A microdrip set calibrated at **60 gtt/mL** is being used. Calculate the infusion time.

• **Calculate the mL/min infusing first**

60 gtt : 1 mL = 45 gtt : X mL   or $\dfrac{60 \text{ gtt}}{1 \text{ mL}} : \dfrac{45 \text{ gtt}}{X \text{ mL}} = \textbf{0.75 mL/min}$
X = **0.75 mL/min**

• **Divide the total volume by the mL/min rate**

40 mL ÷ 0.75 mL/min = 53.3 = **53 min**

The infusion time is 53 min

EXAMPLE 2   An IV medication of **60 mL** is to infuse at **50 gtt/min** using a set calibrated at **10 gtt/mL**. How long will it take to infuse?

• **Calculate the mL/min infusing**

10 gtt : 1 mL = 50 gtt : X mL   or $\dfrac{10 \text{ gtt}}{1 \text{ mL}} : \dfrac{50 \text{ gtt}}{X \text{ mL}} = \textbf{5 mL/min}$
X = **5 mL/min**

• **Divide the total volume by the mL/min rate**

60 mL ÷ 5 mL/min = **12 min**

The infusion time is 12 min

EXAMPLE 3   An IV medication with a volume of **20 mL** is to infuse at a rate of **30 gtt/min** using a **15 gtt/mL** infusion set. Calculate the infusion time.

• **Calculate the mL/min infusing**

15 gtt : 1 mL = 30 gtt : X mL   or $\dfrac{15 \text{ gtt}}{1 \text{ mL}} : \dfrac{30 \text{ gtt}}{\text{X mL}} = \textbf{2 mL/min}$
X = **2 mL/min**

• **Divide the total volume by the mL/min rate**

20 mL ÷ 2 mL/min = **10 min**

The infusion time is 10 min

PROBLEM

Calculate the infusion time for the following IV medications.

1. A medication with a volume of 25 mL to infuse at 30 gtt/min using a 60 gtt/mL (microdrip) set.   _____

2. A 35 mL volume IV medication to run at 25 gtt/min using a 15 gtt/mL set.   _____

3. A rate of 40 gtt/min ordered for a 70 mL volume of medication using a 20 gtt/mL set.   _____

4. A volume of 55 mL to infuse with a set calibrated at 10 gtt/mL at 45 gtt/min.   _____

5. A 10 mL volume to infuse at 40 gtt/min using a microdrip.   _____

ANSWERS Note: Consider answers which vary by 1-2 min correct. 1. 50 min 2. 21 min 3. 35 min 4. 12 min 5. 15 min

Determining Infusion Completion Time

The reason for calculating infusion times is to know when an IV solution or medication will be completely infused. To obtain the **completion time** for an IV you must now **add the infusion time** you calculated **to the start time**. This is not complicated; it just requires the same care you have been using for the other calculations in this text. The safest way to calculate the completion time is to **add the minutes first**. With them out of the way only the hours are left to add; much less confusing. It's also safer to **write the times down** as you calculate them. So, do that in the following examples and problems. Only the first example will show calculation for military time (0 - 2400), because these calculations are simple additions.

EXAMPLE 1   An IV started at **1450** has an infusion time of **3 hr and 40 min**. What is the completion time?

• **Add the minutes first**

40 min + 50 min = **90 min**

Use 60 min of the 90 min total to change the 14 (hr) to 15; add the additional 30 min for a total of **1530.**

• **Now add the hr**

1530 + 3 hr = **1830**   **Completion time = 1830**

EXAMPLE 2   An IV medication will infuse in **20 minutes**. It is now **6.14 p.m.** When will it be complete?

• **Add the minutes**

6.14 p.m. + **20 min = 6.34 p.m.**   **Completion time = 6.34 p.m.**

Minutes alone are easy to add, even if the answer crosses the a.m./p.m. time change.

EXAMPLE 3   An IV is calculated to infuse in **2 hr 33 min**. It is now **4.43 p.m.** When will it complete?

• **Add the minutes first**

4.43 p.m. + **33 min = 5.16 p.m.**

Now that the minutes are out of the way you only have to add 2 hours; much safer.

• **Add the hr**

5.16 p.m. + **2 hr = 7.16 p.m.**   **The infusion will complete at 7.16 p.m.**

EXAMPLE 4   An IV infusion time is **13 hr 20 min**. What is its completion time if it was started at **10.45 a.m.**?

• **Add the minutes first**

10. 45 a.m. + **20 min = 11.05 a.m.**

You must now **add** the **13 hours** to the **11.05 a.m.** you just calculated. Count on a clock, or on your fingers, whichever you prefer.

• **Add the hr**

11.05 a.m. + **13 hr = 12.05 a.m.**   **The completion time will be 12.05 a.m.**

EXAMPLE 5   An IV with an infusion time of **10 hr 7 min** is started at **9.42 a.m.** When will it complete?

• **Add the min**

9.42 a.m. + **7 min = 9.49 a.m.**

• **Add the hr**

9.49 a.m. + **10 hr = 7.49 p.m.**

The completion time will be 7.49 p.m.

EXAMPLE 6   An IV with an infusion time of **12 hr 30 min** is started at **2.10 a.m.**
When will it complete?

• **Add the min**

2.10 a.m. + **30 min** = **2.40 a.m.**

• **Add the hr**

2.40 a.m. + **12 hr** = **2.40 p.m.**

The completion time will be 2.40 p.m.

PROBLEM

Calculate the completion times for the following infusions.

1. An IV started at 0440 that has an infusion time of
   9 hr 42 min. Use military time.   _____

2. An IV medication started at 7.30 a.m. which has an
   infusion time of 45 min.   _____

3. An IV with an infusion time of 7 hr 7 min which
   was restarted at 10.42 a.m.   _____

4. An IV with a restart time of 9.07 p.m. has an
   infusion time of 6 hr 27 min.   _____

5. An IV with an infusion time of 2 hr 30 min was
   started at 11.49 p.m.   _____

ANSWERS Note: Consider answers which vary by 1-2 min correct. **1.** 1422 **2.** 8.15 a.m. **3.** 5.49 p.m. **4.** 3.34 a.m.
5. 2.19 a.m.

Labeling Solution Bags/Bottles with Infusion and Completion Times

IV bags/bottles are calibrated so that the amount of fluid remaining can be checked at any time. In the majority of hospitals it is routine to label bags/bottles when they are hung with start, progress and finish times, to provide a visual reference of the status of the infusion. Commercially prepared labels are available for this purpose, however you can prepare one using any opaque tape available.

In Figure 90, on page 248, you can see the calibrations on a 1000 mL bag. Notice that each 50 mL is calibrated, but that only the 100 mL calibrations are numbered: 1, 2, 3, (for 100, 200, 300) etc. Notice also that the calibrations on the IV bag are not all the same width: they are somewhat wider at the bottom, because gravity and the pressure of the solution forces more fluid to the bottom of the bag. On an uncomplicated infusion these differences in calibration are relatively unimportant.

The tape on this IV solution bag is for an 8 hour infusion, from 9 a.m. to 5 p.m. The 9A represents the start time of 9 a.m., and the 5P at the bottom represents the completion time of 5 p.m. An 8 hr infusion time for 1000 mL means that 125 mL are to be infused per hour (1000 mL ÷ 8 hr = 125 mL/hr). Each 125 mL is labeled on the calibrated scale with the hour the IV should be at this level. This tape can be read by everyone who cares for this patient, and allows for constant monitoring of the IV. No matter what your responsibility for a patient is you must be aware of IV drip rates, and develop the habit of reading IV labeling, particularly if you have been giving personal care which involves the patient moving around.

Let's look at an example of how you could label an IV which is just being started. You may use a commercial time tape provided by your instructor, or copy the calibrations from one of the photos in this text to make up your own scale on some scratch paper.

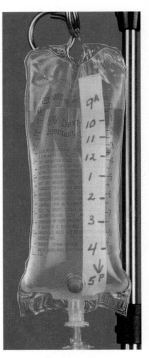

Figure 90

EXAMPLE 1

An IV of **1000 mL** has been ordered to run at **150 mL/hr**. It was started at **1.40 p.m.** Tape the bag with start, progress and completion times.

Add the tape to the bag/bottle so that it is near, but does not cover the calibrations. Enter the start time as 1.40 p.m. at the 1000 mL level. Next, mark each 150 mL from top to bottom with the successive hours the IV will run.

1000 mL − 150 mL = 850 mL	Label 850 mL for 2.40 p.m.
850 mL − 150 mL = 700 mL	Label 700 mL for 3.40 p.m.
700 mL − 150 mL = 550 mL	Label 550 mL for 4.40 p.m.
550 mL − 150 mL = 400 mL	Label 400 mL for 5.40 p.m.
400 mL − 150 mL = 250 mL	Label 250 mL for 6.40 p.m.
250 mL − 150 mL = 100 mL	Label 100 mL for 7.40 p.m.

Calculate the infusion time for the remaining 100 mL.

100 mL ÷ 150 mL/hr = 0.66 = **0.67 hr**

60 min × 0.67 = 40.2 = **40 min**

7.40 p.m. + **40 min** = 8.20 p.m.   **The completion time is 8.20 p.m.**

EXAMPLE 2

An infiltrated IV with **625 mL** remaining is restarted at **5.30 p.m.** to run at **150 mL/hr**. Relabel the bag with the new start, progress and completion times.

Label the 625 mL level with the 5.30 p.m. restart time.

625 mL − 150 mL = 475 mL	Label 475 mL for 6.30 p.m.
475 mL − 150 mL = 325 mL	Label 325 mL for 7.30 p.m.
325 mL − 150 mL = 175 mL	Label 175 mL for 8.30 p.m.
175 mL − 150 mL = 25 mL	Label 25 mL for 9.30 p.m.

Calculate the infusion time for the remaining 25 mL.

25 mL ÷ 150 mL/hr = 0.166 = **0.17 hr**

60 min × 0.17 = 10.2 = **10 min**

9.30 p.m. + **10 min = 9.40 p.m.**   **The completion time is 9.40 p.m.**

EXAMPLE 3   An infiltrated IV with **340 mL** remaining is restarted at **4.15 a.m.** to run at **70 mL/hr.** Relabel the bag with the new start, progress and completion times.

Label the 340 mL level with the 4.15 a.m. restart time.

340 mL – 70 mL = 270 mL	Label 270 mL for 5.15 a.m.
270 mL – 70 mL = 200 mL	Label 200 mL for 6.15 a.m.
200 mL – 70 mL = 130 mL	Label 130 mL for 7.15 a.m.
25 mL – 70 mL = 60 mL	Label 60 mL for 8.15 a.m.

Calculate the infusion time for the remaining 60 mL.

60 mL ÷ 70 mL/hr = 0.857 = **0.86 hr**

60 min × 0.86 = 51.6 = **52 min**

8.15 a.m. + **52 min = 9.17 a.m.**   **The completion time is 9.17 a.m.**

PROBLEM

Calculate the infusion and completion times for the IV's pictured on page 250. Label the IV bags provided with start, progress, and completion time. Have your instructor check your labeling.

1. The IV in Figure 91 of 1000 mL was started at 0710 to run at 75 mL/hr.

    Infusion Time _____   Completion Time _____

2. The 1000 mL IV in Figure 92 has an ordered rate of 125 mL/hr. It was started at 6.30 p.m.

    Infusion Time _____   Completion Time _____

3. The IV in Figure 93 of 1000 mL has an ordered rate of 80 mL/hr. It was started at 5.40 a.m.

    Infusion Time _____   Completion Time _____

ANSWERS   Note: Consider answers which vary by 1-2 min correct. **1.** 13 hr 20 min; 2030 **2.** 8 hr; 2.30 a.m. **3.** 12 hr 30 min; 6.10 p.m.

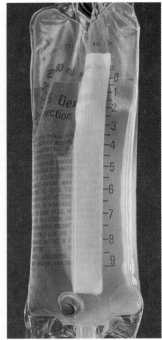

Figure 91

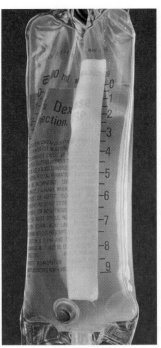

Figure 92

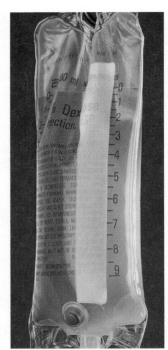

Figure 93

Summary

This concludes the chapter on calculation of infusion and completion times, and labeling of IV bags with start, progress and completion times. The important points to remember from this chapter are:

➡ the infusion time is the time necessary for an IV bag or bottle to infuse completely

➡ the infusion time is calculated by dividing the total volume to infuse by the mL/hr rate ordered

➡ infusion times also may be calculated using the volume of the bag/bottle being hung, the mL/hr or gtt/min rate ordered, and set calibration

➡ the completion time is calculated by adding the infusion time to the start time

➡ when adding the infusion time to the start time it is safer to add the minutes first, then the hours

➡ when the total min are 60 or more an additional hr is added, and 60 min subtracted from the min total

➡ calculating infusion and completion times provides an opportunity to plan ahead and have the next solution ordered ready to hang, or to discontinue the IV when it is completed

➡ it is routine in many hospitals to label IV solution bags with start, finish and progress times to provide a visual record of the infusion status

Summary Self Test

Calculate the infusion and completion times for the following IV's. Don't let the solution abbreviations confuse you; concentrate on locating the information you need for your calculations.

1. The order is for 50 mL D5W to infuse at 50 gtt/min using a microdrip. The infusion was started at 10.10 a.m.

   Infusion Time _____   Completion Time _____

2. An infusion of 1150 mL hyperalimentation is ordered to run at 80 mL/hr. It was started at 8.02 a.m.

   Infusion Time _____   Completion Time _____

3. A total of 280 mL D10W remain in an IV bag. The flow rate is 70 mL/hr. It is now 11.03 a.m.

   Infusion Time _____   Completion Time _____

4. The order is to infuse 500 mL of whole blood at 90 mL/hr. The transfusion was started at 2.40 p.m.

   Infusion Time _____   Completion Time _____

5. An infiltrated IV with 850 mL D5W remaining is restarted at 10 a.m. at a rate of 150 mL/hr.

   Infusion Time _____   Completion Time _____

6. At 4.04 a.m. an IV of 500 mL Intralipids is started at a rate of 50 mL/hr.

   Infusion Time _____   Completion Time _____

7. An IV medication with a volume of 50 mL is started at 1.45 p.m. to infuse at 30 gtt/min using a set calibrated at 15 gtt/mL.

   Infusion Time _____   Completion Time _____

8. An IV of 520 mL RL is restarted at 0420 at a rate of 125 mL/hr.

   Infusion Time _____   Completion Time _____

9. It is 12.00 p.m. and an IV of 900 mL D10NS is infusing at a rate of 100 mL/hr.

   Infusion Time _____   Completion Time _____

10. An antibiotic of 150 mL is started at 7.10 a.m. to infuse at 33 gtt/min with a set calibrated at 10 gtt/mL.

    Infusion Time _____   Completion Time _____

11. An infusion of 250 mL normal saline is started at 11.20 a.m. to infuse at a rate of 20 mL/hr.

    Infusion Time _____   Completion Time _____

12. The flow rate ordered for 1 L of D5W is 80 mL/hr. It was started at 8.07 p.m.

    Infusion Time _____   Completion Time _____

13. One unit of packed cells with a 250 mL volume is started at 3.40 p.m. to be infused at 30 gtt/min using a 20 gtt/mL set.

    Infusion Time _____   Completion Time _____

14. A medication volume of 100 mL is started at 4.00 p.m. to infuse at 42 gtt/min using a microdrip.

    Infusion Time _____   Completion Time _____

15. At 11.00 p.m. 200 mL D5W remain in an IV. The rate is 20 gtt/min and set calibration 10 gtt/mL.

    Infusion Time _____   Completion Time _____

16. An infusion of 350 mL RL is restarted to run at 50 gtt/min using a 10 gtt/mL set. It is now 9.47 a.m.

    Infusion Time _____   Completion Time _____

17. An IV medication of 25 mL is started at 8.17 a.m. using a microdrip, to run at 25 gtt/min.

    Infusion Time _____   Completion Time _____

18. An IV of 425 mL D5 1/4NaCl is restarted at 0814 to infuse at 15 gtt/min using a 10 gtt/mL set.

    Infusion Time _____   Completion Time _____

19. At 10.30 p.m. there are 180 mL left in an IV of D5 0.45%NaCl that is infusing at 25 mL/hr.

    Infusion Time _____   Completion Time _____

20. At 2 p.m. 500 mL of D5NS is started to run at a rate of 20 gtt/min using a 20 gtt/mL set.

    Infusion Time _____   Completion Time _____

21. An infusion of 250 mL of NS is started at 3.04 a.m. to run at 50 gtt/min using a 15 gtt/mL set.

    Infusion Time _____   Completion Time _____

22. With 525 mL D10W remaining a rate change to 35 gtt/min is ordered. It is 2.10 a.m. and a 10 gtt/mL set is being used.

    Infusion Time _____   Completion Time _____

23. A liter of D5 1/4NaCl with 10 U Regular insulin is started at 8.42 a.m. at a rate of 22 gtt/min using a set calibrated at 20 gtt/mL.

    Infusion Time _____   Completion Time _____

24 An infusion of 1000 mL sodium chloride 0.9% is to run at 200 mL/hr. It is started at 6.40 p.m.

    Infusion Time _____   Completion Time _____

25. An IV medication of 100 mL is started at 7.50 a.m. to run at 33 gtt/min using a 10 gtt/mL set.

    Infusion Time _____   Completion Time _____

26. A volume of 500 mL RL is started at 4.04 p.m. at a rate of 50 gtt/min using a microdrip.

    Infusion Time _____   Completion Time _____

252   MATH FOR MEDS

27. An IV of 950 mL NS is restarted at 2.10 a.m. at 25 gtt/min using a 15 gtt/mL set.

    Infusion Time _____   Completion Time _____

28. An IV medication of 30 mL is started at 0915 at a rate of 10 gtt/min using a 10 gtt/mL set.

    Infusion Time _____   Completion Time _____

29. A medication volume of 90 mL was started at 6.15 a.m. to be infused at 30 gtt/min using a 20 gtt/mL set.

    Infusion Time _____   Completion Time _____

30. A set calibrated at 15 gtt/mL is used at 4.20 p.m. to infuse a medication with a volume of 100 mL. The rate ordered is 45 gtt/min.

    Infusion Time _____   Completion Time _____

31. A 20 gtt/mL set is used for a restart of 750 mL D5W at 3.03 p.m. at a rate of 32 gtt/min.

    Infusion Time _____   Completion Time _____

ANSWERS Note: Answers will vary due to rounding. **1.** 60 min; **11.** 10 a.m. **2.** 14 hr 23 min; 10.25 p.m. **3.** 4 hr; 3.03 p.m. **4.** 5 hr 34 min; 8.14 p.m. **5.** 5 hr 40 min; 3.40 p.m. **6.** 10 hr; 2.04 p.m. **7.** 25 min; 2.10 p.m. **8.** 4 hr 10 min; 0830 **9.** 9 hr; 9 p.m. **10.** 45 min; 7.55 a.m. **11.** 12 hr 30 min; 11.50 p.m. **12.** 12 hr 30 min; 8.37 a.m. **13.** 2 hr 47 min; 6.27 p.m. **14.** 143 min or 2 hr 23 min; 6.23 p.m. **15.** 1 hr 40 min; 12.40 a.m. **16.** 1 hr 10 min; 10.57 a.m. **17.** 60 min; 9.17 a.m. **18.** 4 hr 43 min; 1257 **19.** 7 hr 12 min; 5.42 a.m. **20.** 8 hr 20 min; 10.20 p.m. **21.** 1 hr 15 min; 4.19 a.m. **22.** 2 hr 30 min; 4.40 a.m. **23.** 15 hr 9 min; 11.51 p.m. **24.** 5 hr; 11.40 p.m. **25.** 30 min; 8.20 a.m. **26.** 10 hr; 2.04 a.m. **27.** 9 hr 19 min; 11.29 a.m.; or 9 hr 29 min; 11:39 a.m. **28.** 30 min; 0945 **29.** 60 min; 7.15 a.m. **30.** 33 min; 4.53 p.m. **31.** 7 hr 48 min; 10.51 p.m.

DIRECTIONS

Label the following solution bags for the times and rates indicated. Have your instructor check your labeling.

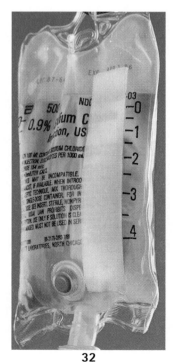

32
Started: 10:47 a.m.
Rate: 80 mL/hr

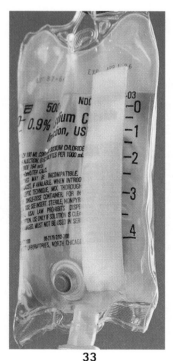

33
Started: 1315
Rate: 100 mL/hr

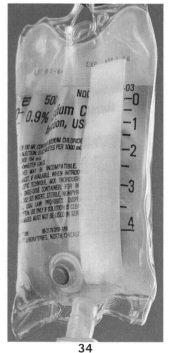

34
Started: 2:10 p.m.
Rate: 90 mL/hr

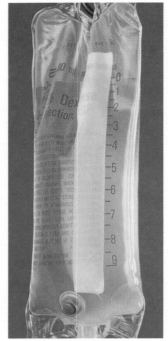

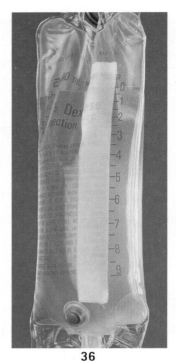

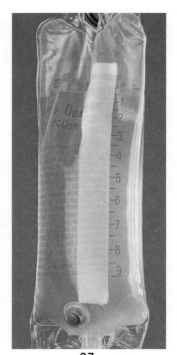

35
Started: 0440
Rate: 75 mL/hr

36
Started: 0730
Rate: 50 mL/hr

37
Started: 6:20 p.m.
Rate: 25 mL/hr

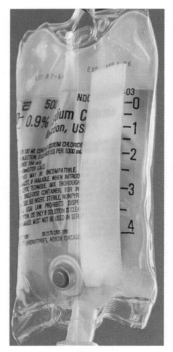

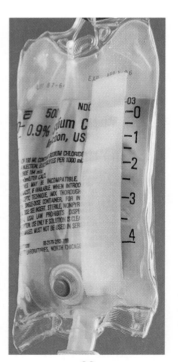

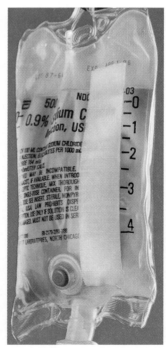

38
Started: 3:03 a.m.
Rate: 50 mL/hr

39
Started: 0744
Rate: 125 mL/hr

40
Started: 2140
Rate: 100 mL/hr

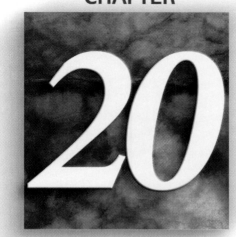

IV Medication and Titration Calculations

OBJECTIVES
The student will calculate
1. flow rates to infuse ordered dosages
2. dosages and flow rates based on kg body weight
3. dosage infusing from flow rate and solution strength
4. dosage and flow rate ranges for titrated medications

Many IV drugs are used in critical and life threatening situations to alter or maintain vital physiologic functions, for example heart rate, cardiac output, blood pressure, respirations and renal function. In general, these drugs have a very rapid action and short duration. They may be administered by IV push or bolus, but also diluted in 250-500 mL of IV solution, most commonly D5W.

Intravenous medications may be ordered by flow rate (mL/hr or gtt/min), by dosage (mcg/mg/U per min/hr), or based on a patient's weight (mcg/mg/U per kg per min/hr). They may also be ordered to infuse within a specific dosage range, for example 1-3 mcg/min, to elicit a measurable physiologic response; an example would be to maintain a systolic BP above 100 mm Hg. This adjustment of rate is called **titration**, and dosage increments are made within the ordered range until the desired response has been established. Most IV drugs require close and continuous monitoring. When available an electronic infusion device (EID), either volumetric pump, controller, or syringe pump is used for their administration. If an EID is not available, a microdrip set calibrated at 60 gtt/mL, or dosage controlled Soluset/Buretrol/Volutrol, is routinely used. All calculations in this chapter are for an EID or microdrip, and the mL/hr and gtt/min rates are interchangeable.

The calculations in this chapter include 1) converting ordered dosages to the flow rates necessary to administer them, and 2) using flow rates to calculate the dosage infusing at any given moment. A patient's weight is often a critical factor in IV dosages, and its use in calculations will also be covered. A variety of EID's display dosage and flow rate equivalents, but you must know how to do these calculations yourself, because you are likely to encounter situations where you will have to do so. IV drugs which alter a basic physiologic function generally have narrow margins of safety, and accuracy is imperative in their calculation. Double checking of math is both mandatory, and routine. As a general rule, dosages are calculated to the nearest tenth, while flow rates are rounded to the nearest gtt or mL.

All calculations in this chapter assume the use of an EID or microdrip infusion set, therefore the mL/hr and gtt/min rates are identical, and interchangeable.

Calculating mL/hr Rate from Dosage Ordered

One of the most common IV drug calculations is to determine the mL/hr flow rate for a specific drug dosage ordered. So, let's start by looking at some examples of these.

EXAMPLE 1 A solution of Cardizem **125 mg/100 mL** D5W is to infuse at a rate of **20 mg/hr**. Calculate the **mL/hr** flow rate.

- **Use the solution strength available to calculate the mL/hr rate for 20 mg/hr**

$$125 \text{ mg} : 100 \text{ mL} = 20 \text{ mg} : X \text{ mL} \quad \text{or} \quad \frac{125 \text{ mg}}{100 \text{ mL}} : \frac{20 \text{ mg}}{X \text{ mL}} = \textbf{16 mL/hr}$$
$$125 \text{ X} = 100 \times 20$$
$$X = \textbf{16 mL/hr}$$

To infuse 20 mg/hr set the flow rate at 16 mL/hr

EXAMPLE 2 A maintenance dose of Levophed **2 mcg/min** has been ordered using an **8 mg in 250 mL** D5W solution. Calculate the **mL/hr** flow rate.

- **Calculate the dosage per hr first**

2 mcg/min × 60 min = **120 mcg/hr**

The solution strength is in mg, so a mcg to mg conversion is now needed.

- **Convert 120 mcg to mg to match the mg solution strength**

120 mcg = **0.12 mg**

- **Use the solution strength available to calculate the mL/hr rate**

$$8 \text{ mg} : 250 \text{ mL} = 0.12 \text{ mg} : X \text{ mL} \quad \text{or} \quad \frac{8 \text{ mg}}{250 \text{ mL}} : \frac{0.12 \text{ mg}}{X \text{ mL}} = \textbf{4 mL/hr}$$
$$8X = 250 \times 0.12$$
$$X = 3.75 = \textbf{4 mL/hr}$$

To infuse 2 mcg/min set the flow rate at 4 mL/hr

 Conversions may be made in either direction, solution strength to dosage ordered, or dosage ordered to solution strength.

EXAMPLE 3 Neosynephrine **50 mg in 250 mL** D5W is used to infuse a dosage of **200 mcg/min**. Calculate the flow rate in **mL/hr**.

- **Calculate the dosage per hr**

200 mcg/min × 60 min = **12,000 mcg/hr**

- **Convert 12,000 mcg to mg to match the mg solution strength**

12,000 mcg = **12 mg**

- **Calculate the mL/hr flow rate**

$$50 \text{ mg} : 250 \text{ mL} = 12 \text{ mg} : X \text{ mL} \quad \text{or} \quad \frac{50 \text{ mg}}{250 \text{ mL}} : \frac{12 \text{ mg}}{X \text{ mL}} = \textbf{60 mL/hr}$$
$$50X = 250 \times 12$$
$$X = \textbf{60 mL/hr}$$

To infuse 200 mcg/min set the flow rate at 60 mL/hr

EXAMPLE 4   Isuprel has been ordered for a cardiac patient at the rate of **3 mcg/min** using a **1 mg/250 mL** D5W solution. Calculate the **mL/hr** flow rate.

• **Calculate the dosage per hr**

3 mcg/min × 60 min = **180 mcg/hr**

• **Convert 180 mcg to mg to match the mg solution strength**

180 mcg = **0.18 mg**

• **Calculate the mL/hr flow rate**

$$1 \text{ mg} : 250 \text{ mL} = 0.18 \text{ mg} : X \text{ mL} \qquad \text{or} \qquad \frac{1 \text{ mg}}{250 \text{ mL}} : \frac{0.18 \text{ mg}}{X \text{ mL}} = \textbf{45 mL/hr}$$
$$X = 250 \times 0.18$$
$$X = \textbf{45 mL/hr}$$

To infuse 3 mcg/min set the flow rate at 45 mL/hr

EXAMPLE 5   A **500 mL** D5W solution with **2 g** Pronestyl is to be infused at a rate of **1 mg/min** via volumetric pump. Calculate the **mL/hr** flow rate.

• **Calculate the dosage per hr**

1 mg/min × 60 min = **60 mg/hr**

• **Convert g to mg in the solution strength**

2 g = 2000 mg

• **Calculate mL/hr rate**

$$2000 \text{ mg} : 500 \text{ mL} = 60 \text{ mg} : X \text{ mL} \qquad \text{or} \qquad \frac{2000 \text{ mg}}{500 \text{ mL}} : \frac{60 \text{ mg}}{X \text{ mL}} = \textbf{15 mL/hr}$$
$$2000X = 500 \times 60$$
$$X = \textbf{15 mL/hr}$$

Set the pump at 15 mL/hr to infuse 1 mg/min

PROBLEM

Calculate the mL/hr flow rates to administer the following IV dosages. Round answers to the nearest mL.

1. Trandate 20 mg/hr is ordered using a 100 mg/100 mL solution.   _____

2. Levophed is ordered at the rate of 3 mcg/min. The solution strength is 8 mg Levophed in 250 mL D5W.   _____

3. A solution of 2 g Pronestyl in 500 mL D5W is used to administer a dosage of 2 mg/min.   _____

4. Isuprel 2 mcg/min is ordered. The solution strength is 1 mg/250 mL.   _____

5. An initial dose of Cardizem 25 mg/hr is ordered. The solution strength is 125 mg/100 mL.   _____

ANSWERS   1. 20 mL/hr   2. 6 mL/hr   3. 30 mL/hr   4. 30 mL/hr   5. 20 mL/hr

Calculating mL/hr Rate from Dosage per kg Ordered

Many drug dosages are calculated based on a patient's weight, for example 5 mg/kg/hr. **Body weight, to the nearest tenth kg,** is used for these calculations. **A preliminary step** of calculating the dosage for the patient based on her/his weight is necessary before the flow rate can be calculated.

All of the following rates are for mL/hr controller/pump/syringe pump infusion (the gtt/min microdrip rate will be identical). **Express fractional dosage answers to the nearest tenth, and mL rates to the nearest whole mL.**

EXAMPLE 1 Dopamine is ordered at the rate of **3 mcg/kg/min** for a patient weighing **95.9 kg**. The solution strength is **400 mg** dopamine in **250 mL** D5W. Calculate the mL/hr flow rate.

• **Calculate the dosage per min first**

3 mcg/kg/min $\times$ 95.9 kg = **287.7 mcg/min**

• **Convert mcg/min to mcg/hr**

287.7 mcg/min $\times$ 60 min = **17,262 mcg/hr**

• **Convert mcg/hr to mg/hr**

17,262 mcg/hr = 17.26 = **17.3 mg/hr**

• **Calculate the flow rate**

400 mg : 250 mL = 17.3 mg : X mL   or $\dfrac{400 \text{ mg}}{250 \text{ mL}} : \dfrac{17.3 \text{ mg}}{X \text{ mL}} = 10.8 = $ **11 mL/hr**
400X = 250 $\times$ 17.3
X = 10.8 = **11 mL/hr**

To infuse 3 mcg/kg/min set the rate at 11 mL/hr

EXAMPLE 2 Esmolol **2.5 g in 250 mL** D5W has been ordered at a rate of **100 mcg/kg/min** for a patient weighing **104.6 kg**. Calculate the mL/hr flow rate.

• **Calculate the dosage per min**

100 mcg/kg/min $\times$ 104.6 kg = **10,460 mcg/min**

• **Convert mcg/min to mg/min**

10,460 mcg $\div$ 1000 = 10.46 = **10.5 mg/min**

• **Convert mg/min to mg/hr**

10.5 mg/min $\times$ 60 min = **630 mg/hr**

• **Calculate the flow rate**

2500 mg : 250 mL = 630 mg : X mL   or $\dfrac{2500 \text{ mg}}{250 \text{ mL}} : \dfrac{630 \text{ mg}}{X \text{ mL}} = $ **63 mL/hr**
2500X = 250 $\times$ 630
X = **63 mL/hr**

To infuse 100 mcg/kg/min set the rate at 63 mL/hr

EXAMPLE 3

Nipride has been ordered at **4 mcg/kg/min** from a solution of **50 mg** Nipride in **250 mL** D5W. The patient weighs **107.3 kg**. Calculate the mL/hr flow rate.

- **Calculate the dosage per min**

4 mcg/kg/min $\times$ 107.3 kg = **429.2 mcg/min**

- **Convert mcg/min to mcg/hr**

429.2 mcg/min $\times$ 60 min = **25,752 mcg/hr**

- **Convert mcg/hr to mg/hr**

25,752 $\div$ 1000 = 25.75 = **25.8 mg/hr**

- **Calculate the flow rate**

$$50 \text{ mg} : 250 \text{ mL} = 25.8 \text{ mg} : \text{X mL} \quad \text{or} \quad \frac{50 \text{ mg}}{250 \text{ mL}} : \frac{25.8 \text{ mg}}{\text{X mL}} = \textbf{129 mL/hr}$$
$$50\text{X} = 250 \times 25.8$$
$$\text{X} = \textbf{129 mL/hr}$$

To infuse 4 mcg/kg/min set the rate at 129 mL/hr

EXAMPLE 4

Dobutrex **5 mcg/kg/min** has been ordered using a **500 mg/250 mL** D5W strength solution. The patient weighs **99.4 kg**. Calculate the mL/hr flow rate.

- **Calculate the dosage per min**

5 mcg/kg/min $\times$ 99.4 kg = **497 mcg/min**

- **Convert mcg/min to mcg/hr**

497 mcg/min $\times$ 60 min = **29,820 mcg/hr**

- **Convert mcg/hr to mg/hr**

29,820 mcg $\div$ 1000 = 29.82 = **29.8 mg/hr**

- **Calculate the flow rate**

$$500 \text{ mg} : 250 \text{ mL} = 29.8 \text{ mg} : \text{X mL} \quad \text{or} \quad \frac{500 \text{ mg}}{250 \text{ mL}} : \frac{29.8 \text{ mg}}{\text{X mL}} = \textbf{15 mL/hr}$$
$$500\text{X} = 250 \times 29.8$$
$$\text{X} = 14.9 = \textbf{15 mL/hr}$$

To infuse 5 mcg/kg/min set the rate at 15 mL/hr

EXAMPLE 5

Breviblock **100 mcg/kg/min** has been ordered using a **5 g/500 mL** D5W solution. The patient weighs **77.6 kg**. Calculate the mL/hr flow rate.

- **Calculate the dosage per min**

100 mcg/kg/min $\times$ 77.6 kg = **7760 mcg/min**

- **Convert mcg/min to mg/min**

7760 mcg/min $\div$ 1000 = 7.76 = **7.8 mg/min**

• **Convert mg/min to mg/hr**

7.8 mg/min $\times$ 60 min = **468 mg/hr**

• **Calculate the flow rate**

5000 mg : 500 mL = 468 mg : X mL   or $\dfrac{5000 \text{ mg}}{500 \text{ mL}} : \dfrac{468 \text{ mg}}{\text{X mL}} = 46.8 = \textbf{47 mL/hr}$
        5000X = 500 $\times$ 468
           X = 46.8 = **47 mL/hr**

To infuse 100 mcg/kg/min set the rate at 47 mL/hr

PROBLEM

Calculate the dosage per min, and mL/hr flow rate for the following infusions.

1. Nipride 3 mcg/kg/min has been ordered for an 87.4 kg patient. The solution has a strength of 50 mg Nipride in 250 mL D5W.   _____ _____

2. Dopamine has been ordered at 4 mcg/kg/min using a 400 mg/250 mL D5W solution. The patient weighs 92.4 kg.   _____ _____

3. Dobutamine 2.5 mcg/kg/min has been ordered. The solution is 500 mg/250 mL D5W. The patient weighs 80.7 kg.   _____ _____

4. Esmolol 150 mcg/kg/min has been ordered for a 92.1 kg patient. The solution strength is 2.5 g/250 mL D5W.   _____ _____

5. Propofol 5 mcg/kg/min is ordered for an 80.3 kg patient. The solution strength is 1 g/100 mL D5W.   _____ _____

ANSWERS 1. 262.2 mcg/min; 79 mL/hr **2.** 369.6 mcg/min; 14 mL/hr **3.** 201.8 mcg/min; 6 mL/hr **4.** 13,815 mcg or 13.8 mg/min; 83 mL/hr **5.** 401.5 mcg/min; 2 mL/hr

Calculating Dosage Infusing from Flow Rate

It is possible to calculate the dosage being administered at any moment from the **flow rate infusing**, and the **solution concentration**.

EXAMPLE 1   **500 mL** D5W containing dopamine **800 mg** is infusing at a rate of **25 mL/hr**. Calculate the dosage infusing, in **mg/hr** and **mcg/min**.

• **Calculate the mg/hr infusing first**

500 mL : 800 mg = 25 mL : X mg   or $\dfrac{500 \text{ mL}}{800 \text{ mg}} : \dfrac{25 \text{ mL}}{\text{X mg}} = \textbf{40 mg/hr}$
        500X = 800 $\times$ 25
           X = **40 mg/hr**

• **Convert mg/hr to mcg/hr**

40 mg/hr = **40,000 mcg/hr**

• **Convert mcg/hr to mcg/min**

40,000 mcg $\div$ 60 min = 666.6 = **667 mcg/min**

A dosage of 40 mg/hr and 667 mcg/min are infusing

EXAMPLE 2 A post-op cardiac bypass patient has Nipride infusing at **30 gtt/min** (30 mL/hr). The solution strength is **100 mg** Nipride in **500 mL** D5W. Calculate the **mg/hr** and **mcg/min** infusing.

• **Calculate the mg/hr infusing**

$$500 \text{ mL} : 100 \text{ mg} = 30 \text{ mL} : X \text{ mg} \quad \text{or} \quad \frac{500 \text{ mL}}{100 \text{ mg}} : \frac{30 \text{ mL}}{X \text{ mg}} = 6 \text{ mg/hr}$$
$$500X = 100 \times 30$$
$$X = 6 \text{ mg/hr}$$

• **Convert mg/hr to mcg/hr**

6 mg/hr = **6000 mcg/hr**

• **Convert mcg/hr to mcg/min**

6000 mcg ÷ 60 min = **100 mcg/min**

A dosage of 6 mg/hr and 100 mcg/min is infusing

EXAMPLE 3 A patient with ventricular ectopi is receiving a continuous Lidocaine infusion at a flow rate of **15 mL/hr**. The solution strength is **2 g** Lidocaine in **500 mL** D5W. Calculate the **mg/hr** and **mg/min** being infused. The average dosage of Lidocaine is **1-4 mg/min**. Is the dosage within normal range?

• **Convert the g to mg first**

2 g = **2000 mg**

• **Calculate the mg/hr infusing**

$$500 \text{ mL} : 2000 \text{ mg} = 15 \text{ mL} : X \text{ mg} \quad \text{or} \quad \frac{500 \text{ mL}}{2000 \text{ mg}} : \frac{15 \text{ mL}}{X \text{ mg}} = 60 \text{ mg/hr}$$
$$500X = 2000 \times 15$$
$$X = 60 \text{ mg/hr}$$

• **Calculate the mg/min infusing**

60 mg ÷ 60 min = **1 mg/min**

A dosage of 60 mg/hr or 1 mg/min is infusing. This dosage is within the normal 1-4 mg/min range

EXAMPLE 4 A solution of **5 g (5000 mg)** Breviblock in **500 mL** D5W is infusing at **30 mL/hr.** Calculate the **mg/min** infusing.

• **Calculate the mg/hr infusing**

$$500 \text{ mL} : 5000 \text{ mg} = 30 \text{ mL} : X \text{ mg} \quad \text{or} \quad \frac{500 \text{ mL}}{5000 \text{ mg}} : \frac{30 \text{ mL}}{X \text{ mg}} = 300 \text{ mg/hr}$$
$$500X = 5000 \times 30$$
$$X = 300 \text{ mg/hr}$$

• **Calculate the mg/min infusing**

300 mg/hr ÷ 60 min = **5 mg/min**

A dosage of 5 mg/min is infusing

PROBLEM

Calculate the dosages indicated in the following problems. Express dosages to the nearest tenth.

1. A continuous infusion of Isuprel is ordered for a newly admitted patient in cardiogenic shock. The solution strength is 2 mg in 500 mL D5W, and the rate of infusion is 40 mL/hr. Calculate the mcg/min infusing. _____

   Is this within the normal 1-5 mcg/min rate? _____

2. The order is to infuse dobutamine 500 mg in 250 mL at a rate of 7 mL/hr. Calculate the mg/hr _____

   and mcg/min the patient will receive. _____

3. Pronestyl 2 g in 500 mL D5W is ordered for a patient with frequent PVC's, to run at 30 mL/hr. Calculate the number of mg/min the patient is receiving. _____

   The normal dosage range for this drug is between 1-6 mg/min. Is the dosage within these limits? _____

4. A patient has an order for nitroglycerine 6 mL/hr by volumetric pump. The solution strength is 50 mg/250 mL. How many mcg/min are being infused? _____

5. Esmolol is ordered to control the ventricular rate of a patient during surgery. The solution available has a strength of 2.5 g in 250 mL D5W. The order is to infuse at 32 mL/hr. Calculate the mg/hr and mg/min being infused. _____

   _____

ANSWERS 1. 2.7 mcg/min; yes 2. 14 mg/hr; 233.3 mcg/min 3. 2 mg/min; yes 4. 20 mcg/min 5. 320 mg/hr; 5.3 mg/min

Titration of Infusions

Titration refers to the adjustment of dosage within a specific range to obtain a measurable physiologic response, for example Levophed 2-4 mcg/min to maintain systolic BP> 100. The dosage is increased or decreased within the ordered range until the desired response is obtained. The **lowest dosage is set first**, and adjusted upwards and downwards as necessary. The **upper dosage is never exceeded** unless a new order is obtained.

EID's (pumps, controllers, or syringe pumps) are most often used for administration. Flow rates are calculated in mL/hr for the lowest, and highest dosage ordered, and adjusted within this range to elicit the desired physiologic response. Let's look at some examples.

EXAMPLE 1 Levophed **2-4 mcg/min** has been ordered to maintain systolic BP> 100 mm. The solution being titrated has **8 mg** Levophed in **250 mL** D5W. Calculate the flow rate for the **2-4 mcg range**.

The **lower** 2 mcg/min flow rate is calculated first.

   • **Convert mcg/min to mcg/hr**

   2 mcg/min × 60 min = **120 mcg/hr**

- **Convert mcg/hr to mg/hr**

  120 mcg = **0.12 mg/hr**

- **Calculate the lower mL/hr flow rate**

  8 mg : 250 mL = 0.12 mg : X mL   or $\dfrac{8 \text{ mg}}{250 \text{ mL}} : \dfrac{0.12 \text{ mg}}{X \text{ mL}} = 3.75 = \textbf{4 mL/hr}$
  8X = 250 × 0.12
  X = 3.75 = **4 mL/hr**

The flow rate for the lower 2 mcg/min dosage is 4 mL/hr

The **upper** 4 mcg/min flow rate is calculated next.

- **Convert mcg/min to mcg/hr**

  4 mcg/min × 60 min = **2400 mcg/hr**

- **Convert mcg/hr to mg/hr**

  2400 mcg/hr = **0.24 mg/hr**

- **Calculate the upper mL/hr flow rate**

  8 mg : 250 mL = 0.24 mg : X mL   or $\dfrac{8 \text{ mg}}{250 \text{ mL}} : \dfrac{0.24 \text{ mg}}{X \text{ mL}} = 7.5 = \textbf{8 mL/hr}$
  8X = 250 × 0.24
  X = 7.5 = **8 mL/hr**

The flow rate for the upper 4 mcg/min dosage is 8 mL/hr

The flow rate range to titrate a dosage of 2-4 mcg/min is 4-8 mL/hr

Special Note: Because the range of dosage was 2-4 mcg/min, or exactly double, the calculations could have been done for only the lower 2 mcg/min dosage and simply doubled to obtain the 4 mcg/min rate.

Let's assume that several changes in mL/hr have been made, and that the BP has now stabilized at **5 mL/hr**. Look how simple it is to determine how many **mcg/min** (or per hr) the patient is now receiving.

- **Calculate the dosage infusing at 5 mL/hr**

  250 mL : 8 mg = 5 mL : X mg   or $\dfrac{250 \text{ mL}}{8 \text{ mg}} : \dfrac{5 \text{ mL}}{X \text{ mg}} = \textbf{0.16 mg/hr}$
  250X = 8 × 5
  X = **0.16 mg/hr**

- **Convert mg/hr to mcg/hr**

  0.16 mg/hr = **160 mcg/hr**

- **Convert mcg/hr to mcg/min infusing**

  160 mcg/hr ÷ 60 min = 2.67 = **2.7 mcg/min**

At a flow rate of 5 mL/hr the patient is now receiving 2.7 mcg/min

EXAMPLE 2   Inocor is to be titrated between **415-830 mcg/min** to maintain diastolic BP< 90 mm. The solution concentration is **100 mg** in **40 mL** NS. Calculate the **mL/hr** flow rate range.

The **lower** 415 mcg/min flow rate is calculated first.

- **Convert mcg/min to mcg/hr**

  415 mcg/min × 60 min = **24,900 mcg/hr**

- **Convert mcg/hr to mg/hr**

  24,900 mcg/hr = **24.9 mg/hr**

- **Calculate the lower mL/hr flow rate**

  100 mg : 40 mL = 24.9 mg : X mL   or $\dfrac{100\ mg}{40\ mL} : \dfrac{24.9\ mg}{X\ mL}$ = 9.96 = **10 mL/hr**
  100X = 40 × 24.9
  X = 9.96 = **10 mL/hr**

The **upper** 830 mcg/min dosage is exactly double the lower 415 mcg/min dosage, so the flow rate range for the upper dosage will be double that of the lower.

- **Calculate the upper dosage flow rate**

  10 mL/hr × 2 = **20 mL/hr**

  A dosage of 415-830 mcg/min requires a flow rate of 10-20 mL/hr

The rate is adjusted several times, and the IV is now infusing at **14 mL/hr**. How many **mcg/min** are now infusing?

- **Calculate the mg/hr infusing**

  40 mL : 100 mg = 14 mL : X mL   or $\dfrac{40\ mL}{100\ mg} : \dfrac{14\ mL}{X\ mg}$ = **35 mg/hr**
  40X = 100 × 14
  X = **35 mg/hr**

- **Convert mg/hr to mcg/hr**

  35 mg/hr × 1000 = **35,000 mcg/hr**

- **Convert mcg/hr to mcg/min infusing**

  35,000 mcg/hr ÷ 60 min = 583.33 = **583.3 mcg/min**

  A 14 mL/hr flow rate will infuse 583.3 mcg/min

EXAMPLE 3   A patient weighing **103.1 kg** has orders for Nipride to be titrated between **0.3-3 mcg/kg/min** to sustain BP> 100 mm. The solution concentration is **50 mg** in **250 mL** D5W.

The **dosage range for this weight** is calculated first.

- **Calculate the lower dosage per min**

  0.3 mcg/kg/min × 103.1 kg = 30.93 = **30.9 mcg/min**

- **Calculate the upper dosage per min**

  3 mcg/kg/min × 103.1 kg = **309.3 mcg/min**

  The dosage range for this 103.1 kg patient is 30.9 to 309.3 mcg/min

The flow rate for the **lower** 30.9 mcg/min dosage is now calculated.

- **Convert mcg/min to mcg/hr**

  30.9 mcg/min × 60 min = **1854 mcg/hr**

- **Convert mcg/hr to mg/hr**

  1854 mcg/hr = **1.9 mg/hr**

- **Calculate the lower mL/hr flow rate**

  50 mg : 250 mL = 1.9 mg : X mL   or $\dfrac{50 \text{ mg}}{250 \text{ mL}} : \dfrac{1.9 \text{ mg}}{X \text{ mL}} = 9.5 = $ **10 mL/hr**
  50X = 250 × 1.9
  X = 9.5 = **10 mL/hr**

The flow rate for the **upper** 309.3 mcg/min dosage is now calculated.

- **Convert mcg/min to mcg/hr**

  309.3 mcg/min × 60 min = **18,558 mcg/hr**

- **Convert mcg/hr to mg/hr**

  18,558 mcg/hr = 18.55 = **18.6 mg/hr**

- **Calculate the flow rate**

  50 mg : 250 mL = 18.6 mg : X mL   or $\dfrac{50 \text{ mg}}{250 \text{ mL}} : \dfrac{18.6 \text{ mg}}{X \text{ mL}} = $ **93 mL/hr**
  50X = 250 × 18.6
  X = **93 mL/hr**

To deliver 0.3-3 mcg/kg/min to this 103.1 kg patient the flow rate must be titrated between 9-93 mL/hr

If after several titrations the patient stabilizes at a rate of **22 mL/hr**, how many **mcg/min** will be infusing?

- **Calculate the mg/hr infusing**

  250 mL : 50 mg = 22 mL : X mL   or $\dfrac{250 \text{ mL}}{50 \text{ mg}} : \dfrac{22 \text{ mL}}{X \text{ mg}} = $ **4.4 mg/hr**
  250X = 50 × 22
  X = **4.4 mg/hr**

- **Convert mg/hr to mcg/hr**

  4.4 mg/hr × 1000 = **4400 mcg/hr**

- **Convert mcg/hr to mcg/min infusing**

  4400 mcg/hr ÷ 60 min = **73.3 mcg/min**

A flow rate of 22 mL/hr will infuse 73.3 mcg/min

EXAMPLE 4   Nipride has been ordered to titrate at **3-6 mcg/kg/min**. The solution strength is **50 mg in 250 mL**. Calculate the flow rate range for a **72.4 kg** patient.

The **dosage range for this weight** is calculated first.

• **Calculate the lower dosage per min**

3 mcg/kg/min × 72.4 kg = **217.2 mcg/min**

The **upper** dosage of 6 mcg/kg/min is exactly double the lower rate, so multiply the lower rate by 2 to obtain the upper dosage range.

• **Calculate the upper dosage per min**

217.2 mcg/min × 2 = **434.4 mcg/min**

The dosage range for this patient is 217.2 – 434.4 mcg/min

The flow rate for the **lower** dosage is now calculated.

• **Convert mcg/min to mcg/hr**

217.2 mcg/min × 60 min = **13,026 mcg/hr**

• **Convert mcg/hr to mg/hr**

13,026 mcg/hr = **13 mg/hr**

• **Calculate the lower mL/hr flow rate**

50 mg : 250 mL = 13 mg : X mL   or $\dfrac{50\ mg}{250\ mL} : \dfrac{13\ mg}{X\ mL}$ = **65 mL/hr**
50X = 250 × 13
X = **65 mL/hr**

The **upper flow rate** will be exactly double the lower.

• **Calculate the upper flow rate**

65 mL/hr × 2 = **130 mL/hr**

To deliver 3-6 mcg/kg/min to this 72.4 kg patient, the flow rate must be titrated between 65-130 mL/hr

If after several adjustments upwards the flow rate is stabilized at **75 mL/hr**, what will the **mcg/min** dosage be?

• **Calculate the mg/hr infusing**

250 mL : 50 mg = 75 mL : X mL   or $\dfrac{250\ mL}{50\ mg} : \dfrac{75\ mL}{X\ mg}$ = **15 mg/hr**
250X = 50 × 75
X = **15 mg/hr**

• **Convert mg/hr to mcg/hr**

15 mg/hr = **15,000 mcg/hr**

• **Convert mcg/hr to mcg/min infusing**

15,000 mcg ÷ 60 min = **250 mcg/min**

An infusion rate of 75 mL/hr will deliver Nipride 250 mcg/min

PROBLEM

Calculate the dosage range, mL/hr flow rate, and stabilizing dosages as indicated for the following titrations. Express fractional dosages to the nearest tenth.

1. A 2 g in 500 mL D5W solution of Bretylium is ordered to titrate at 1-2 mg/min for ventricular arrythmias. After several titrations the rate is stabilized at 18 mL/hr.

   Flow rate range _____   Stabilizing dosage/min _____

2. Isuprel is ordered to titrate between 1-3 mcg/min to sustain heart rate at a minimum of 64/min. The solution strength is 1 mg per 250 mL D5W. The patient is stabilized at 35 mL/hr.

   Flow rate range _____   Stabilizing dosage/min _____

3. A stabilizing dosage of Inocor is established at a rate of 14 mL/hr. The dosage range being titrated is 5-8 mcg/kg/min. The patient weighs 103.7 kg, and the solution strength is 100 mg in 40 mL NS.

   Dosage range mcg/min _____   Flow rate range mL/hr _____

   Stabilizing dosage/min _____

4. Esmolol is to titrate between 50-100 mcg/kg/min. The patient weighs 78.7 kg, and the solution strength is 2500 mg in 250 mL D5W. After several titrations the rate is stabilized at 30 mL/hr.

   Dosage range mcg/min _____   Flow rate range mL/hr _____

   Stabilizing dosage/min _____

5. A patient weighing 73.2 kg has a Dobutrex solution of 500 mg in 250 mL D5W ordered to titrate between 3-10 mcg/kg/min. After many adjustments, the rate is stabilized at 27 mL/hr.

   Dosage range mcg/min _____   Flow rate range mL/hr _____

   Stabilizing dosage/min _____

ANSWERS 1. 15-30 mL/hr; 1.2 mg/min 2. 15-45 mL/hr; 2.3 mcg/min 3. 518.5-829.6 mcg/min; 12-20 mL/hr; 583.3 mcg/min 4. 3935-7870 mcg/min; 24-47 mL/hr; 5000 mcg/min 5. 219.6-732 mcg/min; 7-22 mL/hr; 900 mcg/min

---

Summary

This concludes the chapter on titration of IV medications. The important points to remember about these medications are:

➡ they have a rapid action and short duration

➡ they have a narrow margin of safety, and continuous patient monitoring is required in their use

➡ they are frequently titrated within a specific dosage/flow rate to elicit a measurable physiologic response

➡ when titrated they are initiated at the lowest dosage ordered, and increased or decreased slowly to obtain the desired response

➡ they are infused using an EID or 60 gtt/mL microdrip set

➡ the mL/hr flow rate for EID's and the gtt/min microdrip rate are identical and interchangeable

➡ calculations for dosage and flow rates must be double checked

Summary Self Test

DIRECTIONS

Read each question thoroughly, and calculate only the dosages and flow rates indicated.

1. Dobutrex 6 mcg/kg/min is ordered to infuse IV to sustain the blood pressure of a patient weighing 75.4 kg. The solution available is 500 mg in 250 mL D5W.

    mcg/min dosage _____ mL/hr flow rate _____

2. The order is to infuse a Nipride solution of 50 mg in 250 mL D5W at 0.8 mcg/kg/min. Calculate the flow rate in mL/hr for a 65.9 kg patient.

    mcg/min dosage _____ mL/hr flow rate _____

3. A patient with aspiration pneumonia has an order for aminophylline 250 mg in 500 mL D5W to infuse between 0.5 and 0.7 mg/kg/hr. The patient weighs 82.4 kg. He stabilizes at 75 mL/hr.

    mg/hr dosage range _____ mL/hr flow rate range _____

    stabilizing dosage/hr _____

4. A solution of 400 mg dopamine HCl in 250 mL D5W is infusing at 20 gtt/min.

    mcg/min dosage _____

5. Pronestyl 1-6 mg/min is ordered. The solution strength is 2 g/500 mL. The patient stabilizes at a rate of 80 mL/hr.

    mL/hr flow rate range _____

    stabilizing dosage mg/min _____

6. A patient with bigeminy has orders for an infusion of 2 g Lidocaine in 500 mL D5W at 60 mL/hr. Is this dosage within the normal 1-4 mg/min range?

    mg/min dosage _____ mg/hr dosage _____

    normal range? _____

7. A terminal cancer patient has orders for continuous morphine sulfate IV. The solution available is 25 mg in 50 mL. The order is to infuse at 8 mg/hr.

    mL/hr flow rate _____

8. A solution of amrinone lactate 100 mg in 40 mL NS is ordered to infuse at 5 mcg/kg/min for a patient weighing 77.1 kg.

    mL/hr flow rate _____

9. A patient in heart block has Isuprel ordered at 4 mcg/min. The solution available is 1 mg in 250 mL D5W.

    mL/hr flow rate _____

10. A patient weighing 80 kg has an order for intropin to infuse at 8 mcg/kg/min. The solution strength is 800 mg intropin in 500 mL D5W.

    mcg/min dosage _____   mL/hr flow rate _____

11. Dopamine 400 mg is added to 250 mL D5W and infused at 45 gtt/min. Calculate the mcg/min and mg/hr infusing.

    mcg/min dosage _____   mg/hr dosage _____

12. A patient with tetanus has orders for IV Thorazine 1 mg/min. The solution strength is 250 mg in 250 mL D5W.

    mL/hr flow rate _____

13. A patient weighing 77.9 kg is to receive Esmolol 80 mcg/kg/min. The solution strength is 2.5 g in 250 mL D5W.

    mcg/min dosage _____   mL/hr flow rate _____

14. Levophed 4 mcg/min has been ordered using an 8 mg in 250 mL D5W solution.

    mL/hr flow rate _____

15. A patient who weighs 81.7 kg has orders for dopamine 8-10 mcg/kg/min. The solution strength is 400 mg dopamine in 250 mL D5W. The IV is infusing at 25 mL/hr.

    mcg/min dosage range _____   mcg/min infusing _____

    within ordered range? _____

16. Nitroprusside 6 mcg/kg/min has been ordered for a 90.7 kg patient. The solution strength is 50 mg nitroprusside in 250 mL D5W.

    mcg/min dosage _____   mL/hr flow rate _____

17. Dopamine 5 mcg/kg/min is ordered. The solution available is 400 mg dopamine in 250 mL D5W. The patient's weight is 70.7 kg.

    mcg/min dosage _____   mL/hr flow rate _____

18. Pronestyl 3 mg/min is ordered. The solution strength is 2 g in 500 mL D5W.

    mL/hr flow rate _____

19. A nitroglycerine solution of 50 mg/250 mL D5W is infusing at 15 gtt/min.

    mcg/min infusing _____

20. Bretylol 2 g in 500 mL D5W is to infuse at a rate of 2 mg/min.

    mL/hr flow rate _____

21. A patient whose weight is 102.4 kg is to receive Nembutal 2 mg/kg/hr. The solution strength is 1 g in 500 mL D5W.

    mg/hr dosage _____   mL/hr flow rate _____

22. Deprovan 1 g in 100 mL D5W is to infuse at a rate of 15 mcg/kg/min. The patient's weight is 94.4 kg.

    mcg/min dosage _____   mL/hr flow rate _____

23. A patient with severe hypotension is receiving 4 gtt/min of a solution of Levophed that contains 8 mg in 250 mL D5W. Is this within the normal range of 2-4 mcg/min?

mcg/min infusing _____ normal range? _____

24. Inocor is ordered to titrate between 5-10 mcg/kg/min. The patient's weight is 97.1 kg, and the solution strength is 100 mg/40 mL NS. The stabilizing flow rate is 17 mL/hr.

mcg/min range _____ mL/hr flow rate range _____

mcg/min stabilizing dosage _____

25. Dobutrex 500 mg in 250 mL D5W is ordered for a 101.2 kg patient to titrate between 3-10 mcg/kg/min. The patient stabilizes at 23 mL/hr.

mcg/min dosage range _____ mL/hr flow rate range _____

mcg/min stabilizing dosage _____

26. An infusion of dobutamine 500 mg in 250 mL D5W has a stabilizing rate of 14 mL/hr.

mcg/min infusing _____

27. Amrinone 5-10 mcg/kg/min is to be titrated for a patient weighing 79.6 kg. The solution strength is 100 mg in 40 mL NS. The patient stabilizes at 12 mL/hr.

mcg/min dosage range _____ mL/hr flow rate range _____

mcg/min stabilizing dosage _____

28. Dopamine 400 mg in 250 mL D5W is to be titrated at 2-20 mcg/kg/min to maintain systolic BP>110. The patient's weight is 62.3 kg. The BP stabilizes at 32 mL/hr.

mcg/min dosage range _____ mL/hr flow rate range _____

mcg/min stabilizing dosage _____

29. Dobutamine has been ordered for a patient weighing 84.9 kg to titrate at 2.5-10 mcg/kg/min. The solution strength is 500 mg dobutamine in 250 mL D5W. The patient stabilizes at a rate of 18 mL/hr.

mcg/min dosage range _____ mL/hr flow rate range _____

mcg/min stabilizing dosage _____

30. Lidocaine is ordered at a rate of 1-4 mg/min. The solution strength is 2 g in 500 mL D5W.

mL/hr flow rate range _____

31. A 10 mcg/min dosage of Levophed is ordered using an 8 mg/250 mL D5W solution.

mL/hr flow rate _____

32. Pronestyl 2 g in 500 mL D5W is to infuse at 3 mg/min. A microdrip is used.

mL/hr flow rate _____

33. A 250 mL D5W solution with 1 mg Isuprel is to be
    infused at 5 mcg/min.

    mL/hr flow rate _____

34. A 4 mcg/min maintenance dosage of Isuprel is ordered.
    The solution is 250 mL D5W with 8 mg Isuprel.

    mL/hr flow rate _____

35. Pronestyl 2 g in 500 mL D5W is ordered to infuse at a
    rate of 6 mg/min.

    mL/hr flow rate _____

36. A 2 g in 500 mL D5W solution of Pronestyl is ordered
    to infuse at 4 mg/min.

    gtt/min flow rate _____

37. A 12 mcg/min dosage of Levophed from an 8 mg in 250 mL
    D5W solution is ordered.

    mL/hr flow rate _____

38. A 40 mg/hr dosage of Trandate from a 100 mg in 100 mL
    D5W solution is ordered.

    mL/hr flow rate _____

39. The order is for Isuprel 4 mcg/min from a 250 mL
    D5W with 1 mg solution.

    mL/hr flow rate _____

40. Cardizem 10 mg/hr from a 125 mg/100mL D5W solution
    has been ordered.

    mL/hr flow rate _____

ANSWERS 1. 452.4 mcg/min; 14 mL/hr 2. 52.7 mcg/min; 16 mL/hr 3. 41.2-57.7 mg/hr; 82-115 mL/hr; 37.5 mg/hr 4. 533.3 mcg/min 5. 15-90 mL/hr; 5.3 mg/min 6. 4 mg/min; 240 mg/hr; yes 7. 16 mL/hr 8. 9 mL/hr 9. 60 mL/hr 10. 640 mcg/min; 24 mL/hr 11. 1200 mcg/min; 72 mg/hr 12. 60 mL/hr 13. 6232 mcg/min; 37 mL/hr 14. 8 mL/hr 15. 653.6-817 mcg/min; 666.7 mcg/min; yes 16. 544.2 mcg/min; 163 mL/hr 17. 353.5 mcg/min; 13 mL/hr 18. 45 mL/hr 19. 50 mcg/min 20. 30 mL/hr 21. 204.8 mg/hr; 102 mL/hr 22. 1416 mcg/min; 9 mL/hr 23. 2.1 mcg/min; yes 24. 485.5-971 mcg/min; 12-23 mL/hr; 708.3 mcg/min 25. 303.6-1012 mcg/min; 9-30 mL/hr; 766.7 mcg/min 26. 466.7 mcg/min 27. 398-796 mcg/min; 10-19 mL/hr; 500 mcg/min 28. 124.6-1246 mcg/min; 5-47 mL/hr; 853.3 mcg/min 29. 212.3-849 mcg/min; 6-25 mL/hr; 600 mcg/min 30. 15-60 mL/hr 31. 19 mL/hr 32. 45 mL/hr 33. 75 mL/hr 34. 8 mL/hr 35. 90 mL/hr 36. 60 mL/hr 37. 23 mL/hr 38. 40 mL/hr 39. 60 mL/hr 40. 8 mL/hr

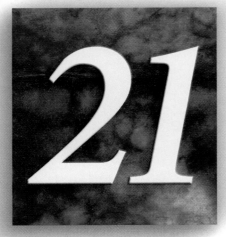

Heparin Infusion Calculations

The student will calculate the

1. amount of heparin to be added to prepare IV solutions
2. mL/hr flow rates for an EID
3. gtt/min flow rates for microdrip and macrodrip sets
4. hourly dosage infusing from mL/hr and gtt/min rates

Heparin is an anticoagulant drug which inhibits new blood clot formation, or the extension of already existing clots. Heparin dosages are expressed in USP units (U), and are commonly administered intravenously. Dosages may be ordered on the basis of U/hour, or, if a standard concentration of IV solution is used, by mL/hr flow rate. Heparin dosages are ordered on a very individualized basis, and blood tests to monitor coagulation times are essential.

 The normal heparinizing dosage for adults is 20,000 – 40,000 U every 24 hours.

This means that the average patient will receive a daily dosage that falls within these 20,000 U to 40,000 U parameters. Dosages larger or smaller may be ordered based on a patient's coagulation time, but dosages markedly different from the average may need to be questioned.

In this chapter you will be introduced to several of the commercially prepared IV solutions containing heparin, as well as to heparin vial labels, which you will use to calculate the preparation of a variety of IV heparin solution strengths using standard solutions. You will also practice calculating heparin flow rates; calculating hourly dosage being administered; and assessing the accuracy of prescribed heparin dosages. The calculations are identical to those you have already practiced in previous chapters except that heparin is measured in units (U). Heparin is most frequently administered using a microdrip and/or an EID (controller, pump), but the examples and exercises which follow will provide practice in calculations using all IV set calibrations: 10, 15, 20 and 60 gtt/mL, as well as mL/hr rates.

Reading Heparin Labels and Preparing IV Solutions

Commercially prepared IV solutions containing heparin are available in several strengths. Refer to the IV bag labeling in Figure 94, and notice the blue "Heparin Sodium 1,000 units in 0.9% Sodium Chloride Injection" on this 500 mL bag. Then refer to the additional red dosage labeling "Heparin 1,000 units (2 units/mL)", and the "Heparin 25,000 units (50 units/mL)" in Figure 95. The red dosages draw particular attention to the fact that these bags contain heparin, acting to make the bags instantly recognizable. They serve as an important safety factor in solution identification.

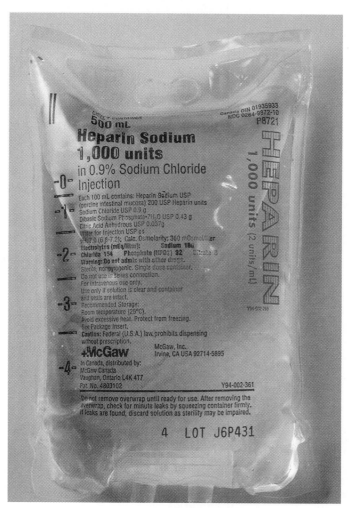

Figure 94

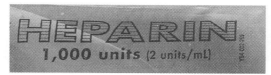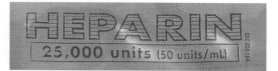

Figure 95

If a commercially prepared heparin dosage strength that you require is not available, you may be required to prepare the solution yourself from **a number of available vial dosage strengths**. Let's stop and look at several vial labels now, so that you can refresh your memory with some typical calculations.

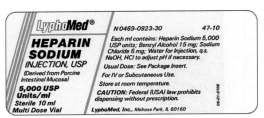

Figure 96

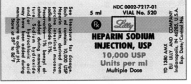
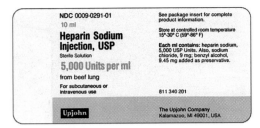

Figure 97

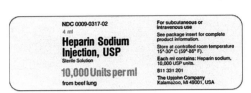

Figure 98

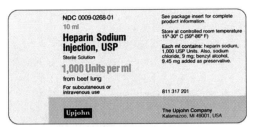

Figure 99

Figure 100

PROBLEM

Read the heparin labels provided and determine how many mL of heparin will be necessary to prepare the solutions indicated.

1. Refer to the label in Figure 96 and determine how many mL will be required to add 20,000 U to an IV solution. _____

2. Refer to the label in Figure 97 and determine how many mL will be required to add 30,000 U to an IV solution. _____

3. Refer to the label in Figure 98 and determine how many mL will be required to add 20,000 U to an IV solution. _____

4. Refer to the label in Figure 99 and determine how many mL of heparin will be required to add 25,000 U to an IV solution. _____

5. Refer to the label in Figure 100 and determine how many mL will be required to add 10,000 U to an IV solution. _____

ANSWERS   1. 4 mL   2. 3 mL   3. 2 mL   4. 5 mL   5. 10 mL

Calculating mL/hr Flow Rate from U/hr Ordered

21

Since heparin is most frequently ordered in U/hr to be administered, for example, 1000 U/hr, and infused using an EID, a common calculation will be the mL/hr flow rate. Let's look at these calculations first, keeping in mind that the mL/hr flow rate for an EID is identical to the gtt/min rate for a microdrip.

EXAMPLE 1   The order is to infuse heparin **1000 U/hr** from a solution of **20,000 U in 500 mL** D5W.

• **Calculate the mL/hr flow rate**

$$20,000 \text{ U} : 500 \text{ mL} = 1000 \text{ U} : X \text{ mL} \quad \text{or} \quad \frac{20,000 \text{ U}}{500 \text{ mL}} : \frac{1000 \text{ U}}{X \text{ mL}} = \textbf{25 mL/hr}$$
$$20,000X = 500 \times 1000$$
$$X = \textbf{25 mL/hr}$$

The flow rate to infuse 1000 U/hr from a solution of 20,000 U in 500 mL is 25 mL/hr

EXAMPLE 2   The order is for heparin **800 U/hr**. The solution available is **40,000 U in 1000 mL** D5W.

• **Calculate the mL/hr flow rate**

$$40,000 \text{ U} : 1000 \text{ mL} = 800 \text{ U} : X \text{ mL} \quad \text{or} \quad \frac{40,000 \text{ U}}{1000 \text{ mL}} : \frac{800 \text{ U}}{X \text{ mL}} = \textbf{20 mL/hr}$$
$$40,000X = 1000 \times 800$$
$$X = \textbf{20 mL/hr}$$

The flow rate to infuse 800 U/hr from a solution of 40,000 U in 1000 mL is 20 mL/hr

EXAMPLE 3   The order is to infuse heparin **1100 U/hr** from a solution strength of **60,000 U in 1 L** D5W.

• **Calculate the mL/hr flow rate**

$$60,000 \text{ U} : 1000 \text{ mL} = 1100 \text{ U} : X \text{ mL} \quad \text{or} \quad \frac{60,000 \text{ U}}{1000 \text{ mL}} : \frac{1100 \text{ U}}{X \text{ mL}} = 18.3 = \textbf{18 mL/hr}$$
$$60,000X = 1000 \times 1100$$
$$X = 18.3 = \textbf{18 mL/hr}$$

The flow rate to infuse 1100 U/hr from a solution of 60,000 U in 1 L is 18 mL/hr

PROBLEM

Calculate the mL/hr flow rates for the following heparin infusions.

1. The order is to infuse 1000 U heparin per hour from an available solution strength of 25,000 U in 500 mL D5W. _____

2. A patient with deep vein thrombosis has orders for heparin 2500 U per hour. The solution strength is 50,000 U in 1000 mL D5W. _____

3. The order is to infuse 1100 U per hour from a 15,000 U in 1 L D5W solution. _____

4. A newly admitted patient has orders for 50,000 U of heparin in 1000 mL D5W to infuse at a rate of 2000 U per hour. _____

5. Administer 1500 U per hour of heparin from an available strength of 40,000 U in 1 L. _____

ANSWERS 1. 20 mL/hr 2. 50 mL/hr 3. 73 mL/hr 4. 40 mL/hr 5. 38 mL/hr

HEPARIN INFUSION CALCULATIONS 275

Calculating gtt/min Flow Rate from U/hr Ordered

When a gtt/min rate is calculated for a 10, 15, 20 or 60 gtt/mL set the calculation will include the set calibration.

EXAMPLE 1

A heparin solution with a strength of **40,000 U per 1000 mL** D5W is ordered to infuse at a rate of **1000 U/hr.** A **15 gtt/mL** set is used.

• **Calculate the mL/hr to be infused first**

$$40,000 \text{ U} : 1000 \text{ mL} = 1000 \text{ U} : X \text{ mL} \quad \text{or} \quad \frac{40,000 \text{ U}}{1000 \text{ mL}} : \frac{1000 \text{ U}}{X \text{ mL}} = \textbf{25 mL/hr}$$
$$X = \textbf{25 mL/hr}$$

• **Calculate the flow rate in gtt/min**

The division factor for a 15 gtt/mL set is 4 (60 ÷ 15)

$$25 \div 4 = 6.2 = \textbf{6 gtt/min}$$

To infuse 1000 U/hr from a 40,000 U/1000 mL solution using a 15 gtt/mL set the rate will be 6 gtt/min

EXAMPLE 2

A solution of heparin **20,000 U in 500 mL** D5W is ordered to infuse at a rate of **800 U** per hour using a **10 gtt/mL** set.

• **Calculate the mL/hr to be infused**

$$20,000 \text{ U} : 500 \text{ mL} = 800 \text{ U} : X \text{ mL} \quad \text{or} \quad \frac{20,000 \text{ U}}{500 \text{ mL}} : \frac{800 \text{ U}}{X \text{ mL}} = \textbf{20 mL/hr}$$
$$X = \textbf{20 mL/hr}$$

• **Calculate the flow rate in gtt/min**

The division factor for a 10 gtt/mL set is 6 (60 ÷ 10)

$$20 \div 6 = 3.3 = \textbf{3 gtt/min}$$

To infuse 800 U/hr from a 20,000 U in 500 mL solution using a 10 gtt/mL set the rate will be 3 gtt/min

EXAMPLE 3

The order is for heparin to infuse at **1200 U per hour.** The solution strength is **60,000 U in 1L D5W.** A **20 gtt/mL** set is used.

• **Calculate the mL/hr to be infused**

$$60,000 \text{ U} : 1000 \text{ mL} = 1200 \text{ U} : X \text{ mL} \quad \text{or} \quad \frac{60,000 \text{ U}}{1000 \text{ mL}} : \frac{1200 \text{ U}}{X \text{ mL}} = \textbf{20 mL/hr}$$
$$X = \textbf{20 mL/hr}$$

• **Calculate the flow rate in gtt/min**

The division factor for a 20 gtt/mL set is 3 (60 ÷ 20)

$$20 \div 3 = 6.6 = \textbf{7 gtt/min}$$

To infuse 1200 U/hr from a 60,000 U in 1 L solution using a 20 gtt/mL set the rate will be 7 gtt/min

EXAMPLE 4 An IV of **500 mL** D5W with **25,000 U** heparin is to infuse at **1500 U/hr** using a **microdrip**.

• Calculate the mL/hr to be infused

$$25{,}000 \text{ U} : 500 \text{ mL} = 1500 \text{ U} : X \text{ mL} \quad \text{or} \quad \frac{25{,}000 \text{ U}}{500 \text{ mL}} : \frac{1500 \text{ U}}{X \text{ mL}} = \textbf{30 mL/hr}$$
$$X = \textbf{30 mL/hr}$$

• Calculate the flow rate in gtt/min

The division factor for a 60 gtt/mL set is 1 (60 ÷ 60)

$$30 \div 1 = \textbf{30 gtt/min}$$

To infuse 1500 U/hr from a 25,000 U in 500 mL solution using a microdrip the rate will be 30 gtt/min

---

PROBLEM

Calculate the gtt/min flow rates to administer the following heparin dosages.

1. A solution of 25,000 U heparin in 500 mL D5W to infuse at a rate of 1000 U per hour using a 10 gtt/mL set. _____

2. Heparin 2500 U per hour using a 20 gtt/mL set. The solution strength is 50,000 U in 1000 mL D5W. _____

3. A solution strength of heparin 15,000 U per 1 L to infuse at 1100 U/hr using a 15 gtt/mL set. _____

4. Heparin 2000 U per hour using a 20 gtt/mL set. The solution strength is 50,000 U in 1000 mL D5W. _____

5. A 30,000 U in 500 mL heparin solution to infuse at 1500 U/hr with a 10 gtt/mL set. _____

6. A 500 mL D5W with 20,000 U heparin to infuse at 1000 U/hr using a microdrip. _____

ANSWERS 1. 3 gtt/min 2. 17 gtt/min 3. 18 gtt/min 4. 13 gtt/min 5. 4 gtt/min 6. 25 gtt/min

Calculating U/hr Infusing from mL/hr Infusing

If a heparin order specifies infusion at a predetermined mL/hr flow rate, the doctor has already calculated the dosage per hour/day the patient is to receive. However, it remains a nursing responsibility to double check dosages to determine if they are within **the normal heparinizing range of 20,000-40,000 U per day.** Here's how you would do this.

EXAMPLE 1 An IV of **1000 mL** D5W containing **40,000 U** of heparin has been ordered to infuse at **30 mL/hr.**

• Calculate the U/hr infusing first

$$1000 \text{ mL} : 40{,}000 \text{ U} = 30 \text{ mL} : X \text{ U} \quad \text{or} \quad \frac{1000 \text{ mL}}{40{,}000 \text{ U}} : \frac{30 \text{ mL}}{X \text{ U}} = \textbf{1200 U/hr}$$
$$X = \textbf{1200 U/hr}$$

An IV of 1000 mL containing 40,000 U heparin infusing at 30 mL/hr is administering 1200 U/hr.

• **Assess for heparinizing range**

$$1200 \text{ U/hr} \times 24 \text{ hr} = \textbf{28,800 U/24 hr}$$

This dosage is within the 20,000 to 40,000 U in 24 hr heparinizing range.

EXAMPLE 2 The order is to infuse a solution of heparin **20,000 U to 1 L** D5W at **80 mL/hr**. Calculate the **U/hr** infusing and assess the accuracy of the order.

• **Calculate the U/hr infusing first**

$$1000 \text{ mL} : 20,000 \text{ U} = 80 \text{ mL} : \text{X U} \quad \text{or} \quad \frac{1000 \text{ mL}}{20,000 \text{ U}} : \frac{80 \text{ mL}}{\text{X U}} = \textbf{1600 U/hr}$$
$$\text{X} = \textbf{1600 U/hr}$$

An IV of 1 L containing 20,000 U heparin infusing at 80 mL/hr is administering 1600 U/hr

• **Assess for heparinizing range**

$$1600 \text{ U/hr} \times 24 \text{ hr} = \textbf{38,400 U/24 hr}$$

This dosage is within the 20,000 to 40,000 U in 24 hr heparinizing range.

EXAMPLE 3 An IV of D5W **500 mL** with **10,000 U** heparin is infusing at **30 mL/hr**. Calculate the **U/hr** dosage and determine if this dose is within the normal range.

• **Calculate U/hr infusing first**

$$500 \text{ mL} : 10,000 \text{ U} = 30 \text{ mL} : \text{X U} \quad \text{or} \quad \frac{500 \text{ mL}}{10,000 \text{ U}} : \frac{30 \text{ mL}}{\text{X U}} = \textbf{600 U/hr}$$
$$\text{X} = \textbf{600 U/hr}$$

An IV of 500 mL containing 10,000 U heparin infusing at 30 mL/hr is administering 600 U/hr

• **Assess for heparinizing range**

$$600 \text{ U/hr} \times 24 \text{ hr} = \textbf{14,400 U/day}$$

This dosage is less than the 20,000 to 40,000 U in 24 hr heparinizing range, so the order should be reconfirmed.

PROBLEM

Calculate the following U/hr heparin dosages, and determine if they are within the normal daily range.

1. The order is to add 30,000 U heparin to 750 mL D5W and infuse at 25 mL/hr.

   U/hr _____ U/day _____ Within normal range? _____

2. A solution of 20,000 U heparin in 500 mL D5W is to be infused at 30 mL/hr.

   U/hr _____ U/day _____ Within normal range? _____

3. One liter of D5NS with heparin 60,000 U is ordered to infuse at 40 mL/hr.

   U/hr _____ U/day _____ Within normal range? _____

4. The order is to add 20,000 U heparin to 1 L D5W and infuse at 30 mL/hr.

   U/hr _____ U/day _____ Within normal range? _____

5. A 25,000 U in 500 mL D5W heparin solution is infusing at 30 mL/hr.

   U/hr _____ U/day _____ Within normal range? _____

ANSWERS 1. 1000 U/hr; 24,000 U/day; yes **2.** 1200 U/hr; 28,800 U/day; yes **3.** 2400 U/hr; 57,600 U/day; high **4.** 600 U/hr; 14,400 U/day; low **5.** 1500 U/hr; 36,000 U/day; yes

Calculating U/hr Infusing from Solution Strength, Set Calibration and gtt/min Rate

The U per hour dosage can also be calculated from a solution ordered or infusing as gtt/min. The solution strength, gtt/min rate, and set calibration will be used for the calculation.

EXAMPLE 1   An IV of **10,000 U** heparin in **1000 mL** D5W is infusing at **40 gtt/min** using a **20 gtt/mL** set. Calculate U/hr infusing.

• **Convert gtt/min to mL/min infusing first**

   20 gtt : 1 mL = 40 gtt : X mL   or $\dfrac{20\ gtt}{1\ mL} : \dfrac{40\ gtt}{X\ mL} = 2\ mL/min$
         X = **2 mL/hr**

• **Calculate the mL/hr infusing**

   2 mL/min × 60 min = **120 mL/hr**

• **Calculate the U/hr infusing**

   1000 mL : 10,000 U = 120 mL : X U   or $\dfrac{1000\ mL}{10,000\ U} : \dfrac{120\ mL}{X\ U} = $ **1200 U/hr**
         X = **1200 U/hr**

The patient is receiving 1200 U/hr from this 10,000 U in 1000 mL heparin solution infusing at 40 gtt/min on a 20 gtt/mL set.

EXAMPLE 2 A heparin solution with a strength of **15,000 U in 500 mL** is infusing at a rate of **10 gtt/min** using a **10 gtt/mL** set. Calculate **U/hr** infusing.

• **Convert the gtt/min rate to mL/min infusing**

$$10 \text{ gtt} : 1 \text{ mL} = 10 \text{ gtt} : X \text{ mL} \quad \text{or} \quad \frac{10 \text{ gtt}}{1 \text{ mL}} : \frac{10 \text{ gtt}}{X \text{ mL}} = \textbf{1 mL/min}$$
$$X = \textbf{1 mL/min}$$

• **Calculate the mL/hr infusing**

$$1 \text{ mL/min} \times 60 \text{ min} = \textbf{60 mL/hr}$$

• **Calculate U/hr infusing**

$$500 \text{ mL} : 15,000 \text{ U} = 60 \text{ mL} : X \text{ U} \quad \text{or} \quad \frac{500 \text{ mL}}{15,000 \text{ U}} : \frac{60 \text{ mL}}{X \text{ U}} = \textbf{1800 U/hr}$$
$$X = \textbf{1800 U/hr}$$

The patient is receiving 1800 U/hr from this 15,000 U in 500 mL heparin solution infusing at 10 gtt/min on a 10 gtt/mL set.

EXAMPLE 3 A **15 gtt/mL** set is used to infuse a **20,000 U/1000 mL** heparin solution at **25 gtt/min**. Calculate the **U/hr** infusing.

• **Convert the gtt/min rate to mL/min infusing**

$$15 \text{ gtt} : 1 \text{ mL} = 25 \text{ gtt} : X \text{ mL} \quad \text{or} \quad \frac{15 \text{ gtt}}{1 \text{ mL}} : \frac{25 \text{ gtt}}{X \text{ mL}} = \textbf{1.6 mL/min}$$
$$X = \textbf{1.6 mL/min}$$

• **Calculate the mL/hr infusing**

$$1.6 \text{ mL/min} \times 60 \text{ min} = \textbf{96 mL/hr}$$

• **Calculate U/hr infusing**

$$1000 \text{ mL} : 20,000 \text{ U} = 96 \text{ mL} : X \text{ U} \quad \text{or} \quad \frac{1000 \text{ mL}}{20,000 \text{ U}} : \frac{96 \text{ mL}}{X \text{ U}} = \textbf{1920 U/hr}$$
$$X = \textbf{1920 U/hr}$$

The patient is receiving 1920 U/hr from this 15,000 U in 500 mL heparin solution infusing at 10 gtt/min on a 10 gtt/mL set.

PROBLEM

Calculate the U/hr of heparin infusing in the following.

1. A solution strength of 40,000 U in 1000 mL infusing at a rate of 35 gtt/min using a 60 gtt/mL microdrip.   _____

2. A set calibrated at 15 gtt/mL infusing a 30,000 U/1000 mL heparin solution at 8 gtt/min.   _____

3. A 25,000 U in 1000 mL strength heparin solution infusing at 15 gtt/min using a 20 gtt/mL set.   _____

4. An IV running at 20 gtt/min using a 20 gtt/mL set with a solution strength of heparin 10,000 U in 500 mL.   _____

5 A 20,000 U/500 mL heparin solution infusing at 22 gtt/min using a 60 gtt/mL set.   _____

ANSWERS 1. 1400 U/hr 2. 960 U/hr 3. 1125 U/hr 4. 1200 U/hr 5. 880 U/hr

21

Summary

This concludes the chapter on heparin administration. The important points to remember are:

➡ heparin is a potent anticoagulant which is frequently added to IV solutions

➡ it is measured in USP units, abbreviated U

➡ the normal heparinizing dosage is 20,000 – 40,000 U/day

➡ the patient on heparin therapy will have frequent blood tests to check coagulation times

➡ heparin may be ordered by mL/hr flow rate, or by U/hr to infuse

➡ if an EID or microdrip is used for infusion the mL/hr and gtt/min rate will be identical

➡ gtt/min rates are calculated from set calibration, IV solution strength and dosage ordered

➡ the dosage infusing at any moment can be calculated from the flow rate, set calibration and solution strength

➡ commercially prepared IV solutions are available for several heparin strengths

➡ additional strengths may require the preparation of heparin from a variety of available vial strengths

Summary Self Test

DIRECTIONS

Calculate the heparin flow rates and hourly dosages as indicated in the following questions.

1. A patient is to receive heparin 1000 U/hr. The IV solution available has 25,000 U in 1 L D5W, and a controller will be used. Flow rate _____

2. A solution of 25,000 U heparin in 1 L D5 1/4NS is infusing at 15 gtt/min using a 10 gtt/mL set. Dosage per hr _____

3. A solution of 35,000 U heparin in 1 L D5 1/2NS is to infuse via volumetric pump at 1200 U/hr. Flow rate _____

4. A patient has orders for 20,000 U heparin in 500 mL D5W to infuse at 40 mL/hr. Dosage per hr _____

5. A solution of 1 L D5W with 50,000 U heparin is to be administered at 1250 U/hr using a 15 gtt/mL set. Flow rate _____

6. A patient with pulmonary emboli has orders for 2500 U heparin per hour. The solution strength is 40,000 U in 1 L D5W and a 10 gtt/mL set is used. Flow rate _____

7. Calculate the flow rate to administer heparin at a rate of 1000 U/hr using a set calibrated at 10 gtt/mL and a solution strength of 25,000 U in 1000 mL D5W. Flow rate _____

8. Calculate the U/hr of heparin infusing at 35 gtt/min from a solution strength of 40,000 U in 1 L D5W. A microdrip is being used. Dosage per hour _____

   Within normal daily range? _____

9. Calculate the hourly heparin dosage infusing at 50 mL/hr from a 35,000 U heparin in 1 L D5W solution. Dosage per hour _____

10. A recent open heart patient has an IV of 500 mL D5W with 20,000 U heparin infusing at 20 gtt/min using a microdrip. Dosage per hr _____

11. A patient is to receive 2000 U heparin per hour from a solution of 50,000 U in 1000 mL D5NS using a 10 gtt/mL set. Flow rate _____

12. An IV of 1000 mL D5W with 20,000 U heparin is infusing at 12 gtt/min using a 10 gtt/mL set. Dosage per hour _____

13. A patient with a fractured pelvis has orders for 1 L D5 1/2NS with 60,000 U heparin to infuse at 30 mL/hr. Dosage per hour _____

    Within normal range? _____

14. The order is for 1000 U heparin per hour. The solution strength is 20,000 U in 500 mL D5NS. A microdrip is used. Flow rate _____

15. A newly admitted patient has an order for 1250 U/hr heparin from a solution strength of 15,000 U in 500 mL D5W. A controller is used to monitor the infusion. Flow rate _____

16. Calculate the hourly dosage infusing with a 25 mL/hr rate from a 1 L D5 1/4NS with 45,000 U heparin solution. Dosage _____

17. A solution of 10,000 U heparin in 500 mL D5W is ordered to infuse at 1000 U/hr via a controller. Flow rate _____

18. A liter of D5W containing 15,000 U heparin is infusing at 20 gtt/min using a 10 gtt/mL set. Dosage per hour _____

19. During morning rounds, you time a patient's IV at 20 gtt/min. The solution is heparin 25,000 U in 1 L D5W, and the set calibration 10 gtt/mL. An hourly dosage of 1500 U was ordered. Is this flow rate correct? _____

20. A patient has an IV of 25,000 U heparin in 1 L D5W infusing at 10 gtt/min using a 15 gtt/mL set. Dosage per hour _____

21. A solution of 500 mL D5NS with 30,000 U heparin is infusing at 25 mL/hr. Dosage per hour _____

    Within normal limits? _____

22. A patient with multiple fractures has an order for 2 L D5 1/2NS each to contain 20,000 U heparin to infuse at 50 mL/hr using a microdrip. Dosage per hour _____

23. A patient is receiving 500 mL D5W with 10,000 U heparin at 20 gtt/min using a 10 gtt/mL set. Dosage per hour _____

24. An IV of 1000 mL D5 1/4NS with 40,000 U heparin is to infuse at 1200 U/hr via pump. Flow rate _____

25. A patient is receiving 900 U/hr of heparin from a 500 mL D5W with 20,000 U solution. The infusion set is calibrated at 20 gtt/mL. Flow rate _____

26. The order is to infuse 500 mL D5 1/4NS with 25,000 U heparin at 1500 U/hr. A microdrip is used. Flow rate _____

27. A liter of D5W with 40,000 U heparin is infusing at 25 mL/hr. Dosage per hour _____

28. A 500 mL IV with 25,000 U heparin is infusing at 30 mL/hr. Dosage per hour _____

29. 500 mL D5W with 30,000 U heparin is to infuse via controller at 1500 U/hr. Flow rate _____

30. The order is to infuse 1 L D5 1/2NS with 45,000 U heparin at 1875 U/hr using a controller. Flow rate _____

31. The order is to infuse 1400 U/hr from a 1 L D5W with 35,000 U heparin solution using a 15 gtt/mL set. Flow rate _____

32. A patient is receiving 1 L of D5W with 12,500 U heparin at 30 gtt/min using a set calibrated at 20 gtt/mL. Dosage per hour _____

ANSWERS 1. 40 mL/hr 2. 2250 U/hr 3. 34 mL/hr 4. 1600 U/hr 5. 6 gtt/min 6. 10 gtt/min 7. 7 gtt/min 8. 1400 U/hr; yes 9. 1750 U/hr 10. 800 U/hr 11. 7 gtt/min 12. 1440 U/hr 13. 1800 U/hr; high 14. 25 gtt/min 15. 42 mL/hr 16. 1125 U/hr 17. 50 mL/hr 18. 1800 U/hr 19. no, double the dose is infusing 20. 1000 U/hr 21. 1500 U/hr; yes 22. 1000 U/hr 23. 2400 U/hr 24. 30 mL/hr 25. 8 gtt/min 26. 30 gtt/min 27. 1000 U/hr 28. 1500 U/hr 29. 25 mL/hr 30. 42 mL/hr 31. 10 gtt/min 32. 1125 U/hr

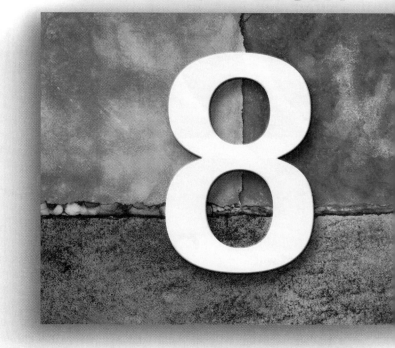

Pediatric Medication Calculations

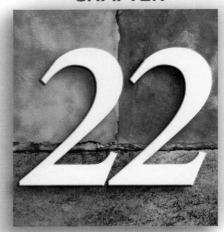

Pediatric Oral and Parenteral Medications

Two differences between adult and pediatric dosages will be immediately apparent: **most oral drugs are prepared as liquids** because infants and small children cannot be expected to swallow tablets easily, if at all, and **dosages are dramatically smaller**. The oral route is used whenever possible, but when a child cannot swallow, or the drug is ineffective given orally, drugs will be administered by a parenteral route.

Both the subcutaneous and intramuscular routes may be used depending on the type of drug to be administered. However, the small muscle size of infants and children limits the use of the intramuscular route, as does the nature of the drug being used. For example, most antibiotics are administered intravenously rather than intramuscularly.

Oral Medications

Most oral pediatric drugs are prepared as liquids to facilitate ease in swallowing. If the child is old enough to cooperate these dosages may be measured in a medication cup. Solutions may also be measured using oral syringes, such as the ones shown in Figure 101. Notice that oral syringes have the same metric calibrations as hypodermic syringes, but also include household measures, for example tsp. Oral syringes have different sized tips to prevent use with hypodermic needles. On some oral syringes the tip is positioned off center (termed eccentric), to further distinguish them from hypodermic syringes, or they may be amber colored, as in the Figure 101 illustration.

If oral syringes are not available, hypodermic syringes (**without the needle**) can also be used for dosage measurement. In addition to accuracy, syringes provide an excellent method of administering oral liquid drugs to infants and small children. Some oral liquids are prepared using a calibrated medication dropper which is an integral part of the medication bottle. These may be calibrated in mL like the dropper shown in Figure 102, or in actual dosage, for example 25 mg, or 50 mg. Animal shaped measures such as those shown in Figure 103 are also helpful in enticing reluctant toddlers to take necessary medications. In each instance the goal is to be sure the infant or child actually swallows the total dosage.

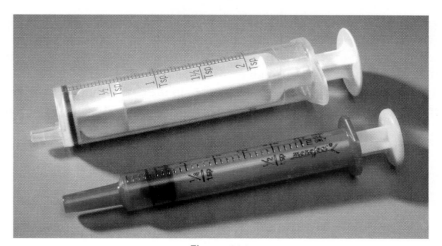

Figure 101

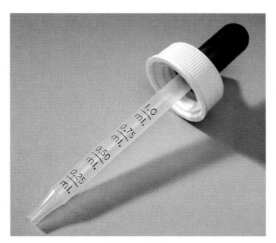

Figure 102

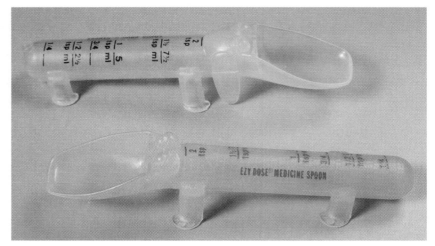

Figure 103

Care must be taken with liquid oral drugs to identify those prepared as **suspensions**. A suspension consists of an insoluble drug in a liquid base, as for example in the Augmentin® suspension in Figure 104. The drug in a suspension settles to the bottom of the bottle between uses, and **thorough mixing immediately prior to pouring is mandatory**. Suspensions must also be administered to the child promptly after measurement to prevent the drug settling out again, and an incomplete dosage being administered.

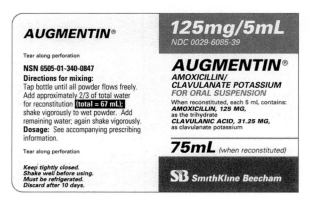

AUGMENTIN®

Tear along perforation

NSN 6505-01-340-0847
Directions for mixing:
Tap bottle until all powder flows freely.
Add approximately 2/3 of total water
for reconstitution (total = 67 mL);
shake vigorously to wet powder. Add
remaining water; again shake vigorously.
Dosage: See accompanying prescribing
information.

Tear along perforation

Keep tightly closed.
Shake well before using.
Must be refrigerated.
Discard after 10 days.

125mg/5mL
NDC 0029-6085-39

AUGMENTIN®
AMOXICILLIN/
CLAVULANATE POTASSIUM
FOR ORAL SUSPENSION
When reconstituted, each 5 mL contains:
AMOXICILLIN, 125 MG,
as the trihydrate
CLAVULANIC ACID, 31.25 MG,
as clavulanate potassium

75mL *(when reconstituted)*

SB SmithKline Beecham

Figure 104

 Suspensions must be thoroughly mixed before measurement and promptly administered, to prevent settling out of their insoluble drugs.

When a tablet or capsule is administered the child's mouth must be checked to be certain it has actually been swallowed. If swallowing is a problem, some tablets can be crushed and given in a small amount of applesauce, ice cream or juice, if the child has no dietary restrictions which would contraindicate this. Keep in mind however, that **enteric coated and timed release tablets or capsules cannot be crushed** since this would destroy the coating which allows them to function on a delayed action basis.

IM and s.c. Medications

The drugs most often given subcutaneously are insulin, and immunizations which specifically require the subcutaneous route. Any site with sufficient subcutaneous tissue may be used, with the upper arm being the site of choice for immunizations. The intramuscular route is used most frequently for preoperative and postoperative medications for sedation and pain, and for immunizations such as DPT (diphtheria, pertussis, tetanus) which must be administered deep IM. The intramuscular site of choice for infants and small children is the vastus lateralis or rectus femoris of the thigh, because the gluteal muscles do not develop until a child has learned to walk. Usually not more than 1 mL is injected per site, and sites are rotated regularly.

Dosage calculation is the same as for adults, except **dosages are sometimes calculated to the nearest hundredth, and measured using a tuberculin syringe** (refer to Chapter 7 if you need to review the calibrations and use of a TB syringe). There is less margin for error in pediatric dosages, and calculations and measurements are routinely double checked.

Summary

This concludes the introduction to pediatric oral and IM, s.c. medication administration. The important points to remember are:

→ care must be taken when administering oral drugs to be positive the child has actually swallowed the dosage

➡ if liquid medications are prepared as suspensions, mix thoroughly prior to measurement, and administer promptly to prevent settling out of their insoluble drugs

➡ care must be taken not to confuse oral syringes which are unsterile, with hypodermic syringes which are sterile

➡ the IM site of choice for infants and small children is the vastus lateralis or rectus femoris of the thigh

➡ usually not more than 1 mL is injected per IM or s.c. site, and sites are rotated regularly

➡ pediatric dosages are frequently calculated to the nearest hundredth and measured using a TB syringe

Summary Self Test

DIRECTIONS

Use the pediatric medication labels provided to measure the following oral dosages. Indicate if the medication is a suspension.

PART I

1. Prepare a 125 mg dosage of Augmentin®. _____ _____

2. Prepare a 125 mg dosage of amoxicillin. _____ _____

3. Prepare a 0.1 mg dosage of digoxin. _____ _____

4. Prepare 3 mg of Proventil®. _____ _____

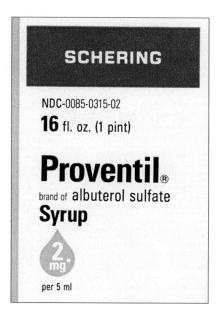

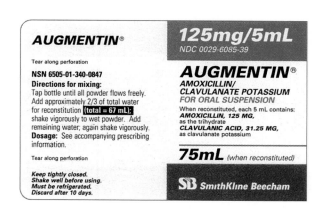

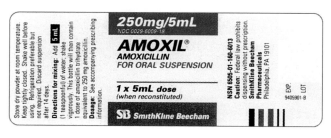

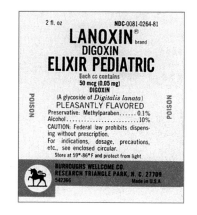

5. Prepare 400,000 U of oral penicillin V.   _____ _____

6. Prepare 40 mg of theophylline.   _____ _____

7. Prepare 62.5 mg of Dilantin®.   _____ _____

8. Prepare 250 mg of tetracycline.   _____ _____

9. Peri-Colace® 3 tsp is ordered. How many mL will this be?   _____ _____

10. Prepare 300 mg of erythromycin.   _____ _____

11. Prepare 120 mg of acetaminophen.   _____ _____

12. Prepare 12.5 mg Benadryl®.   _____ _____

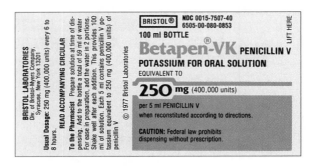

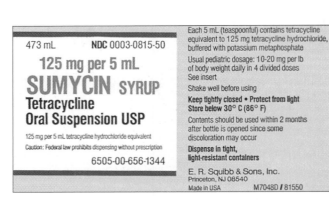

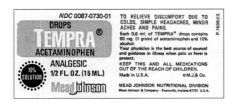

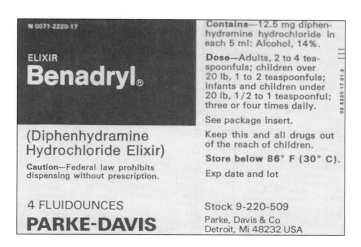

ELIXIR
Benadryl.

(Diphenhydramine
Hydrochloride Elixir)

Caution—Federal law prohibits
dispensing without prescription.

4 FLUIDOUNCES

PARKE-DAVIS

Contains—12.5 mg diphen-
hydramine hydrochloride in
each 5 ml: Alcohol, 14%.

Dose—Adults, 2 to 4 teaspoonfuls; children over
20 lb, 1 to 2 teaspoonfuls;
infants and children under
20 lb, 1/2 to 1 teaspoonful;
three or four times daily.

See package insert.

Keep this and all drugs out
of the reach of children.

Store below 86° F (30° C).

Exp date and lot

Stock 9-220-509

Parke, Davis & Co
Detroit, Mi 48232 USA

N 0071-2220-17

Gentle laxative and stool softener for
treating temporary constipation.
Usual dose: (preferably at bedtime).
Children over 3: 1 to 3 teaspoons.
Adults: 1 to 2 tablespoons.
Warning: Not to be used when ab-
dominal pain, nausea, or vomiting are
present.
Frequent or prolonged use of this preparation may result in dependence on
laxatives.

**Keep this and all medication out
of reach of children.**

NDC 0087-0721-01

SYRUP
PERI-COLACE®
CASANTHRANOL AND DIOCTYL SODIUM SULFOSUCCINATE
LAXATIVE PLUS STOOL SOFTENER

8 FL. OZ. (1/2 PT.)

Mead Johnson

Each tablespoon (15 ml., 3 teaspoons)
contains 30 mg. Peristim® (casanthranol, Mead Johnson) and 60 mg.
COLACE® (dioctyl sodium sulfosuccinate, Mead Johnson).

Contains alcohol 10%.

**PERI-COLACE is also available in 1-
pint bottles of syrup and in bottles
of 30 and 60 capsules.**

Made in U.S.A.   © M. J. & Co.

Mead Johnson
PHARMACEUTICAL DIVISION
Mead Johnson & Company
Evansville, Indiana 47721 U.S.A.

P 7160-04

Ⓟ **PARKE-DAVIS**
People Who Care

N 0071-2214-20
Dilantin-125®
(Phenytoin Oral
Suspension, USP)

125 mg per 5 mL potency

Important—Another strength available;
verify unspecified prescriptions.

Caution—Federal law prohibits
dispensing without prescription.

**IMPORTANT—SHAKE WELL
BEFORE EACH USE**

8 fl oz (237 mL)

BERLEX

NDC 50419-121-16

473 ml

Each 15ml
(tablespoonful)
contains 80mg
anhydrous
theophylline.
Alcohol 20%.

Elixophyllin®
(theophylline)

Store at controlled
room temperature.
Dispense in
tight container.

Dosage: Should be
individualized.
See package insert.

Elixir
80mg/15ml

Caution: Federal law prohibits
dispensing without prescription.

45154-1

BERLEX
Laboratories, Inc.
Wayne, NJ 07470

Use the labels provided to calculate the following IM/s.c. dosages. Calculate to hundredths.

PART II

13. Prepare a 20 mg dosage of meperidine. _____

14. A dosage of morphine 10 mg has been ordered. _____

15. Prepare a 0.1 mg dosage of atropine. _____

16. Draw up a 100 mg dosage of clindamycin. _____

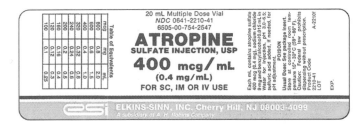

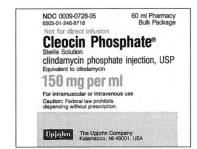

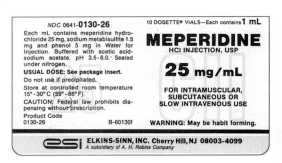

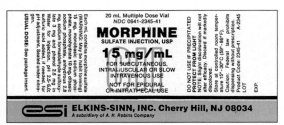

PART III

17. Prepare a 40 mg dosage of meperidine. _____

18. Draw up a 75 mg dosage of kanamycin. _____

19. A dosage of Garamycin® 15 mg has been ordered. _____

20. Prepare a 6 mg dosage of morphine. _____

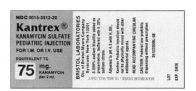

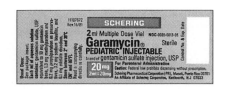

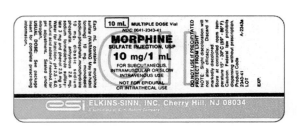

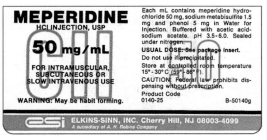

ANSWERS 1. 5 mL, suspension 2. 2.5 mL, suspension 3. 2 cc 4. 7.5 mL 5. 5 mL 6. 7.5 mL 7. 2.5 mL, suspension 8. 10 mL, suspension 9. 15 mL 10. 7.5 mL, suspension 11. 1.2 mL 12. 5 mL 13. 0.8 mL 14. 0.67 mL 15. 0.25 mL 16. 0.67 mL 17. 0.8 mL 18. 2 mL 19. 1.5 mL 20. 0.6 mL

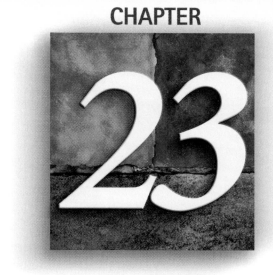

CHAPTER 23

Pediatric Intravenous Medications

Pediatric IV medication administration involves a challenge and a responsibility that is multi-faceted. Infants and children, particularly under the age of four, are incompletely developed physiologically and drug tolerance, absorption and excretion are ongoing concerns. In addition infants and acutely ill children can tolerate only a narrow range of hydration, making administration of IV drugs, which are diluted for administration, a critical and exact skill. Drug dilution protocols may specify a range for dilution, and on many occasions the smallest possible volume may have to be used in order not to overhydrate a child. Dosage and dilution decisions may have to be made on a day to day or even dose to dose basis, and will involve the team effort of nurse, physician and pharmacist. In addition the suitability of any flow rate calculated for administration must be made on an individual basis. For example a calculated flow rate of 100 gtt/min for a 2 year old child is too high a rate to administer.

The fragility of infants' and children's veins, and the irritating nature of many medications, mandates careful site inspection for signs of inflammation and infiltration. This should be done immediately before, during, and after each infusion. Signs of inflammation would include redness, heat, swelling, and tenderness. Signs of infiltration include swelling, coldness, pain, and lack of blood return. Either complication necessitates discontinuance of the IV and a restart at a new site.

IV Medication Guidelines or Protocols are always used to determine drug dosages, dilutions, and administration rates. In this chapter, all examples and problems are representative of actual protocols.

Let's start by looking at the different methods of IV medication administration.

Methods of IV Medication Administration

Intravenous medications may be administered over a period of several hours, for example aminophylline; or on an **intermittent** basis involving several dosages in a 24 hour period, for example antibiotics. When ordered to infuse over several hours medications are usually added to an IV solution bag. Adding the drug to the IV bag may be a hospital pharmacy or staff nurse responsibility, but in any event it is not a complicated procedure. The steps for adding the drug to the solution are as follows:

STEP 1: Locate the type and volume of IV solution ordered.

STEP 2: Measure the dosage of drug to be added.

STEP 3: Use strict aseptic technique to add the drug to the solution bag through the medication port.

OBJECTIVES

The student will
1. list the steps in preparing and administering IV medications from a solution bag/bottle
2. list the steps in preparing and administering IV medications using a calibrated burette
3. explain why a flush is included in IV medication administration
4. calculate flow rates for administration of pediatric IV medications
5. use normal daily and hourly dosage ranges to calculate and assess dosages ordered

PREREQUISITES

Chapters 15, 16, 17, and 18

STEP 4:   Mix the drug thoroughly in the solution.

STEP 5:   Label the IV solution bag with the name and dosage of the drug added.

STEP 6:   Add your initials with the time and date you added the drug.

STEP 7:   Hang the IV and set the flow rate for the infusion. Chart the administration when it has completed.

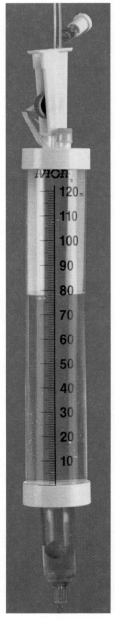

Figure 105

For intermittent administrations the medication may also be prepared in small volume solution bags, or using a **calibrated burette**, such as the one illustrated in Figure 105. Because the total capacity of burettes is between 100 to 150 mL, calibrated in 1 mL increments, exact measurement of small volumes is possible.

Regardless of the method of intermittent administration, the medication infusion is **routinely followed by a flush**, to make sure the medication has cleared the tubing, and that the total dosage has been administered. The volume of the flush will vary depending on the length of IV tubing from the medication source, i.e. burette or syringe, to the infusion site. If a primary line exists, the medication may be administered IVPB (IV piggyback) via a secondary line. If no IV is infusing, a saline or heparin lock (heplock) is frequently in place and used for intermittent administration.

When IV medications are diluted for administration it is necessary to determine hospital policy on **inclusion of the medication volume as part of the volume specified for dilution**. For example if 20 mg has a volume of 2 mL, and it is to be diluted in 30 mL, does this mean you must add 28 mL of diluent to the burette, or 30 mL?

Hospital policies may vary, but in all examples and problems in this chapter **the drug volume will be treated as part of the total diluent volume**. The sequencing of medication and flush administration covered next for burette use is also representative of the procedure which might be followed for IVPB administrations.

Medication Administration via Burette

When a burette is used for medication administration the entire preparation is usually done by staff nurses. Electronic controllers and pumps are used extensively to administer intermittent IV medications to infants and children. When these are used the alarm will sound each time the burette empties to signal when each successive step is necessary. For example it will alarm when the medication has infused and the flush must be started, and again when the flush is completed.

Let's look at some sample orders and go step-by-step through one procedure which may be used.

EXAMPLE 1

A dosage of 250 mg in **15 mL** D5 1/2NS is to be infused over **30 minutes**. It is to be followed with a 5 mL D5 1/2NS flush. An infusion **controller** will be used, and the tubing is a **microdrip** burette.

STEP 1:   Read the drug label and determine what volume the 250 mg dosage is contained in. Let's assume this is 1 mL.

STEP 2:   The dilution is to be 15 mL. Run a total of 14 mL D5 1/2NS into the burette, then add the 1 mL containing the dosage of 250 mg. This gives the ordered volume of 15 mL. Roll the burette between your hands to mix the drug thoroughly with the solution.

STEP 3:   Calculate the flow rate for this microdrip.

Total volume = **15 mL**   Infusion time = **30 min**

Use ratio and proportion to calculate mL/hr rate

$$15 \text{ mL} : 30 \text{ min} = X \text{ mL} : 60 \text{ min} \quad \text{or} \quad \frac{15 \text{ mL}}{30 \text{ min}} = \frac{X \text{ mL}}{60 \text{ min}}$$
$$30X = 60 \times 15 \qquad\qquad\qquad$$
$$X = \textbf{30 mL/hr} \qquad\qquad X = \textbf{30 mL/hr}$$

STEP 4:   Set the controller to infuse 30mL/hr.

STEP 5:   Label the burette to identify the drug and dosage added. Attach a label which states "medication infusing." This makes it possible for others to know the status of the administration if you are not present when the infusion is complete and the controller alarms.

STEP 6:   When the medication has infused add the 5 mL D5 1/2NS flush. Remove the "medication infusing" label and attach a "flush infusing" label. Continue to infuse at 30 mL/hr rate until the burette empties for the second time.

STEP 7:   When the flush has been completed restart the primary IV, or disconnect from the saline/heparin lock. Remove the "flush infusing" label. Chart the dosage and time.

EXAMPLE 2

An antibiotic dosage of **125 mg in 1 mL** is to be **diluted in 20 mL** D5 1/4NS and infused over **30 min**. A **flush of 15 mL** D5 1/4NS is to follow. A **volumetric pump** will be used.

STEP 1:   125 mg has a volume of 1 mL. Add 19 mL of D5 1/4NS to the burette, add the 1 mL of medication and mix thoroughly.

STEP 2:   Calculate the mL/hr flow rate.

Total volume = **20 mL**   Infusion time = **30 min**

$$20 \text{ mL} : 30 \text{ min} = X \text{ mL} : 60 \text{ min} \quad \text{or} \quad \frac{20 \text{ mL}}{30 \text{ min}} = \frac{X \text{ mL}}{60 \text{ min}}$$
$$30X = 60 \times 20 \qquad\qquad\qquad$$
$$X = \textbf{40 mL/hr} \qquad\qquad X = \textbf{40 mL/hr}$$

STEP 3:   Set the pump to infuse 40 mL/hr.

STEP 4: Label the burette with the drug and dosage, and attach a "medication infusing" label.

STEP 5: When the medication has infused start the 15 mL flush. Remove the "medication infusing" label and add the "flush infusing" label.

STEP 6: When the flush has completed restart the primary IV or disconnect from the saline lock. Remove the "flush infusing" label. Chart the dosage and time.

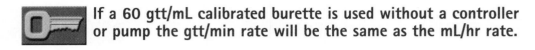 If a 60 gtt/mL calibrated burette is used without a controller or pump the gtt/min rate will be the same as the mL/hr rate.

EXAMPLE 3

An antibiotic dosage of **50 mg** has been ordered diluted in **20 mL** of D5W to infuse over **20 min**. A **15 mL flush** of D5W is to follow. A **microdrip** will be used, but an infusion control device will not be used.

STEP 1: Read the medication label to determine what volume contains 50 mg. You determine that 50 mg is contained in 2 mL.

STEP 2: Run 18 mL of D5W into the burette and add the 2 mL containing 50 mg of drug. Roll between hands to mix thoroughly.

STEP 3: Calculate the flow rate in gtt/min necessary to deliver the medication.

Total volume = **20 mL**   Infusion time = **20 min**

20 mL : 20 min = X mL : 60 min   or $\frac{20 \text{ mL}}{20 \text{ min}} = \frac{X \text{ mL}}{60 \text{ min}}$
20X = 20 × 60
X = **60 mL/hr**   X = **60 mL/hr**

STEP 4: The mL/hr and gtt/min rate is identical for a microdrip. Set the rate at 60 gtt/min.

STEP 5: Label the burette with drug name and dosage, and "medication infusing" label.

STEP 6: When the medication has cleared the burette, add the 15 mL of D5W flush. Continue to run at 60 gtt/min. Remove the "medication infusing" label and replace with a "flush infusing" label.

STEP 7: When the burette empties for the second time, restart the primary IV, or disconnect from the saline lock. Remove the "flush infusing" label. Chart the dosage and time administered.

EXAMPLE 4

An IV medication dosage of 100 mcg has been ordered diluted in **35 mL** NS, and infused in **50 min**. A **10 mL** flush is to follow. A **microdrip** burette will be used.

STEP 1: Read the medication label to determine what volume contains 100 mcg: 100 mcg = 1.5 mL.

STEP 2: Run 33.5 mL of NS into the burette, and add the 1.5 mL of medication. Roll the burette between your hands to mix thoroughly.

STEP 3: Calculate the gtt/min flow rate.

Total volume = **35 mL**   Infusion time = **50 min**

$$35 \text{ mL} : 50 \text{ min} = X \text{ mL} : 60 \text{ min} \quad\quad \text{or} \quad\quad \frac{35 \text{ mL}}{50 \text{ min}} = \frac{X \text{ mL}}{60 \text{ min}}$$
$$50X = 35 \times 60 \quad\quad\quad\quad\quad\quad\quad\quad\quad\quad$$
$$X = \textbf{42 mL/hr} \quad\quad\quad\quad\quad\quad\quad\quad X = \textbf{42 mL/hr}$$
$$= \textbf{42 gtt/min} \quad\quad\quad\quad\quad\quad\quad\quad = \textbf{42 gtt/min}$$

STEP 4: Set the flow rate at 42 gtt/min.

STEP 5: Label the burette with drug name and dosage, and "medication infusing" label.

STEP 6: When the medication has cleared the burette, add the 10 mL flush. Continue to run at 42 gtt/min. Replace the "medication infusing" label with the "flush infusing" label.

STEP 7: When the burette empties of the flush solution, restart the primary IV, or disconnect from the saline lock. Remove the "flush infusing" label, and chart the dosage and time administered.

PROBLEM

Determine the volume of solution which must be added to the burette to mix the following IV drugs. Then calculate the flow rate in gtt/min for each administration using a microdrip, and indicate the mL/hr setting for a controller.

1. An IV medication of 75 mg in 3 mL is ordered diluted to 55 mL to infuse over 45 min.

   Dilution volume _____ gtt/min _____ mL/hr _____

2. A dosage of 100 mg in 2 mL is diluted to 30 mL D5W to infuse in 20 min.

   Dilution volume _____ gtt/min _____ mL/hr _____

3. The volume of a 10 mg dosage of medication is 1 cc. Dilute to 40 mL and administer over 50 min.

   Dilution volume _____ gtt/min _____ mL/hr _____

4. A dosage of 15 mg with a volume of 3 mL is to be diluted to 70 mL and administered in 50 min.

   Dilution volume _____ gtt/min _____ mL/hr _____

5. A medication of 1 g in 4 mL is to be diluted to 60 mL and infused over 90 min.

   Dilution volume _____ gtt/min _____ mL/hr _____

ANSWERS 1. 52 mL; 73 gtt/min; 73 mL/hr   2. 28 mL; 90 gtt/min; 90 mL/hr   3. 39 mL; 48 gtt/min; 48 mL/hr   4. 67 mL; 84 gtt/min; 84 mL/hr   5. 56 mL; 40 gtt/min; 40 mL/hr

Comparing IV Dosages Ordered with Protocols

Knowing how to compare dosages ordered with the dosage protocols for a particular medication is a nursing responsibility.

 Dosages of IV medications are calculated on the basis of body weight, or BSA.

Protocols may list dosages in terms of mg, mcg, or U per day, or per hour. BSA in m^2 is most often used to calculate chemotherapeutic drugs, which are administered only by certified nursing staff. The following examples will demonstrate how to use protocols to check dosages ordered.

EXAMPLE 1

A child weighing **22.6 kg** has an order for **500 mg** of medication in 100 mL D5W **q.12.h.** The normal dosage range is **40–50 mg/kg/day**. Determine if the dosage ordered is within the normal range.

STEP 1:   **Calculate the normal daily dosage range for this child.**

40 mg/day × 22.6 kg = **904 mg**
50 mg/day × 22.6 kg = **1130 mg**

STEP 2:   **Calculate the dosage infusing in 24 hr.**

500 mg in 12 hr = **1000 mg in 24 hr**

STEP 3:   **Assess the accuracy of the dosage ordered.**

The 500 mg in 12 hr is within the 904-1130 mg/day dosage range.

EXAMPLE 2

A child with a body weight of **18.4 kg** is to receive a medication with a dosage range of **100–150 mg/kg/day**. The order is for **600 mg** in 75 mL D5W **q.6.h.** Determine if the dosage is within normal range.

STEP 1:   **Calculate the normal daily dosage range.**

100 mg/kg × 18.4 kg = **1840 mg/day**
150 mg/kg × 18.4 kg = **2760 mg/day**

STEP 2:   **Calculate the daily dosage ordered.**

The dosage ordered is 600 mg q.6.h. (4 doses).
600 mg × 4 = **2400 mg/day**

STEP 3:   **Assess the accuracy of the dosage ordered.**

The dosage ordered, 2400 mg/day, is within the normal range of 1840–2760 mg/day.

EXAMPLE 3

A child weighing **17.7 kg** is receiving an IV of **250 mL** D5W containing **2000 U** heparin, which is to infuse at **50 mL/hr**. The dosage range of heparin is **10–25 U/kg/hr**. Assess the accuracy of this dosage.

STEP 1:   Calculate the normal dosage range per hour.

10 U/kg/hr $\times$ 17.7 kg = **177 U/hr**
25 U/kg/hr $\times$ 17.7 kg = **442.5 U/hr**

STEP 2:   Calculate the dosage infusing per hour.

2000 U : 250 mL = X U : 50 mL   or $\dfrac{2000\ U}{250\ mL} = \dfrac{X\ U}{50\ mL}$
250X = 2000 $\times$ 50   250 mL   50 mL
X = **400 U/hr**   X = **400 U/hr**

STEP 3:   Access the accuracy of the dosage ordered.

The IV is infusing at a rate of 50 mL per hour, which is 400 U/hr. The normal dosage range is 177–442.5 U/hr. The dosage is within normal range.

EXAMPLE 4

A child weighing **32.7 kg** has an IV of **250 mL** D5 1/4S containing **400 mcg** of medication to infuse over **5 hours**. The normal range for this drug is **1–3 mcg/kg/hr**. Determine if this dosage is within the normal dosage range.

STEP 1:   Calculate the hourly dosage range.

1 mcg/kg/hr $\times$ 32.7 kg = **32.7 mcg/hr**
3 mcg/kg/hr $\times$ 32.7 kg = **98.1 mcg/hr**

STEP 2:   Calculate the dosage infusing per hour.

400 mcg $\div$ 5 hr = **80 mcg/hr**

STEP 3:   Access the accuracy of the dosage ordered.

The dosage of 80 mcg/hr infusing is within the normal range of 32.7–98.1 mcg/hr.

PROBLEM

Calculate the normal dosage range to the nearest tenth, and the dosage being administered for the following medications. Assess the dosages ordered.

1. A child weighing 24.4 kg has an IV of 250 mL D5W containing 2500 U of a drug. The dosage range for this drug is 15–25 U/kg/hr. The infusion controller is set to deliver 50 mL/hr.

   Dosage range per hr _____   Dosage infusing per hr _____

   Assessment _____

2. A solution of D5W containing 25 mg of a drug is to infuse in 30 min. The dosage range is 4–8 mg/kg/day, q.6.h. The child weighs 18.7 kg.   Dosage range per day _____

   Daily dosage ordered _____   Assessment _____

3. An IV solution containing 125 mg of medication is infusing. The dosage range is 5–10 mg/kg/dose, and the child weighs 14.2 kg.

   Dosage range per dose _____   Assessment _____

4. A child weighing 14.3 kg is to receive an IV drug with a dosage range of 50–100 mcg/kg/day in two divided doses. An infusion of 50 mL D5W containing 400 mcg to run 30 min has been ordered. Daily dosage range _____

   Daily dosage ordered _____ Assessment _____

5. A dosage of 4 mg (4000 mcg) of drug in 500 mL of D5 1/2S is to infuse over 4 hours. The dosage range of the drug is 24–120 mcg/kg/hr, and the child weighs 16.1 kg.

   Dosage range per hr _____ Dosage infusing per hr _____

   Assessment _____

6. A child weighing 20.9 kg is to receive a medication with a normal dosage range of 80–160 mg/kg/day, in divided doses q.6.h. The IV ordered contains 500 mg.

   Dosage range per day _____ Daily dosage ordered _____

   Assessment _____

7. A child weighing 22.3 kg is to receive 750 mL of D5 1/4S containing 6 g of a drug, which is to run over 24 hours. The dosage range of the drug is 200–300 mg/kg/day.

   Dosage range per day _____ Assessment _____

8. An IV of 50 mL D5W containing 55 mcg of a drug is infusing over a 30 min period. The child weighs 14.9 kg and the dosage range is 6–8 mcg/kg/day, q.12.h. Dosage range per day _____

   Daily dosage ordered _____ Assessment _____

9. A child weighing 27.1 kg is to receive a medication with a normal range of 0.5–1 mg/kg/dose. An IV containing 20 mg of medication has been ordered.

   Dosage per dose _____ Assessment _____

10. An IV medication of 60 mcg in 200 mL is ordered to infuse over 2 hr. The normal dosage range is 1.5–3 mcg/kg/hr. The child weighs 16.7 kg. Dosage range per hr _____

   Dosage infusing per hr _____ Assessment _____

ANSWERS 1. 366–610 U/hr; 500 U/hr; normal range 2. 74.8–149.6 mg/day; 100 mg/day; normal range 3. 71–142 mg/dose; normal range 4. 715–1430 mcg/day; 800 mg; normal range 5. 386.4–1932 mcg/hr; 1000 mcg; normal range 6. 1672–3344 mg/day; 2000 mg; normal range 7. 4460–6690 mg/day; normal range 8. 89.4–119.2 mcg/day; 110 mcg; normal range 9. 13.6–27.1 mg/dose; normal range 10. 25.1–50.1 mcg/hr; 30 mcg; normal range

Summary

This concludes the chapter on administration of IV drugs to infants and children. The important points to remember from this chapter are:

➡ IV medications may be ordered to infuse over a period of several hours, or minutes

➡ IV medications are diluted for administration, and it is important to determine hospital policy on inclusion of the medication volume as part of the total dilution volume

➡ a flush is used following medication administration to make sure the medication has cleared the tubing and the total dosage has been administered

➡ the volume of flush solution on intermittent infusions will vary depending on the amount needed to clear the infusion line

➡ drug protocols are used to calculate normal dosage ranges, and to assess dosages ordered

➡ pediatric IV medication administration requires constant assessment of the child's ability to tolerate dosage, dilution and rate of administration

➡ children's veins are very fragile, and intravenous sites must be checked for inflammation and infiltration immediately before, during and following each medication administration

Summary Self Test

DIRECTIONS

Determine the volume of solution which must be added to a calibrated burette to mix the following IV drugs. The medication volume is included in the total dilution volume. Calculate the flow rate in gtt/min for each infusion. A microdrip with a calibration of 60 gtt/mL is used.

	Volume of diluent	gtt/min rate
1. An IV antibiotic of 750 mg in 3 mL has been ordered diluted to a total of 25 mL D5W to infuse over 40 minutes.		
2. A dosage of 500,000 U of a penicillin preparation with a volume of 4 mL has been ordered diluted to 50 mL D5 1/2NS to infuse in 60 min.		
3. A dosage of 1.5 g/2 mL of an antibiotic is to be diluted to a total of 40 mL D5W and administered over 40 min.		
4. An antibiotic dosage of 200 mg in 4 mL is to be diluted to 50 mL and administered over 70 min.		
5. A dosage of 20 mg in 2 mL has been ordered diluted to 30 mL, to be infused over 35 min.		
6. A dosage of 25 mg in 5 mL has been ordered diluted to 40 mL and administered in 50 min.		

	Volume of diluent	gtt/min rate

7. A 10 mg in 2 mL dosage has been ordered diluted to 20 mL to infuse over 30 min.   _____ _____

8. A medication dosage of 800 mg in 4 mL is to be diluted to 60 mL and infused over 80 min.   _____ _____

9. A dosage of 0.5 g in 2 mL is to be diluted to 40 mL and run in 30 min.   _____ _____

10. A medication of 1000 mg in 1 mL is to be diluted to 15 mL and administered over 20 min.   _____ _____

DIRECTIONS

The following IV drugs are to be administered using a volumetric or syringe pump. Determine the amount of diluent to be added, and the flow rate in mL/hr to set the pumps.

	Volume of diluent	mL/hr rate

11. A dosage of 40 mg in 4 mL is to be diluted to 50 mL and administered in 90 min.   _____ _____

12. A 2 g in 5 mL dosage has been ordered diluted to a total of 90 mL and administered in 45 min.   _____ _____

13. An 80 mg dosage with a volume of 2 mL is to be diluted to 80 mL and administered in 60 min.   _____ _____

14. A 60 mg dosage with a volume of 4 mL is ordered diluted to 30 mL and run over 20 min.   _____ _____

15. A 5 mg per 2 mL dosage is to be diluted to 80 mL and administered in 50 min.   _____ _____

16. The dosage ordered is 0.75 g in 3 mL to be diluted to 30 mL. Run in over 40 min.   _____ _____

17. A medication of 100 mg in 2 mL is ordered diluted to 30 mL and run in 25 min.   _____ _____

18. The dosage ordered is 100 mg in 1 mL to be diluted to 50 mL. Run in over 45 min.   _____ _____

19. A 30 mg dosage in 1 mL has been ordered diluted to 10 mL to infuse in 10 min.   _____ _____

20. A dosage of 250 mg in 5 mL has been ordered diluted to 40 mL and infused in 60 min.   _____ _____

DIRECTIONS

Calculate the normal dosage range to the nearest tenth, and the dosage being administered for the following medications. Assess the dosages ordered.

21. A child weighing 15.4 kg is to receive a dosage with a range of 5–7.5 mg/kg/dose. The solution bag is labeled 100 mg.

Dosage range _____ Assessment _____

22. The order is for 200 U in 75 mL. The child weighs 13.1 kg and the dosage range is 15–20 U/kg per dose.

Dosage range _____ Assessment _____

23. A dosage of 1.5 mg in 20 mL has been ordered. The normal dosage
range is 0.1–0.3 mg/kg/day in 2 divided doses. The child's weight
is 12.4 kg.　　　　　　　　　　　Dosage range per day ＿＿＿＿＿＿

　　　　Daily dosage ordered ＿＿＿＿＿＿　Assessment ＿＿＿＿＿＿

24. A dosage of 400 mg in 75 mL of medication is to be infused q.8.h.
The normal range is 15–45 mg/kg/day, and the child weighs 27.9 kg.

　　　Dosage range per day ＿＿＿＿＿＿　Daily dosage ordered ＿＿＿＿＿＿

　　　　　　　　　　　　　　　　　　Assessment ＿＿＿＿＿＿

25. A child weighing 15.7 kg is to receive a medication with a normal
hourly range of 3–7 mcg/kg. A 250 mL solution bag containing
350 mcg is infusing at a rate of 50 mL/hr.　　Dosage range per hr ＿＿＿＿＿＿

　　　　Dosage infusing per hour ＿＿＿＿＿＿　Assessment ＿＿＿＿＿＿

26. A child weighing 19.6 kg is to receive a medication with a normal dosage
range of 60–80 mg/kg/day. A 90 mL infusion containing 375 mg has
been ordered q.6.h.　　　　　　　　Dosage range per day ＿＿＿＿＿＿

　　　　Daily dosage ordered ＿＿＿＿＿＿　Assessment ＿＿＿＿＿＿

27. Two infusions of 250 mL each containing 300 mg of medication are
to infuse continuously over a 24 hr period (250 mL q.12.h.). The child
receiving the infusion weighs 11.7 kg, and the normal dosage range
of the drug is 50–100 mg/kg/day.　　　Dosage range per day ＿＿＿＿＿＿

　　　　Daily dosage ordered ＿＿＿＿＿＿　Assessment ＿＿＿＿＿＿

28. The order is for 100 mL D5W containing 150 mg of medication
to infuse q.8.h. The normal dosage range is 3–12 mg/kg/day,
and the child weighs 40.1 kg.　　　　Dosage range per day ＿＿＿＿＿＿

　　　　Daily dosage ordered ＿＿＿＿＿＿　Assessment ＿＿＿＿＿＿

29. A child has an infusion of 250 mL containing 500 U of medication to
run at 50 mL/hr. The normal dosage range is 10–25 U/hr. The child
weighs 10.3 kg.　　　　　　　　　Dosage range per hour ＿＿＿＿＿＿

　　　　Dosage infusing per hour ＿＿＿＿＿＿　Assessment ＿＿＿＿＿＿

30. The normal dosage range of a drug is 0.5–1.5 U/hr. A child weighing
10.7 kg has a 150 mL volume of solution containing 45 U infusing at
a rate of 20 mL/hr.　　　　　　　Normal dosage range per hr ＿＿＿＿＿＿

　　　　Dosage infusing per hour ＿＿＿＿＿＿　Assessment ＿＿＿＿＿＿

31. A child weighing 12.5 kg is receiving an IV of 2500 U heparin in
250 mL D5W at 40 mL/hr. The normal dosage range for heparin
is 10–25 U/kg/hr.　　　　　　　　Normal dosage range per hour ＿＿＿＿＿＿

　　　　Dosage infusing per hour ＿＿＿＿＿＿　Assessment ＿＿＿＿＿＿

32. A child with a weight of 10 kg is to receive a medication with a normal
dosage range of 60–80 mg/kg/day. The order is for 200 mg q.6.h.

　　　　　　　　　　　　Normal dosage range per day ＿＿＿＿＿＿

　　　　Daily dosage ordered ＿＿＿＿＿＿　Assessment ＿＿＿＿＿＿

33. Order: 0.5 g naficillin in 100 mL D5W q.6.h. Normal dosage range is 100–200 mg/kg/day. Child weighs 15 kg.

Normal dosage range per day _____

Daily dosage ordered _____ Assessment _____

34. A continuous IV of 500 mL with 20 mEq KCl is infusing at 30 mL/hr. The dosage for potassium chloride is not to exceed 40 mEq/day. Dosage infusing per hour _____

Dosage infusing per day _____ Assessment _____

35. A 24 kg child is receiving 116 mg per hr of rifampin IV for 3 hours. Dosage range for this drug is 10–20 mg/kg/day.

Normal dosage range per day _____

Dosage received after 3 hours _____ Assessment _____

36. A 25% solution of serum Albumin is infusing at 15 mL/hr for a total of 6 hours. Normal dosage for children is 5–25 g/day.

Grams infused after 6 hr _____ Assessment _____

37. The usual dosage of chloramphenicol for children is 50 mg/kg/24 hr in equally divided doses. Order: infuse 50 mL with 290 mg chloramphenicol q.6.h. The child weighs 51 lbs.

Normal dosage per day _____ Daily dosage ordered _____

Assessment _____

38. Order: 500 mL D5RL with 30 mEq KCl to infuse at 40 mL/hr. A maximum of 10 mEq/hr of KCl should not be exceeded and the total 24 hr dosage should not exceed 40 mEq/day.

Dosage infusing per hr _____ Dosage infusing per day _____

Assessment _____

39. A child weighing 30 kg has an IV of 100 mL D5W containing 600 mcg of medication to infuse over 2 hours. The normal range for this drug is 2–4 mcg/kg/hr. Normal dosage range per hour _____

Dosage infusing per hour _____ Assessment _____

40. 150 mL with 18 mg of medication is ordered to infuse over 10 hours. The normal range for this drug is 0.2 mg–0.6 mg/kg/hr. Child weighs 9 kg. Normal dosage range per hr _____

Dosage infusing per hour _____ Assessment _____

ANSWERS   1. 22 mL; 38 gtt/min   2. 46 mL; 50 gtt/min   3. 38 mL; 60 gtt/min   4. 46 mL; 43 gtt/min   5. 28 mL; 51 gtt/min   6. 35 mL; 48 gtt/min   7. 18 mL; 40 gtt/min   8. 56 mL; 45 gtt/min   9. 38 mL; 80 gtt/min   10. 14 mL; 45 gtt/min   11. 46 mL; 33 mL/hr   12. 85 mL; 120 mL/hr   13. 78 mL; 80 mL/hr   14. 26 mL; 90 mL/hr   15. 78 mL; 96 mL/hr   16. 27 mL; 45 mL/hr   17. 28 mL; 72 mL/hr   18. 49 mL; 67 mL/hr   19. 9 mL; 60 mL/hr   20. 35 mL; 40 mL/hr   21. 77–115.5 mg/dose; normal   22. 196.5–262 U/dose; normal   23. 1.2–3.7 mg/day; 3 mg; normal   24. 418.5–1255.5 mg/day; 1200 mg; normal   25. 47.1–109.9 mcg/hr; 70 mcg; normal   26. 1176–1568 mg/day; 1500 mg; normal   27. 585–1170 mg/day; 600 mg; normal   28. 120.3–481.2 mg/day; 450 mg; normal   29. 103–257.5 U/hr; 100 U/hr; normal   30. 5.4–16.1 U/hr; 6 U/hr; normal   31. 125–312.5 U/hr; 400 U/hr; too high   32. 600–800 mg/day; 800 mg; normal   33. 1500–3000 mg/day; 2000 mg; normal   34. 1.2 mEq/hr; 28.8 mEq/day; normal   35. 240–480 mg/day; 348 mg; normal   36. 22.5 g/6 hr; normal   37. 1160 mg/day; 1160 mg; normal   38. 2.4 mEq/hr; 58 mEq/day; too high   39. 60–120 mcg/hr; 300 mcg; too high   40. 1.8–5.4 mg/hr; 1.8 mg; normal

INDEX

VACATION HOMES AND LOG CABINS

16 COMPLETE PLANS

Prepared by the
United States Department
of Agriculture

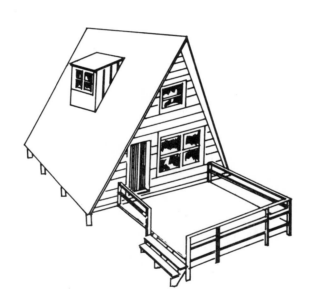

DOVER PUBLICATIONS, INC.
NEW YORK

INTRODUCTION

These sixteen building plans, compiled by the Cooperative Farm Building Plan Exchange, were developed by the cooperative effort of Extension Service (USDA), State Extension Service, State Experiment Stations, Cooperative State Research Service (USDA), and Agricultural Engineering Research Division, Agricultural Research Service (USDA).

The building plans, their purpose, and some of the construction details are shown in the illustrations and are described in the brief text for each plan.

Economy of material and labor has been given particular emphasis. The structures are efficient and useful for the purposes intended.

The buildings range from a 10-foot x 14-foot one-room cabin to much larger buildings with two or more bedrooms that make suitable year-round houses as well as comfortable vacation homes. Several different basic construction techniques (conventional wood-frame, A-frame, pole-frame, concrete masonry, log cabin) are represented.

Published in Canada by General Publishing Company, Ltd., 30 Lesmill Road, Don Mills, Toronto, Ontario.

This Dover edition, first published in 1978, is an abridged and slightly altered republication of portions of Agriculture Handbook No. 438, *Recreational Buildings and Facilities,* published by the Agricultural Research Service of the United States Department of Agriculture in 1972, and of the following complete working drawings published by the Department of Agriculture: Plan Nos. 5184, 5185, 5186, 5928, 5968, 6013, 5964, 5965, 6003, 5506, 5507, 7013, 6002, 6004, 5997, 7010 (various dates).

International Standard Book Number: 0-486-23631-5
Library of Congress Catalog Card Number: 77-99250

Manufactured in the United States of America
Dover Publications, Inc.
180 Varick Street
New York, N.Y. 10014

CONTENTS

1. ONE-ROOM FRAME CABIN

This low-cost, one-room cabin may be set on pressure-treated post foundations to reduce construction costs. Where termites are a problem, the floor can be made of concrete. If wood is used in such areas, joists and sills should be chemically treated.

Barn boards of random widths and half-round battens can be used for the exterior wall covering and can be painted. Other details of construction are shown on the illustrations.

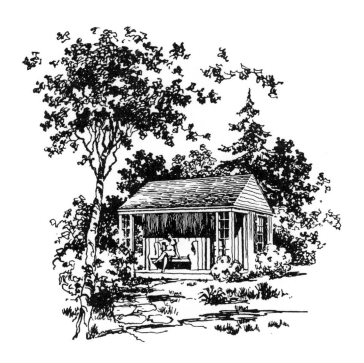

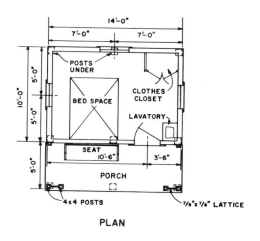

PLAN

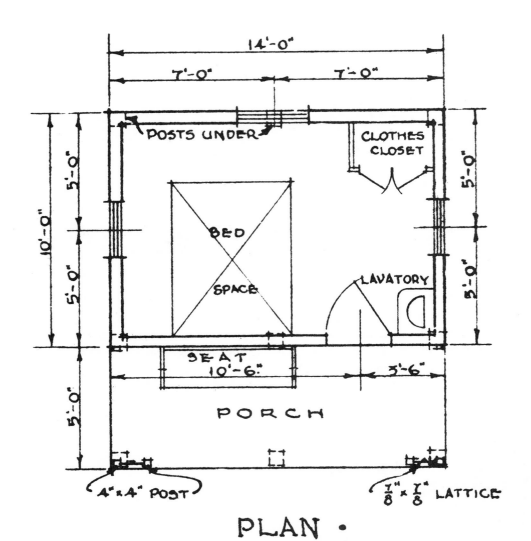

14'-0"

7'-0" · 7'-0"

POSTS UNDER

CLOTHES CLOSET

5'-0" · 5'-0"

10'-0"

5'-0"

BED SPACE

LAVATORY

5'-0"

SEAT 10'-6"

3'-6"

PORCH

5'-0"

4" x 4" POST

$\frac{7"}{8} \times \frac{7"}{8}$ LATTICE

PLAN ·

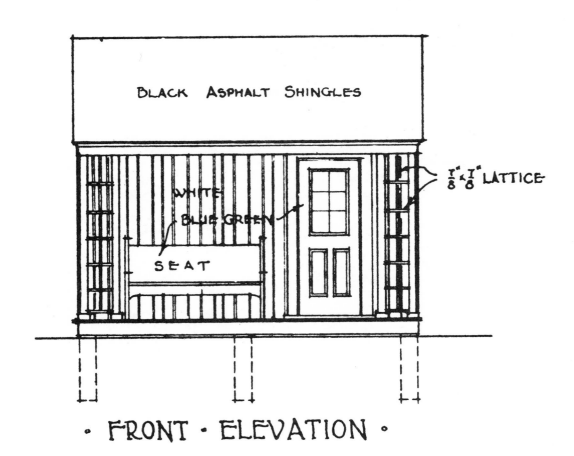

BLACK ASPHALT SHINGLES

WHITE

BLUE GREEN

SEAT

$\frac{7"}{8} \times \frac{7"}{8}$ LATTICE

· FRONT · ELEVATION ·

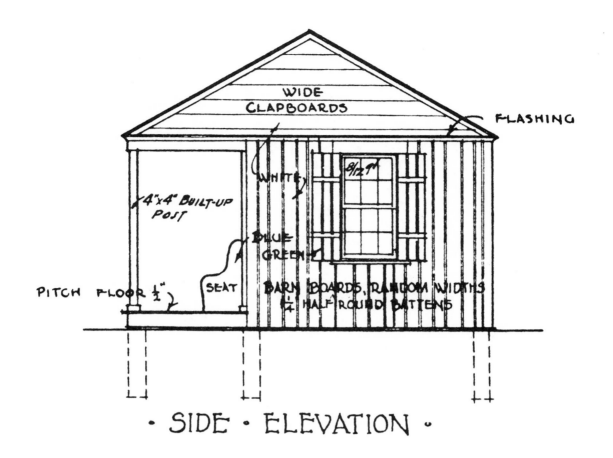

WIDE CLAPBOARDS

FLASHING

WHITE

4"x4" BUILT-UP POST

BLUE GREEN

8/12 T

PITCH FLOOR 1½"

SEAT

BARN BOARDS, RANDOM WIDTHS
1¼" HALF ROUND BATTENS

· SIDE · ELEVATION ·

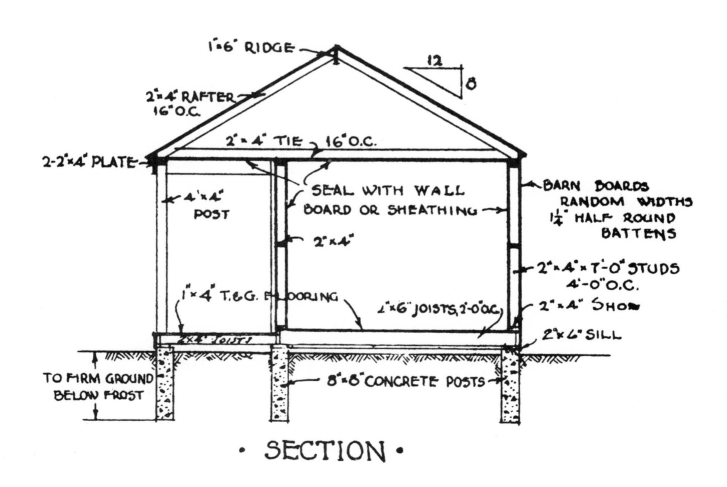

1"x6" RIDGE

12
8

2"x4" RAFTER 16" O.C.

2"x4" TIE 16" O.C.

2-2"x4" PLATE

4"x4" POST

SEAL WITH WALL BOARD OR SHEATHING

2"x4"

BARN BOARDS RANDOM WIDTHS 1¼" HALF ROUND BATTENS

1"x4" T.&G. FLOORING

1"x6" JOISTS, 2'-0" O.C.

2"x4"x7'-0" STUDS 4'-0" O.C.

2"x4" SHOE

2"x4" JOISTS

2"x6" SILL

TO FIRM GROUND BELOW FROST

8"x8" CONCRETE POSTS

· SECTION ·

2. THREE-ROOM FRAME CABIN

This cabin is suitable for camping or could be utilized as a bunkhouse during the harvest season. It could also serve temporarily as living quarters for a family while a permanent farmhouse was being built. The cookstove would furnish heat. In cold climates the cabin should be insulated.

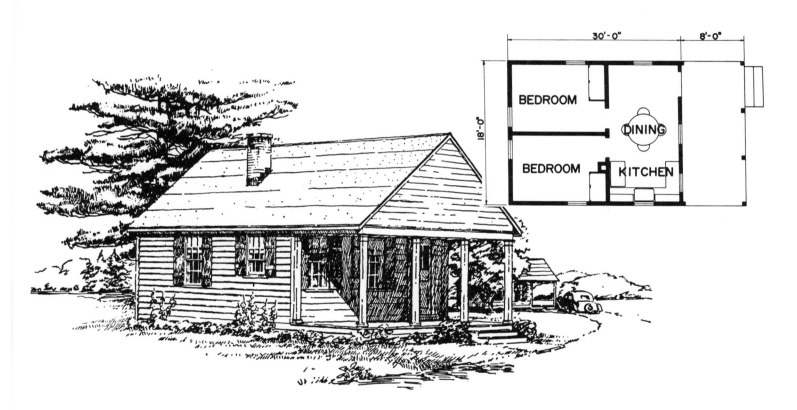

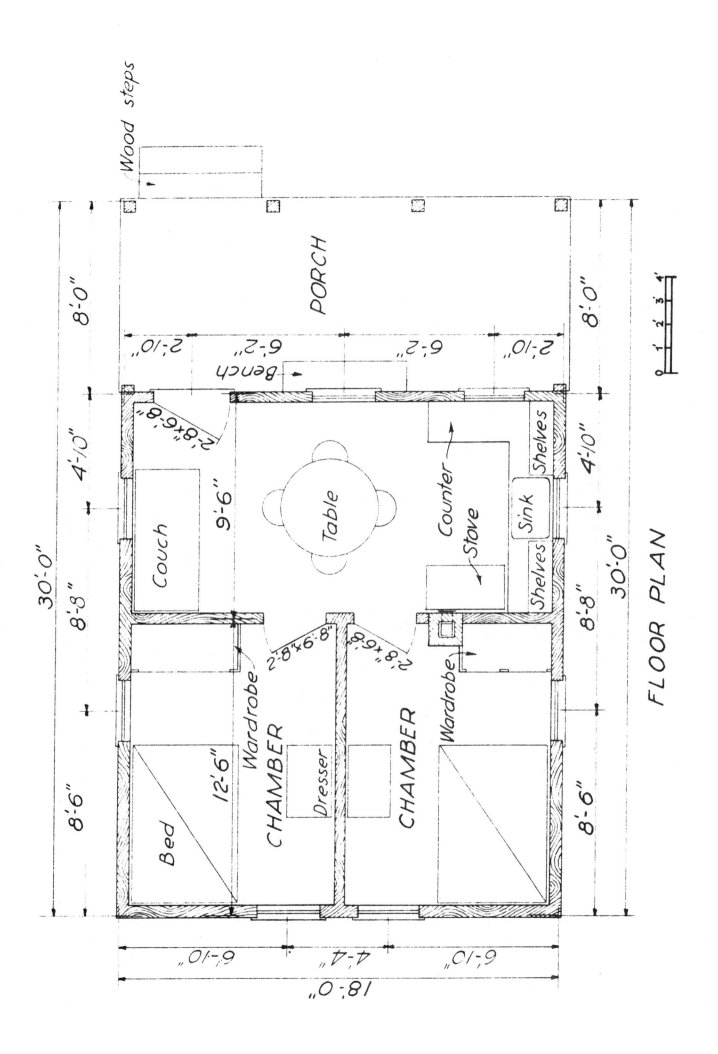

Wood steps

PORCH

Bench

8'-0"   8'-0"

2'-10"   6'-2"   6'-2"   2'-10"

2'-8"×6'-8"

Shelves

Couch

9'-6"

Table

Counter
Stove

Sink

Shelves

30'-0"

4'-0"   8'-8"   8'-8"   4'-0"

30'-0"

Wardrobe

2'-8"×6'-8"   2'-8"×6'-8"

Wardrobe

CHAMBER

Dresser

CHAMBER

8'-6"   12'-6"

8'-6"

Bed

6'-10"   4'-4"   6'-10"

18'-0"

FLOOR PLAN

0 1 2 3 4'

6

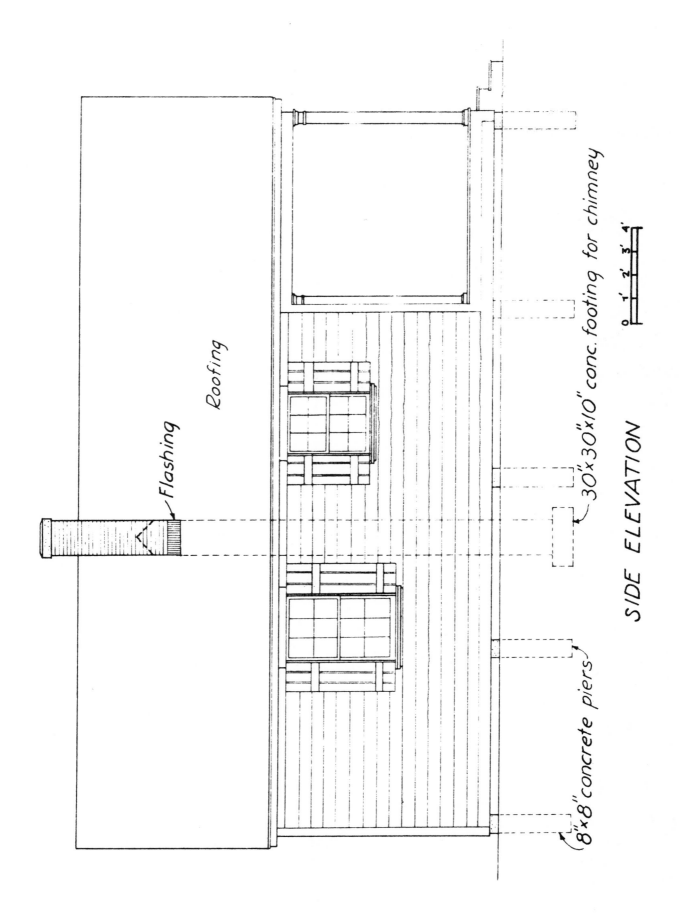

Flashing

Roofing

30"×30"×10" conc. footing for chimney

8"×8" concrete piers

SIDE ELEVATION

0 1' 2' 3' 4'

7

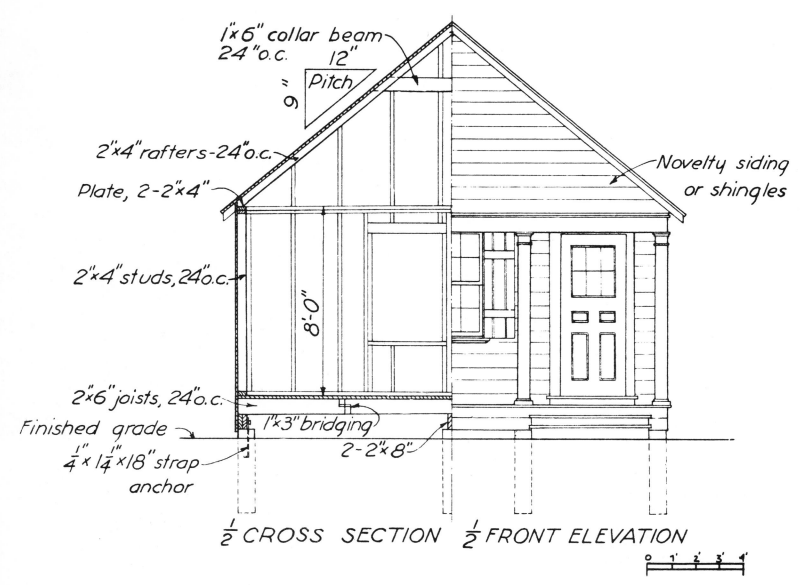

1"x6" collar beam 24" o.c.

Pitch 12" 9"

2"x4" rafters - 24" o.c.

Plate, 2-2"x4"

Novelty siding or shingles

2"x4" studs, 24" o.c.

8'-0"

2"x6" joists, 24" o.c.

Finished grade

$\frac{1}{4}$"x1$\frac{1}{4}$"x18" strap anchor

1"x3" bridging

2-2"x8"

$\frac{1}{2}$ CROSS SECTION $\frac{1}{2}$ FRONT ELEVATION

0 1 2 3 4

BILL OF MATERIALS
CONCRETE - 1:2:4
7 bags cement, $\frac{1}{2}$ cu. yd. sand, 1 cu. yd. gravel, = 1.15 cu. yds. concrete
CHIMNEY
750 brick, 12 lin. ft. 8"x8" flue lining, Mortar = 2 bags lime, 2$\frac{1}{2}$ bags cement, $\frac{1}{2}$ cu. yd. sand.
LUMBER

9 - 2"x8"x16'-0" - girders
7 - 2"x6"x16'-0" - girders & plates
21 - 2"x6"x18'-0" - joists
8 - 2"x6"x12'-0" - plates
36 - 2"x4"x12'-0" - rafters
1 - 2"x10"x8'-0" - step carriage
7 - 1"x6"x14'-0" - collar ties
140 lin. ft. 1"x3" - bridging
875 ft. B.M. 1"x6" - roof sheathing
1050 ft. B.M. 1"x6" - siding
675 ft. B.M. 1"x4" - flooring
760 sq. ft. roof area.
300 sq. ft. wallboard or beaded ceiling (interior partitions)

4 - 6"x6"x7'-0" porch posts
2 - 4"x6"x7'-0" porch pilasters
36 lin. ft. 1"x8" - porch trim
54 lin. ft. 1"x6" - porch trim
350 lin. ft. 1"x4" - trim
36 lin. ft. 2" drip cap moulding
1 double-hung window, 12 lt. 2'-8"x3'-10"
7 double-hung windows, 12 lt. 2'-8"x4'-6"
8 window frames with outside trim and shutters
1 - 2'-8"x6'-8"x1$\frac{3}{4}$" glazed door
1 - door frame with outside trim
2 - 2'-6"x6'-8"x1$\frac{3}{8}$" inside doors

MISCELLANEOUS
16 - $\frac{1}{4}$"x1$\frac{1}{4}$"x18" strap anchors & $\frac{1}{4}$" lag screws
1 - terra-cotta stovepipe thimble
1 - piece sheet metal, 24"x60" - flashing
Hardware, nails, paint, and equipment as selected

3. 14-FOOT × 18-FOOT FRAME CABIN

This economical building provides for Pullman-type berths. If a central heat source is not practical, a chimney should be added to provide for a heater. Space is also provided for a toilet, as shown on the plan.

The sill is steel-strapped to concrete posts that extend below frost line.

Floor joists are framed into the sill and securely anchored with metal fasteners.

Both floor joists and sill should be protected from termite attack.

This building is frame construction with the exterior surface covered with rough-sawn, random-width boards and 1¼-inch, half-round, wood battens.

Interior has tongue-and-groove flooring, with walls and ceiling covered with building board or sheathing.

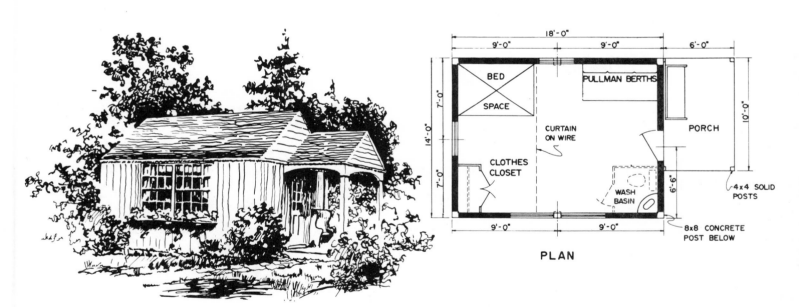

PLAN

9

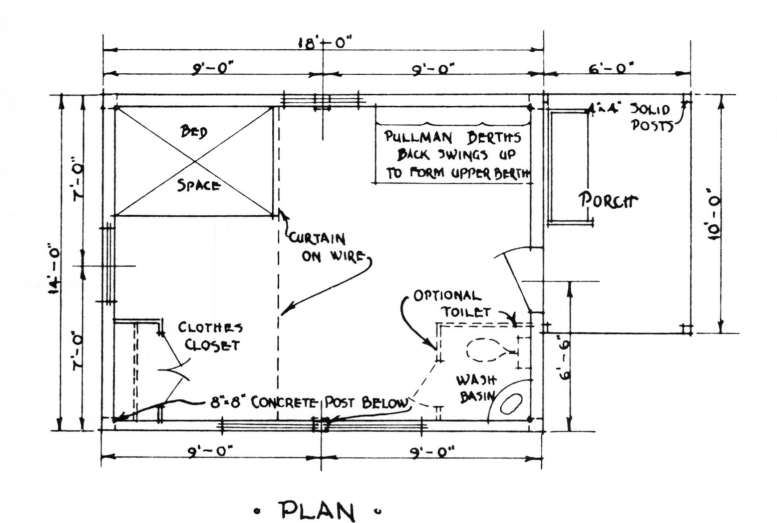

18'-0"

9'-0"   9'-0"   6'-0"

7'-0"

BED
SPACE

PULLMAN BERTHS
BACK SWINGS UP
TO FORM UPPER BERTH

4"x4" SOLID
POSTS

PORCH

14'-0"

10'-0"

CURTAIN
ON WIRE

7'-0"

CLOTHES
CLOSET

OPTIONAL
TOILET

8"x8" CONCRETE POST BELOW

WASH
BASIN

6'-6"

9'-0"   9'-0"

• PLAN •

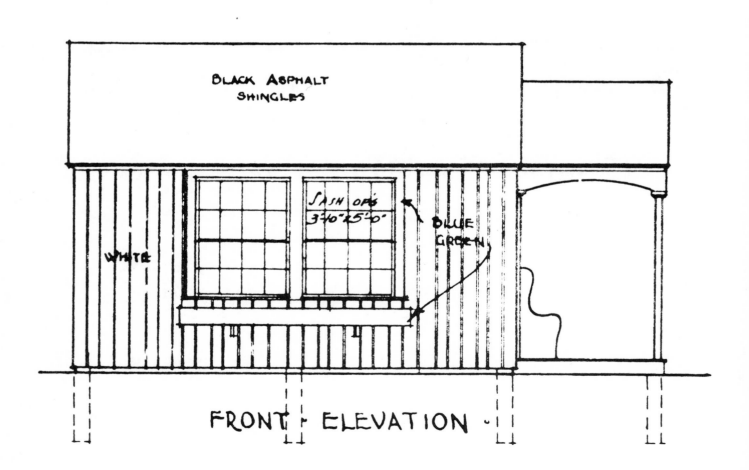

BLACK ASPHALT
SHINGLES

WHITE

SASH OP'G
3'-10"x5'-0"

BLUE
GREEN

• FRONT • ELEVATION •

10

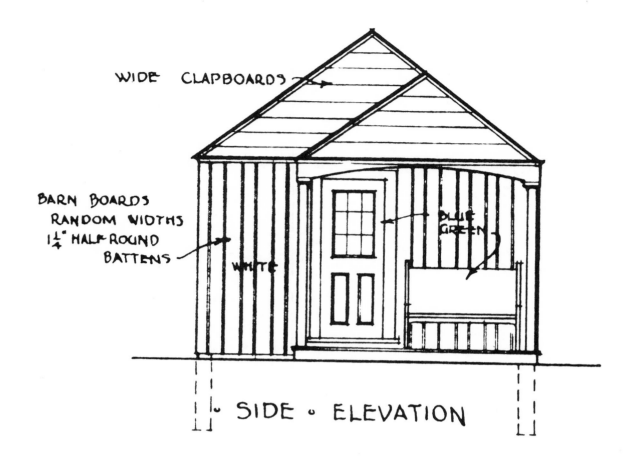

WIDE CLAPBOARDS

BARN BOARDS
RANDOM WIDTHS
1¼" HALF-ROUND
BATTENS

WHITE

BLUE GREEN

· SIDE · ELEVATION

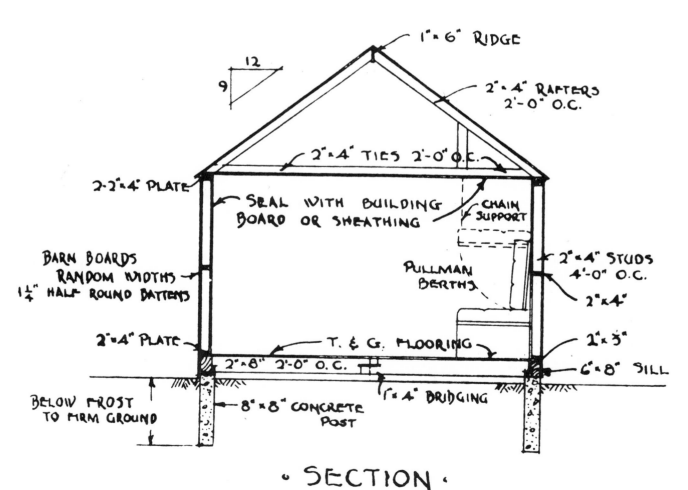

1"× 6" RIDGE

2"× 4" RAFTERS
2'-0" O.C.

2"× 4" TIES 2'-0" O.C.

2-2"×4" PLATE

SEAL WITH BUILDING
BOARD OR SHEATHING

CHAIN
SUPPORT

PULLMAN
BERTHS

2"× 4" STUDS
4'-0" O.C.

2"× 4"

BARN BOARDS
RANDOM WIDTHS
1¼" HALF-ROUND BATTENS

2"× 4" PLATE

T. & G. FLOORING

2"× 3"

2"× 8" 2'-0" O.C.

6"× 8" SILL

BELOW FROST
TO FIRM GROUND

8"× 8" CONCRETE
POST

1"× 4" BRIDGING

· SECTION ·

4. 24-FOOT × 24-FOOT FRAME CABIN

The basic floor plan for this frame cabin is 24 by 24 feet, slab-on-grade construction. The exterior shell can be built and the plumbing roughed in at a reasonably low cost. Interior finish, storage walls, and an addition can be added later.

The simple interior arrangement is flexible and can be adapted to many uses—a beach house, lake or mountain cabin; a low-cost permanent home with one, two, or three bedrooms; or a temporary home. The outside may be rustic or of the finest modern siding. The inside may have rough framing and concrete floor exposed, or it may be highly finished. Thus, the design fits a wide variety of needs.

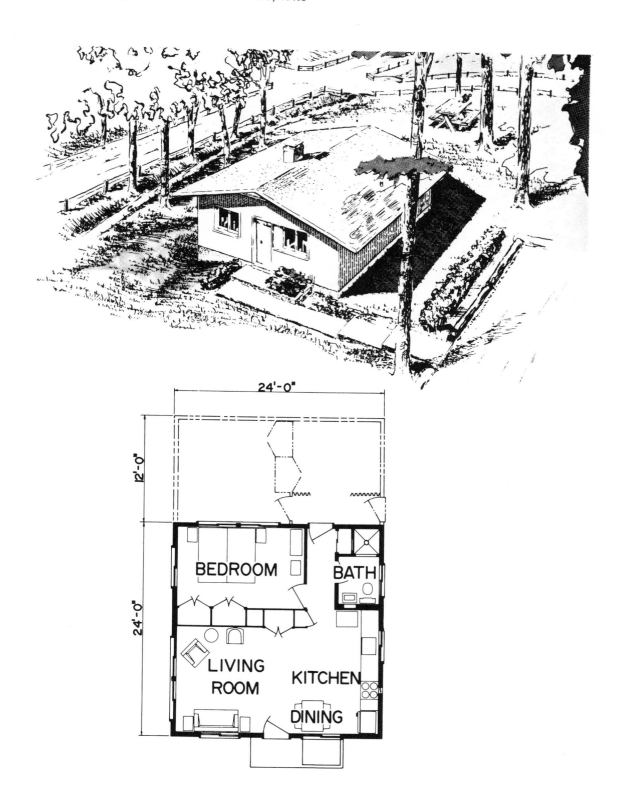

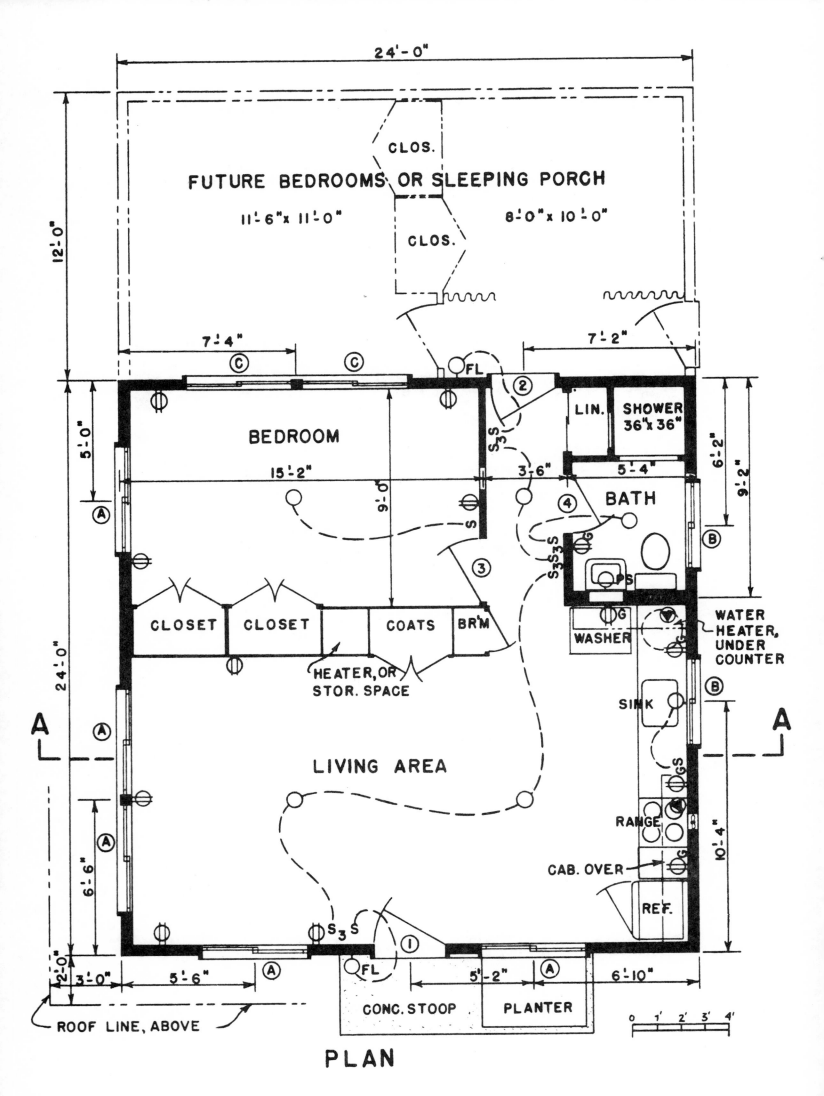

FUTURE BEDROOMS OR SLEEPING PORCH

CLOS.

CLOS.

11'-6" x 11'-0"

8'-0" x 10'-0"

24'-0"

12'-0"

7'-4"

7'-2"

C

C

FL

2

LIN.

SHOWER
36" x 36"

BEDROOM

15'-2"

5'-0"

9'-0"

S₃S

3'-6"

5'-4"

6'-2"

9'-2"

A

S

4

BATH

B

3

S₃S₃S

24'-0"

CLOSET

CLOSET

COATS

BR'M

WATER
HEATER,
UNDER
COUNTER

HEATER, OR
STOR. SPACE

WASHER

G

G

G

B

SINK

G S

A

LIVING AREA

RANGE

G

6'-6"

A

CAB. OVER

G

10'-4"

REF.

2'-0"

3'-0"

5'-6"

A

S₃S

1

FL

5'-2"

A

6'-10"

ROOF LINE, ABOVE

CONC. STOOP

PLANTER

0 1' 2' 3' 4'

PLAN

14

WINDOW SCHEDULE

Ⓐ ... 4'-5" WIDE x 3'-5" HIGH
Ⓑ ... 3'-7" " x 2'-5" "
Ⓒ ... 4'-5" " x 1'-9" "

PACKAGED SLIDING WINDOWS.
TYPE AND TRIM TO BE AS
SELECTED BY OWNER.

ELECTRICAL SYMBOLS

S-----SWITCH
S₃-----THREE-WAY SWITCH
◯-----CEILING FIXTURE, RECESSED
◯PS--WALL FIXTURE, PULL SWITCH
◯FL--FLOODLIGHT
⊕-----DUPLEX CONVENIENCE OUTLET
⊕G---DUP, CONV. OUTLET WITH GROUND
⬤-----230 VOLT, RANGE & WATER HEATER

DOOR SCHEDULE

① ... 3'-0" x 6'-8" EXTERIOR
② ... 2'-8" x 6'-8" "
③ ... 2'-8" x 6'-8" INTERIOR
④ ... 2'-6" x 6'-8" "

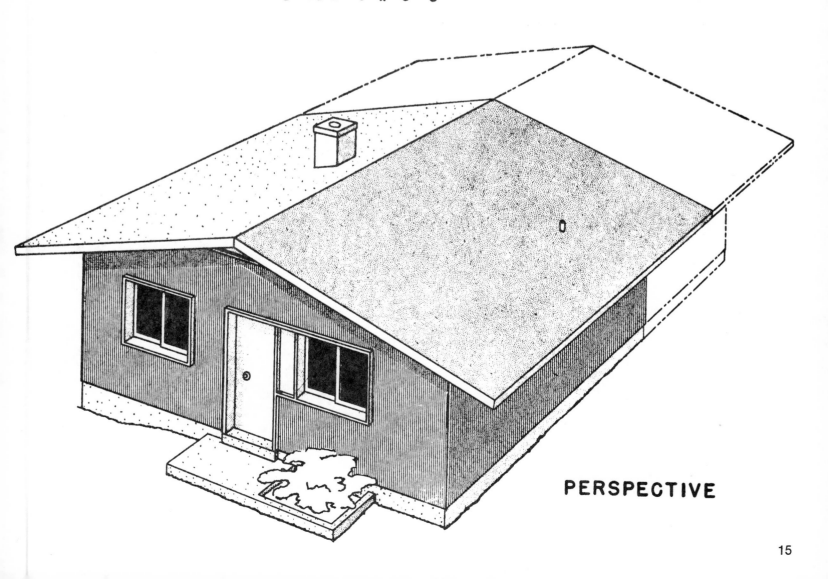

PERSPECTIVE

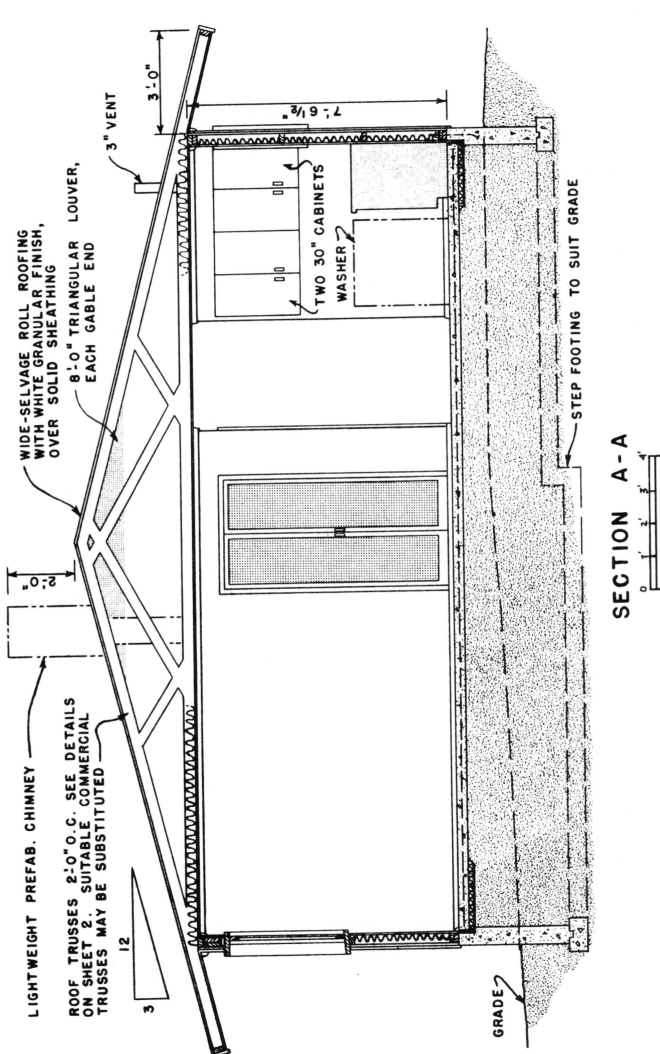

LIGHTWEIGHT PREFAB. CHIMNEY

ROOF TRUSSES 2'-0" O.C. SEE DETAILS ON SHEET 2. SUITABLE COMMERCIAL TRUSSES MAY BE SUBSTITUTED

12
3

WIDE-SELVAGE ROLL ROOFING WITH WHITE GRANULAR FINISH, OVER SOLID SHEATHING

8'-0" TRIANGULAR LOUVER, EACH GABLE END

3" VENT

3'-0"

7'-6 1/2"

2'-0"

TWO 30" CABINETS

WASHER

STEP FOOTING TO SUIT GRADE

GRADE

SECTION A-A

0 1 2 3 4'

FOR ECONOMY AND EASE OF CONSTRUCTION, APPLY THE INTERIOR WALL, CEILING AND FLOOR FINISH BEFORE ERECTING ANY PARTITIONS. THIS WILL ALSO PERMIT FUTURE REMOVAL OR MOVING OF ANY PARTITIONS EXCEPT THOSE WHICH CONTAIN PLUMBING.

THE FINISH GRADE SHOULD SLOPE AWAY FROM THE CABIN ON ALL SIDES.

16

Alternate floor plans

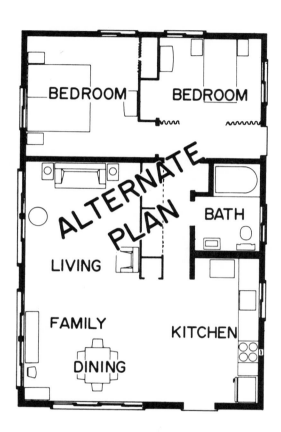

Alternate plans for this cabin can be developed to obtain additional rental income in recreational areas. The basic building can be arranged in several ways, depending on the type of facility and on accommodations needed by vacationers. For example, a screened porch, a bunk room, and/or additional bedrooms can be added.

The working drawings show construction details for storage walls (2 feet wide, 4 feet long, and 8 feet high) which may be built from standard 4- by 8-feet sheets of material. The roof trusses eliminate any need for interior load-bearing walls, so the walls may be located wherever desired. If built lower than ceiling height, they can be moved easily.

If the cabin is to be used as a permanent dwelling, storage space is needed outside. The space should be large enough to accommodate paints, hand and garden tools, lawn mower, outboard motor, gasoline, and similar equipment and supplies. Also, the shed should be large enough to permit handyman activities.

Careful consideration should be given to the heating system. If expansion is planned, the system must be capable of heating the larger unit.

The alternate plan reproduced shows one arrangement that is possible for expansion. Although it has more living, sleeping, and storage space than the basic plan, it also requires outdoor storage if it is to be used as a permanent home. The working drawings show only the expanded building with storage walls.

The roof trusses used in the design are simple lap-nailed construction and have been load-tested. The truss members can be nailed together and trimmed later to eliminate precision marking and cutting. If the details of the working drawings are followed, a reliable roof support can be easily and quickly constructed.

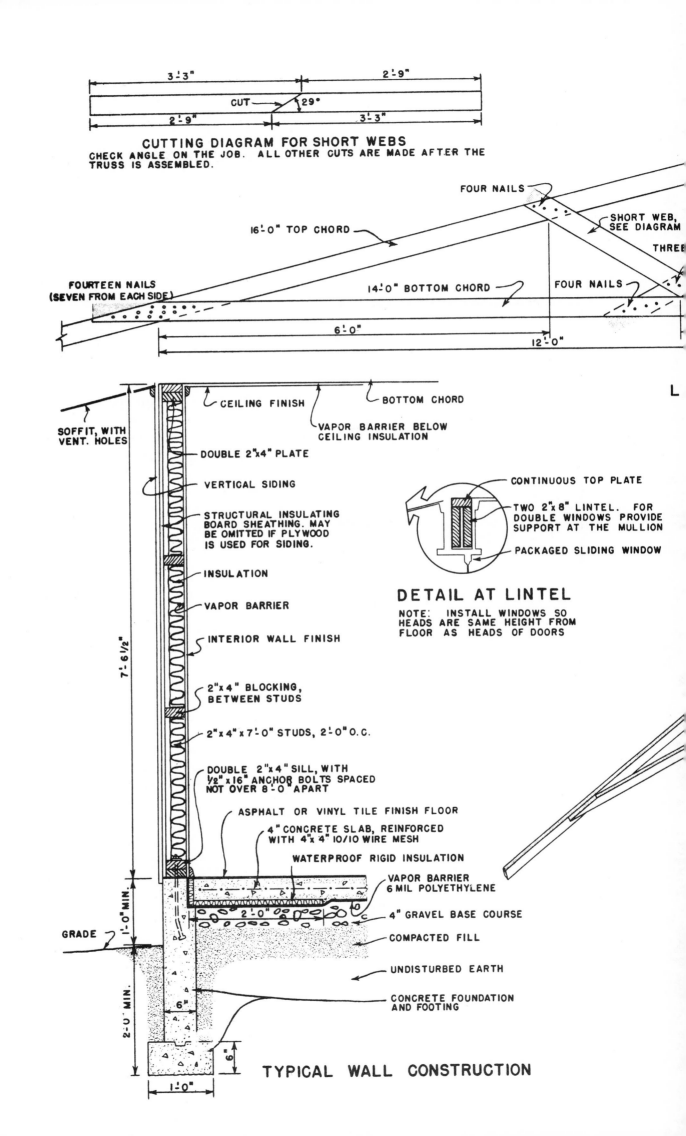

CUTTING DIAGRAM FOR SHORT WEBS

3'-3"   2'-9"

CUT   29°

2'-9"   3'-3"

CHECK ANGLE ON THE JOB. ALL OTHER CUTS ARE MADE AFTER THE
TRUSS IS ASSEMBLED.

FOUR NAILS

SHORT WEB,
SEE DIAGRAM

16'-0" TOP CHORD

THREE

FOURTEEN NAILS
(SEVEN FROM EACH SIDE)

14'-0" BOTTOM CHORD

FOUR NAILS

6'-0"

12'-0"

L

SOFFIT, WITH
VENT. HOLES

CEILING FINISH

BOTTOM CHORD

VAPOR BARRIER BELOW
CEILING INSULATION

DOUBLE 2"x4" PLATE

VERTICAL SIDING

STRUCTURAL INSULATING
BOARD SHEATHING. MAY
BE OMITTED IF PLYWOOD
IS USED FOR SIDING.

INSULATION

VAPOR BARRIER

INTERIOR WALL FINISH

7'-6 1/2"

2"x4" BLOCKING,
BETWEEN STUDS

2"x4"x7'-0" STUDS, 2'-0" O.C.

DOUBLE 2"x4" SILL, WITH
1/2"x16" ANCHOR BOLTS SPACED
NOT OVER 8'-0" APART

ASPHALT OR VINYL TILE FINISH FLOOR

4" CONCRETE SLAB, REINFORCED
WITH 4"x 4" 10/10 WIRE MESH

WATERPROOF RIGID INSULATION

VAPOR BARRIER
6 MIL POLYETHYLENE

2'-0"

4" GRAVEL BASE COURSE

COMPACTED FILL

GRADE

1'-0" MIN.

UNDISTURBED EARTH

CONCRETE FOUNDATION
AND FOOTING

2'-0" MIN.

6"

6"

1'-0"

TYPICAL WALL CONSTRUCTION

CONTINUOUS TOP PLATE

TWO 2"x8" LINTEL. FOR
DOUBLE WINDOWS PROVIDE
SUPPORT AT THE MULLION

PACKAGED SLIDING WINDOW

DETAIL AT LINTEL

NOTE: INSTALL WINDOWS SO
HEADS ARE SAME HEIGHT FROM
FLOOR AS HEADS OF DOORS

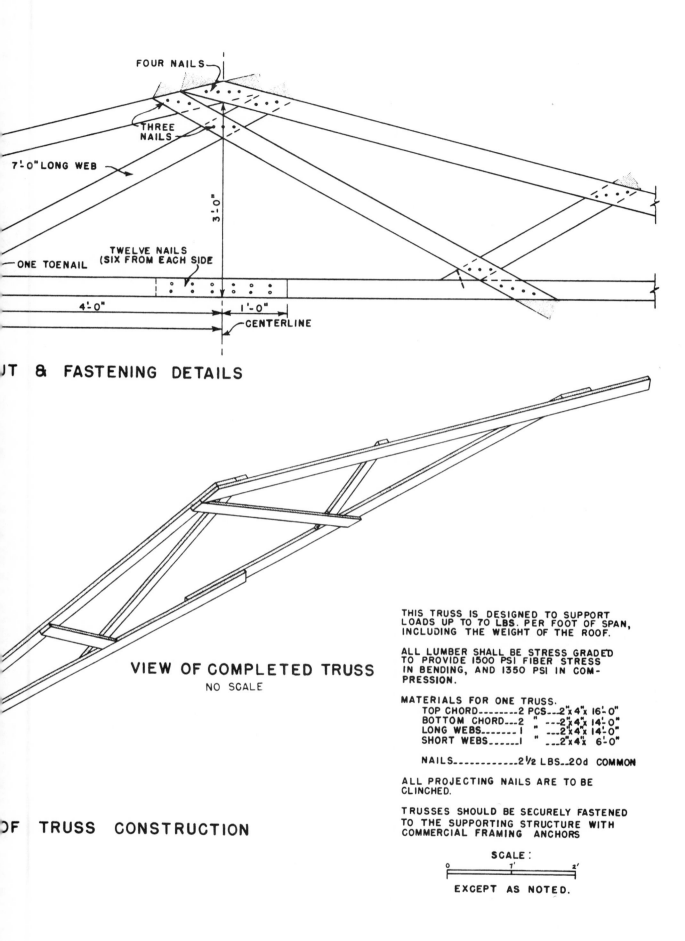

FOUR NAILS

THREE NAILS

7'-0" LONG WEB

3'-0"

ONE TOENAIL

TWELVE NAILS
(SIX FROM EACH SIDE

4'-0"

1'-0"

CENTERLINE

JT & FASTENING DETAILS

VIEW OF COMPLETED TRUSS
NO SCALE

OF TRUSS CONSTRUCTION

THIS TRUSS IS DESIGNED TO SUPPORT
LOADS UP TO 70 LBS. PER FOOT OF SPAN,
INCLUDING THE WEIGHT OF THE ROOF.

ALL LUMBER SHALL BE STRESS GRADED
TO PROVIDE 1500 PSI FIBER STRESS
IN BENDING, AND 1350 PSI IN COM-
PRESSION.

MATERIALS FOR ONE TRUSS.
    TOP CHORD _____ 2 PCS___2"x 4"x 16'-0"
    BOTTOM CHORD ___ 2 " ___2"x 4"x 14'-0"
    LONG WEBS _____ 1 " ___2"x 4"x 14'-0"
    SHORT WEBS _____ 1 " ___2"x 4"x 6'-0"

    NAILS _____ 2½ LBS__20d COMMON

ALL PROJECTING NAILS ARE TO BE
CLINCHED.

TRUSSES SHOULD BE SECURELY FASTENED
TO THE SUPPORTING STRUCTURE WITH
COMMERCIAL FRAMING ANCHORS

SCALE:
0   1'   2'

EXCEPT AS NOTED.

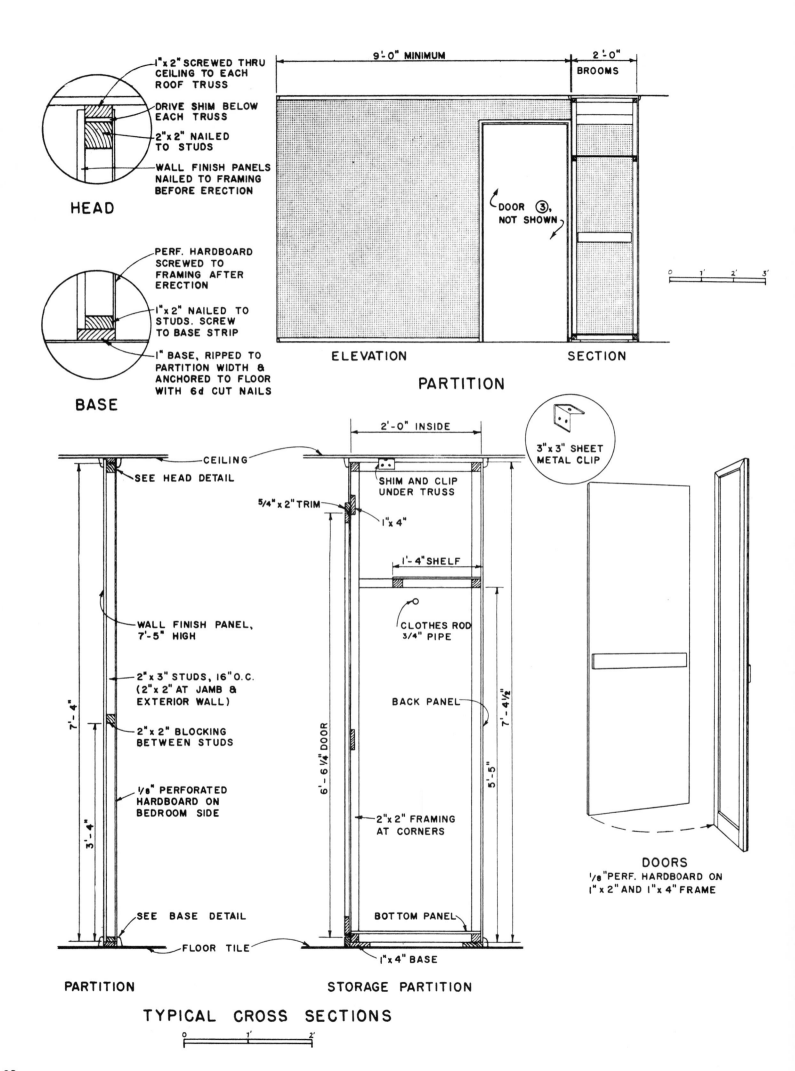

HEAD

1"x 2" SCREWED THRU CEILING TO EACH ROOF TRUSS

DRIVE SHIM BELOW EACH TRUSS

2"x 2" NAILED TO STUDS

WALL FINISH PANELS NAILED TO FRAMING BEFORE ERECTION

BASE

PERF. HARDBOARD SCREWED TO FRAMING AFTER ERECTION

1"x 2" NAILED TO STUDS. SCREW TO BASE STRIP

1" BASE, RIPPED TO PARTITION WIDTH & ANCHORED TO FLOOR WITH 6d CUT NAILS

9'-0" MINIMUM

2'-0"

BROOMS

DOOR ③, NOT SHOWN

ELEVATION

SECTION

PARTITION

0   1'   2'   3'

2'-0" INSIDE

3"x 3" SHEET METAL CLIP

CEILING

SEE HEAD DETAIL

SHIM AND CLIP UNDER TRUSS

5/4"x 2" TRIM

1"x 4"

1'-4" SHELF

WALL FINISH PANEL, 7'-5" HIGH

CLOTHES ROD 3/4" PIPE

BACK PANEL

2"x 3" STUDS, 16"O.C. (2"x 2" AT JAMB & EXTERIOR WALL)

2"x 2" BLOCKING BETWEEN STUDS

1/8" PERFORATED HARDBOARD ON BEDROOM SIDE

7'-4"

3'-4"

6'- 6 1/4" DOOR

7'- 4 1/2"

5'-5"

2"x 2" FRAMING AT CORNERS

SEE BASE DETAIL

BOTTOM PANEL

FLOOR TILE

1"x 4" BASE

PARTITION

STORAGE PARTITION

DOORS
1/8" PERF. HARDBOARD ON 1"x 2" AND 1"x 4" FRAME

TYPICAL CROSS SECTIONS

0   1'   2'

20

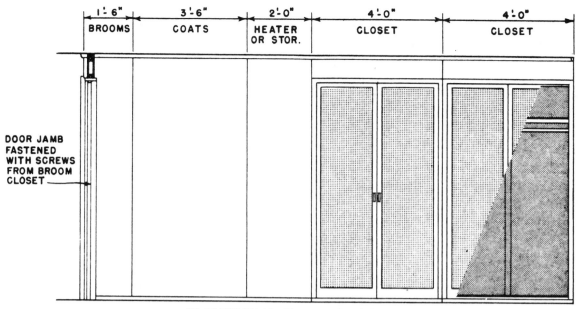

ELEVATION, CUT AWAY TO SHOW INTERIOR

STORAGE PARTITION

DOOR JAMB
FASTENED
WITH SCREWS
FROM BROOM
CLOSET

1'-6"	3'-6"	2'-0"	4'-0"	4'-0"
BROOMS	COATS	HEATER OR STOR.	CLOSET	CLOSET

0   1'   2'   3'

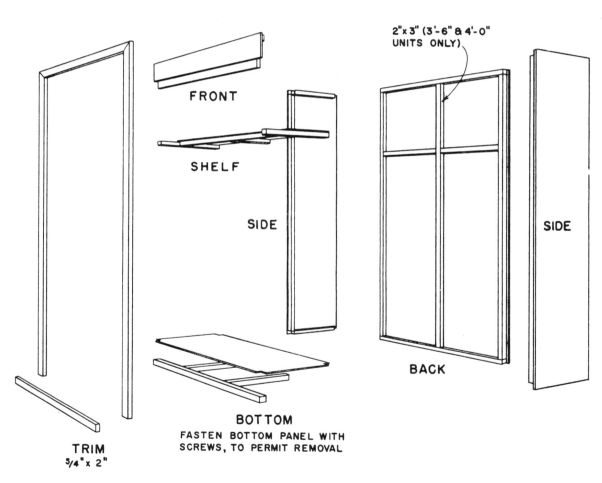

FRONT

SHELF

SIDE

2"x 3" (3'-6" & 4'-0" UNITS ONLY)

SIDE

BACK

TRIM
³⁄₄" x 2"

BOTTOM

FASTEN BOTTOM PANEL WITH
SCREWS, TO PERMIT REMOVAL

EXPLODED VIEW OF TYPICAL CLOSET UNIT
SHOWING COMPONENTS READY FOR ASSEMBLY

THESE BEDROOM PARTITIONS ARE DESIGNED TO PERMIT FUTURE REARRANGEMENT OR REMOVAL.

THE STORAGE PARTITION IS MADE UP OF INDIVIDUAL CLOSET UNITS WHICH ARE SUPPORTED ON CONTINUOUS 1"x 4" BOARDS WHICH SERVE TO PROTECT THE FINISH FLOOR TILE. JOINTS AT THE FLOOR AND CEILING ARE COVERED BY TRIM. USE OF VERTICALLY GROOVED PLYWOOD OR HARDBOARD PANELS WILL AID IN CONCEALING THE JOINTS BETWEEN UNITS.

ALL FRAMING IS 2"x 2" EXCEPT AS NOTED.

CLOSET DOORS SHOULD HAVE MAGNETIC LATCHES AT TOP AND BOTTOM.

PERFORATED HARDBOARD IS USED ON CLOSET DOORS FOR VENTILATION AND ON THE OTHER PARTITION FOR TEXTURE AND TO PERMIT HANGING LIGHT SHELVES, ETC., ON COMMERCIAL BRACKETS.

CONSTRUCTION OF HEATER ENCLOSURE WILL DEPEND ON THE TYPE OF HEATING UNIT TO BE INSTALLED.

5. 24-FOOT × 24-FOOT CONCRETE-BLOCK CABIN

Concrete masonry construction is suggested for this modern cabin because concrete is low-cost, durable, easy to maintain, and attractive.

Complete kitchen facilities in the cabin combine with the living-dining area to form a unified activities center for the family. Though the basic plan calls for one bedroom, the activities center is large enough for a family that would need three bedrooms. The two extra bedrooms may be added at the rear, as suggested in the working drawings, without altera-

tion of the present rooms or equipment. A bath with shower, a space for a washer, and good storage facilities contribute to pleasant and convenient living in this cabin.

Suggestions for block selection, insulation, finishing materials, and paint are given. These ideas, along with personal preference for trim and for paint color combinations, can be used to give warmth and character to the cabin.

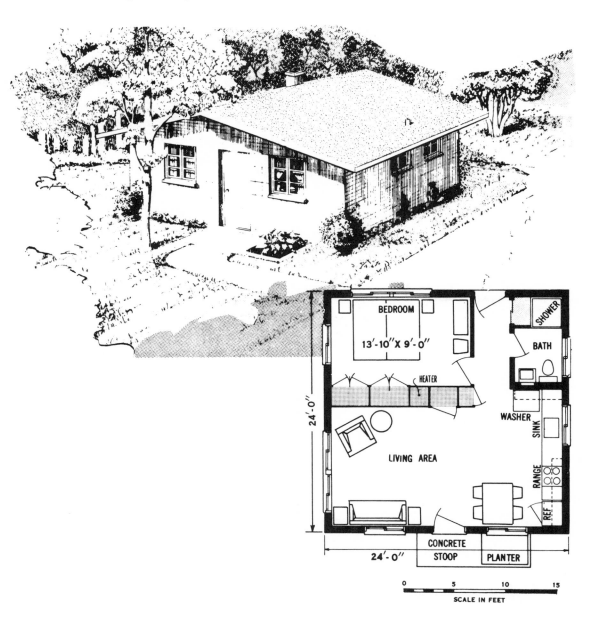

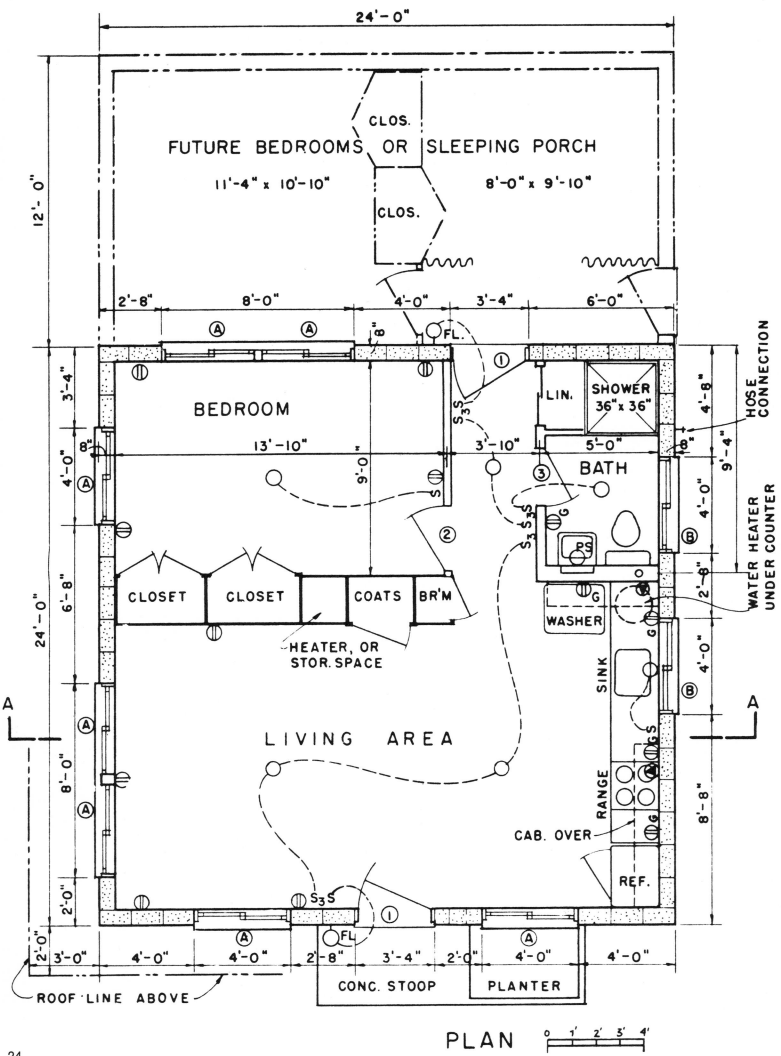

FUTURE BEDROOMS OR SLEEPING PORCH

11'-4" x 10'-10"

8'-0" x 9'-10"

CLOS.

CLOS.

24'-0"

12'-0"

2'-8"   8'-0"   4'-0"   3'-4"   6'-0"

BEDROOM

13'-10"

9'-0"

3'-4"

4'-0"

8"

6'-8"

24'-0"

8'-0"

2'-0"

2'-0"

CLOSET   CLOSET   COATS   BR'M

HEATER, OR
STOR. SPACE

LIVING   AREA

LIN.

SHOWER
36" x 36"

BATH

3'-10"

5'-0"

PS

WASHER

SINK

RANGE

CAB. OVER

REF.

8"

4'-8"

9'-4"

4'-0"

2'-8"

4'-0"

8'-8"

HOSE CONNECTION

WATER HEATER UNDER COUNTER

FL.

S₃S

S

FL.

S₃S

3'-0"   4'-0"   4'-0"   2'-8"   3'-4"   2'-0"   4'-0"   4'-0"

ROOF LINE ABOVE

CONC. STOOP   PLANTER

PLAN   0 1' 2' 3' 4'

24

WINDOW SCHEDULE (OPENINGS)
ROUGH

Ⓐ   4'-0" WIDE X 4'-0" HIGH

Ⓑ   4'-0"   "   X 2'-8"   "

PACKAGED SLIDING WINDOWS
TYPE AND TRIM TO BE AS
SELECTED BY OWNER.

ELECTRICAL SYMBOLS

S   SWITCH

S_3 THREE-WAY SWITCH

◯   CEILING FIXTURE, RECESSED

◯PS   WALL FIXTURE, PULL SWITCH

◯FL   FLOODLIGHT

⊕   DUPLEX CONVENIENCE OUTLET

⊕G   DUP. CONV. OUTLET WITH GROUND

⊛   230 VOLT, RANGE & WATER HEATER

DOOR SCHEDULE

①   3'-0" X 6'-8"   EXTERIOR

②   2'-8" X 6'-8"   INTERIOR

③   2'-6" X 6'-8"   "

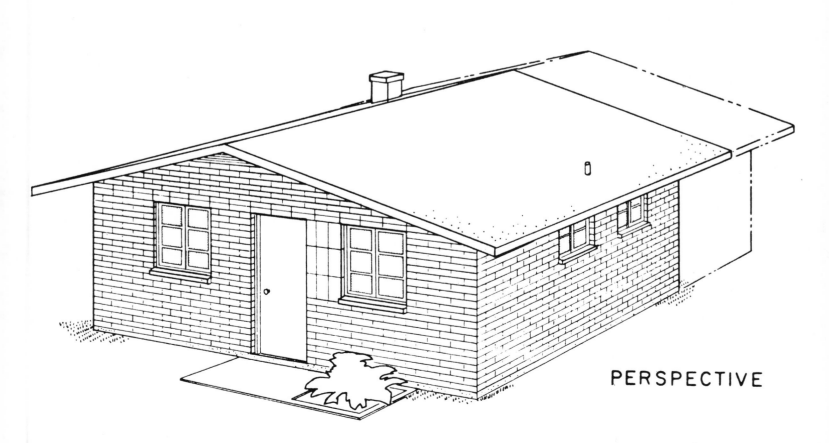

PERSPECTIVE

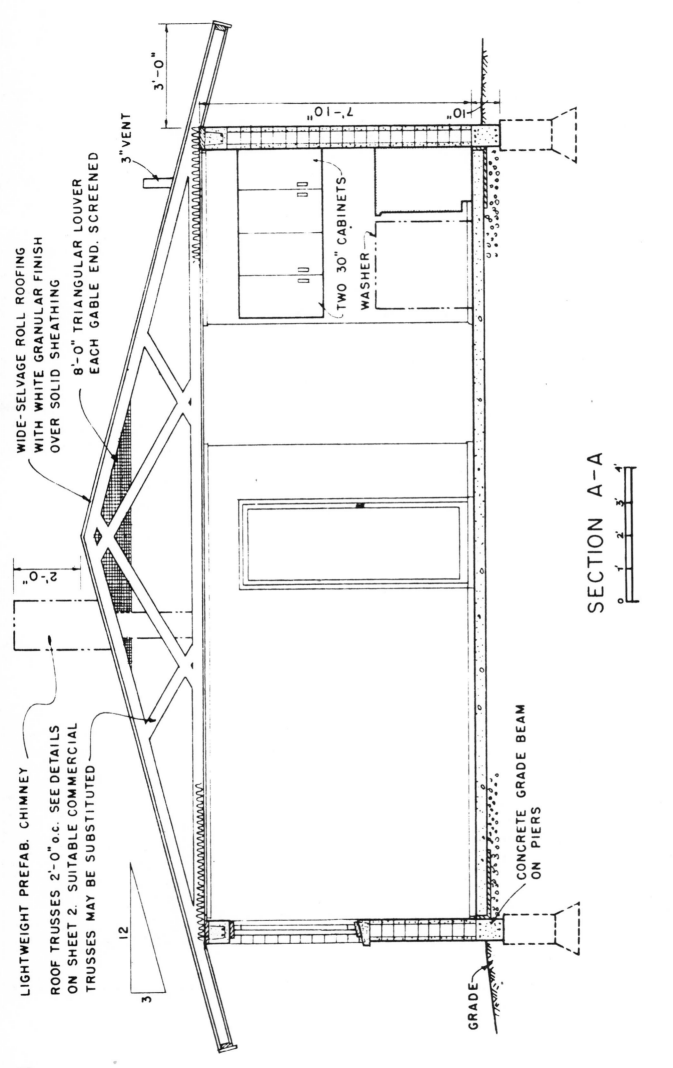

WIDE-SELVAGE ROLL ROOFING
WITH WHITE GRANULAR FINISH
OVER SOLID SHEATHING

8'-0" TRIANGULAR LOUVER
EACH GABLE END. SCREENED

3" VENT

LIGHTWEIGHT PREFAB. CHIMNEY

ROOF TRUSSES 2'-0" o.c. SEE DETAILS
ON SHEET 2. SUITABLE COMMERCIAL
TRUSSES MAY BE SUBSTITUTED

12

3

CONCRETE GRADE BEAM
ON PIERS

GRADE

3'-0"

2'-0"

7'-10"

10"

TWO 30" CABINETS

WASHER

SECTION A-A

0 1 2' 3' 4'

FOR ECONOMY AND EASE OF CONSTRUCTION, APPLY THE
INTERIOR WALL, CEILING AND FLOOR FINISH BEFORE
ERECTING ANY PARTITIONS. THIS WILL ALSO PERMIT
FUTURE REMOVAL OR MOVING OF ANY PARTITIONS
EXCEPT THOSE WHICH CONTAIN PLUMBING.

THE FINISH GRADE SHOULD SLOPE AWAY
FROM THE CABIN ON ALL SIDES.
SEE DETAILS ON SHEET 2 FOR ALTERNATE
FOUNDATION DETAILS.

26

Block selection

The working drawings show 4- x 8- x 16-inch concrete block units, which give horizontal mortar lines at 4-inch intervals. These relatively close-spaced mortar joints have a pleasing appearance, but the finished cost is increased by one-third as compared with that of standard 8- x 8- x 16-inch units.

Properly tooled joints are very important for watertight walls and for overall good appearance. Concave or "v" joints are recommended.

When mortar in joints is "thumb print" hard, it should be firmly pressed into the concave or "v" formation with a tooling device that is wider than the joint and 24 to 36 inches long. This long tooling device makes straight, uniform horizontal joints.

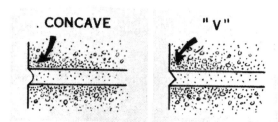

Insulation

Insulation above the ceiling is recommended for cabins built in any climate and for use in any season. Either loose fill or batt-type insulation may be used. Vermiculite fill in the cores of the blocks and foamed semirigid insulation about the perimeter of the floor slab are necessary for winter comfort. Lightweight-aggregate blocks are recommended because insulation is easier to apply to them than to the denser concrete blocks with sand and gravel aggregate. Lightweight blocks are also easier to handle, and nails can be driven into them.

Finishing material

Interior-wall, ceiling, and floor finishes can be applied before partitions are erected. This saves cutting and fitting labor. Ceiling tiles made of insulating board are popular for this type of building because no further finishing is required. Low-cost asphalt tiles serve well over a concrete floor slab.

A latex paint is recommended for the interior walls. Besides being economical and easy to apply, it is well suited for masonry and the other inside materials. The exterior masonry walls should have a base coat of portland cement paint (a special cement powder to be mixed with water) for watertightness. Apply this with a stiff-bristle scrub brush to fill the pores of the block. The second exterior coat should be an acrylic resin, outside latex paint.

Interior partitions

The clear span of the roof trusses permits free placement of interior partitions. If the partitions are not hindered by wiring or plumbing, they can be easily moved for remodeling. Partitions should be slightly less than ceiling height and wedged at the bottom to press them against the ceiling.

The working drawings show construction details of the storage room wall that separates the living area from the bedroom. Built from standard 4- x 8-foot sheets of material, the wall is 2 feet deep by 8 feet high.

Perforated hardboard is suggested for closet doors and backs, for ventilation as well as for its decorative quality. Brackets and hooks can be placed in the perforated board to make the storage space more usable.

Construction of the heater enclosure will depend on the type of heating unit to be installed.

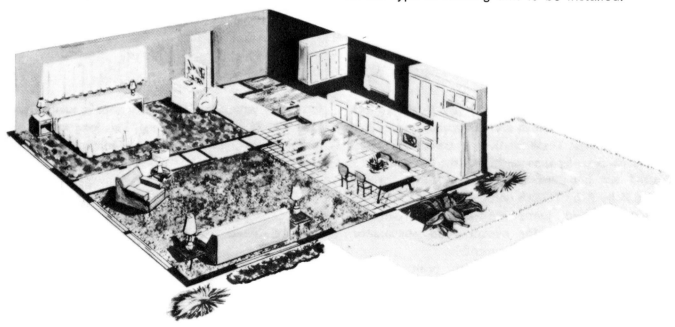

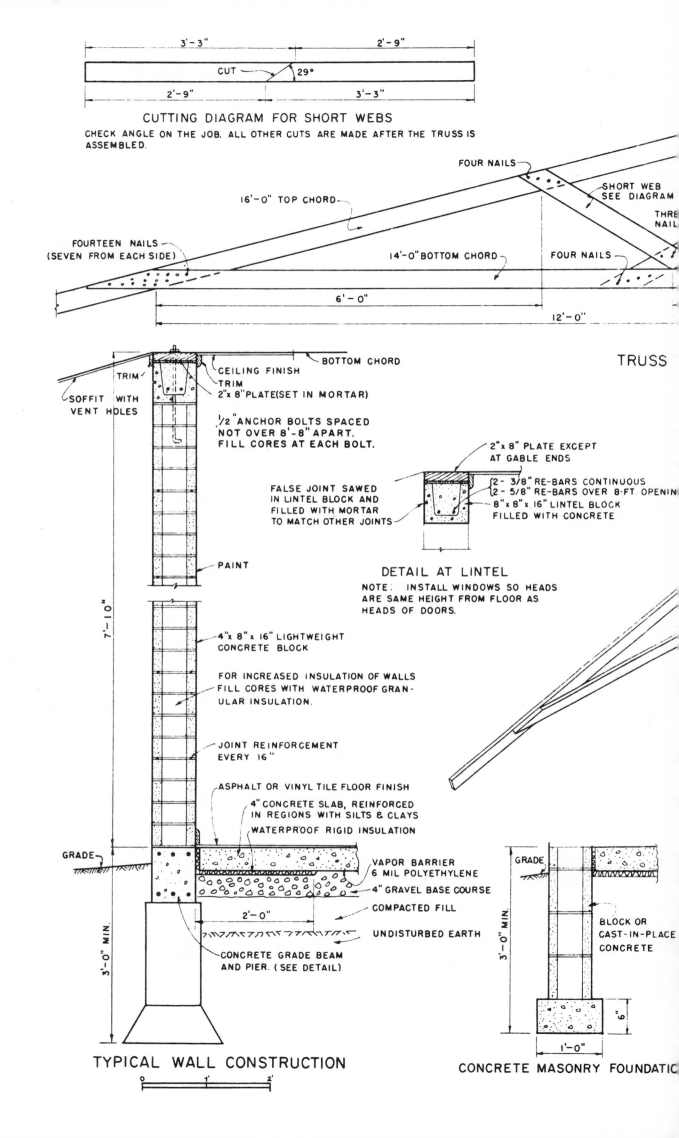

CUTTING DIAGRAM FOR SHORT WEBS

3'-3"   2'-9"

CUT   29°

2'-9"   3'-3"

CHECK ANGLE ON THE JOB. ALL OTHER CUTS ARE MADE AFTER THE TRUSS IS ASSEMBLED.

FOUR NAILS

16'-0" TOP CHORD

SHORT WEB SEE DIAGRAM

THRE NAIL

FOURTEEN NAILS (SEVEN FROM EACH SIDE)

14'-0" BOTTOM CHORD

FOUR NAILS

6'-0"

12'-0"

BOTTOM CHORD

TRUSS

TRIM
SOFFIT WITH VENT HOLES

CEILING FINISH
TRIM
2"x 8" PLATE (SET IN MORTAR)

½" ANCHOR BOLTS SPACED NOT OVER 8'-8" APART. FILL CORES AT EACH BOLT.

2"x 8" PLATE EXCEPT AT GABLE ENDS

2 - 3/8" RE-BARS CONTINUOUS
2 - 5/8" RE-BARS OVER 8-FT OPENIN
8"x 8"x 16" LINTEL BLOCK FILLED WITH CONCRETE

FALSE JOINT SAWED IN LINTEL BLOCK AND FILLED WITH MORTAR TO MATCH OTHER JOINTS

PAINT

DETAIL AT LINTEL

NOTE: INSTALL WINDOWS SO HEADS ARE SAME HEIGHT FROM FLOOR AS HEADS OF DOORS.

4"x 8" x 16" LIGHTWEIGHT CONCRETE BLOCK

FOR INCREASED INSULATION OF WALLS FILL CORES WITH WATERPROOF GRANULAR INSULATION.

JOINT REINFORCEMENT EVERY 16"

7'-10"

ASPHALT OR VINYL TILE FLOOR FINISH
4" CONCRETE SLAB, REINFORCED IN REGIONS WITH SILTS & CLAYS
WATERPROOF RIGID INSULATION

GRADE

GRADE

VAPOR BARRIER 6 MIL POLYETHYLENE
4" GRAVEL BASE COURSE
COMPACTED FILL
UNDISTURBED EARTH

2'-0"

BLOCK OR CAST-IN-PLACE CONCRETE

3'-0" MIN.

3'-0" MIN.

CONCRETE GRADE BEAM AND PIER. (SEE DETAIL)

6"

1'-0"

TYPICAL WALL CONSTRUCTION

0   1   2

CONCRETE MASONRY FOUNDATIC

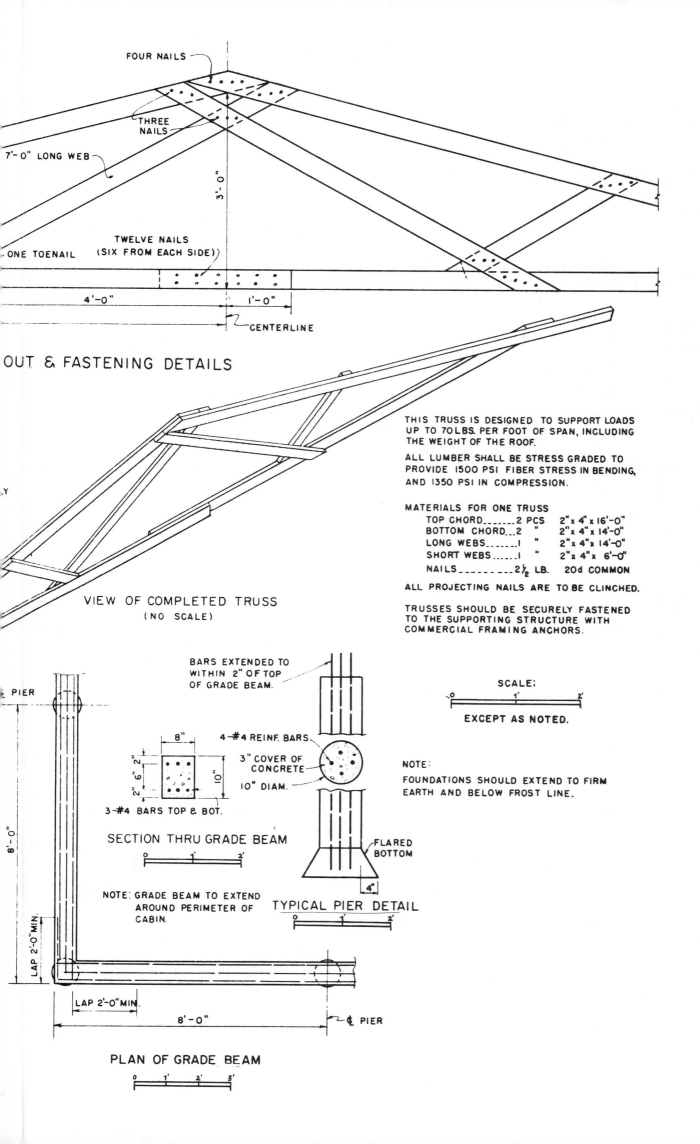

FOUR NAILS

THREE NAILS

7'-0" LONG WEB

3'-0"

ONE TOENAIL

TWELVE NAILS
(SIX FROM EACH SIDE)

4'-0"

1'-0"

CENTERLINE

OUT & FASTENING DETAILS

VIEW OF COMPLETED TRUSS
(NO SCALE)

THIS TRUSS IS DESIGNED TO SUPPORT LOADS
UP TO 70 LBS. PER FOOT OF SPAN, INCLUDING
THE WEIGHT OF THE ROOF.

ALL LUMBER SHALL BE STRESS GRADED TO
PROVIDE 1500 PSI FIBER STRESS IN BENDING,
AND 1350 PSI IN COMPRESSION.

MATERIALS FOR ONE TRUSS
TOP CHORD......2 PCS   2"x 4"x 16'-0"
BOTTOM CHORD..2 "   2"x 4"x 14'-0"
LONG WEBS......1 "   2"x 4"x 14'-0"
SHORT WEBS.....1 "   2"x 4"x 6'-0"
NAILS...........2½ LB.   20d COMMON

ALL PROJECTING NAILS ARE TO BE CLINCHED.

TRUSSES SHOULD BE SECURELY FASTENED
TO THE SUPPORTING STRUCTURE WITH
COMMERCIAL FRAMING ANCHORS.

PIER

BARS EXTENDED TO
WITHIN 2" OF TOP
OF GRADE BEAM.

8"

2" 6" 2"

10"

4 #4 REINF. BARS

3" COVER OF
CONCRETE

10" DIAM.

3 #4 BARS TOP & BOT.

SECTION THRU GRADE BEAM

NOTE: GRADE BEAM TO EXTEND
AROUND PERIMETER OF
CABIN.

FLARED
BOTTOM

4"

TYPICAL PIER DETAIL

SCALE:

0   1'   2'

EXCEPT AS NOTED.

NOTE:

FOUNDATIONS SHOULD EXTEND TO FIRM
EARTH AND BELOW FROST LINE.

8'-0"

LAP 2'-0" MIN.

LAP 2'-0" MIN.

8'-0"

℄ PIER

PLAN OF GRADE BEAM

0   1'   2'   3'

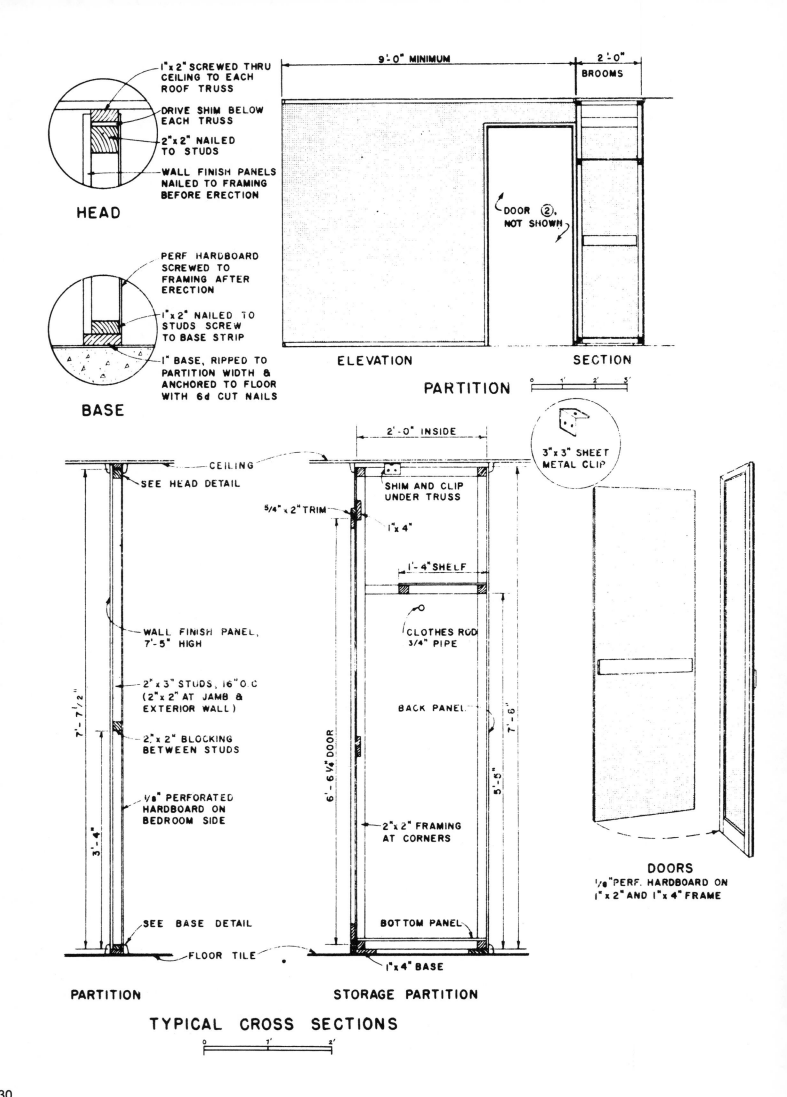

HEAD

- 1"x 2" SCREWED THRU CEILING TO EACH ROOF TRUSS
- DRIVE SHIM BELOW EACH TRUSS
- 2"x 2" NAILED TO STUDS
- WALL FINISH PANELS NAILED TO FRAMING BEFORE ERECTION

BASE

- PERF HARDBOARD SCREWED TO FRAMING AFTER ERECTION
- 1"x 2" NAILED TO STUDS SCREW TO BASE STRIP
- 1" BASE, RIPPED TO PARTITION WIDTH & ANCHORED TO FLOOR WITH 6d CUT NAILS

9'-0" MINIMUM

2'-0" BROOMS

DOOR ② NOT SHOWN

ELEVATION   SECTION

PARTITION

0 1' 2' 3'

3"x 3" SHEET METAL CLIP

PARTITION

- CEILING
- SEE HEAD DETAIL
- WALL FINISH PANEL, 7'-5" HIGH
- 2"x 3" STUDS, 16" O.C (2"x 2" AT JAMB & EXTERIOR WALL)
- 2"x 2" BLOCKING BETWEEN STUDS
- 1/8" PERFORATED HARDBOARD ON BEDROOM SIDE
- SEE BASE DETAIL
- FLOOR TILE

7'-7 1/2"

3'-4"

STORAGE PARTITION

2'-0" INSIDE

- SHIM AND CLIP UNDER TRUSS
- 5/4" x 2" TRIM
- 1"x 4"
- 1'-4" SHELF
- CLOTHES ROD 3/4" PIPE
- BACK PANEL
- 2"x 2" FRAMING AT CORNERS
- BOTTOM PANEL
- 1"x 4" BASE

6'-6 1/4" DOOR

7'-6"

5'-5"

DOORS

1/8" PERF. HARDBOARD ON 1"x 2" AND 1"x 4" FRAME

TYPICAL CROSS SECTIONS

0 1' 2'

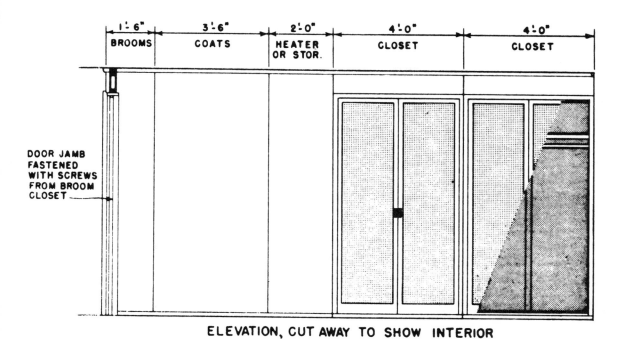

1'-6"	3'-6"	2'-0"	4'-0"	4'-0"
BROOMS	COATS	HEATER OR STOR.	CLOSET	CLOSET

DOOR JAMB
FASTENED
WITH SCREWS
FROM BROOM
CLOSET

ELEVATION, CUT AWAY TO SHOW INTERIOR

STORAGE PARTITION

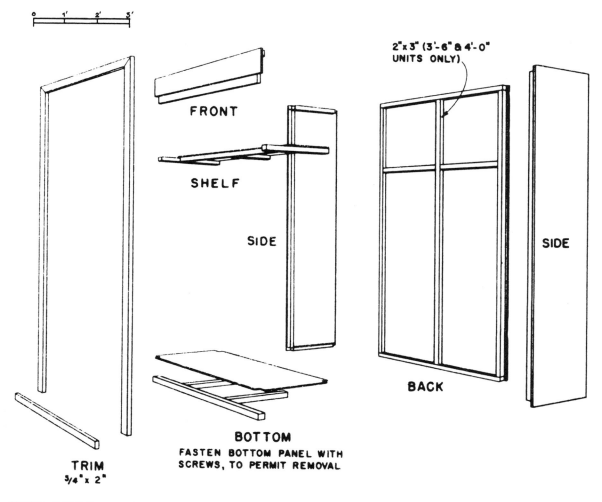

FRONT

SHELF

SIDE

2"x3" (3'-6" & 4'-0"
UNITS ONLY)

SIDE

BACK

BOTTOM
FASTEN BOTTOM PANEL WITH
SCREWS, TO PERMIT REMOVAL

TRIM
3/4" x 2"

EXPLODED VIEW OF TYPICAL CLOSET UNIT
SHOWING COMPONENTS READY FOR ASSEMBLY

THESE BEDROOM PARTITIONS ARE DESIGNED TO PERMIT FUTURE REARRANGEMENT OR REMOVAL.

THE STORAGE PARTITION IS MADE UP OF INDIVID-UAL CLOSET UNITS WHICH ARE SUPPORTED ON CONTINUOUS 1"x4" BOARDS WHICH SERVE TO PROTECT THE FINISH FLOOR TILE JOINTS AT THE FLOOR AND CEILING ARE COVERED BY TRIM. USE OF VERTICALLY GROOVED PLY-WOOD OR HARDBOARD PANELS WILL AID IN CONCEALING THE JOINTS BETWEEN UNITS.

ALL FRAMING IS 2"x2" EXCEPT AS NOTED.

CLOSET DOORS SHOULD HAVE MAGNETIC LATCHES AT TOP AND BOTTOM.

PERFORATED HARDBOARD IS USED ON CLOSET DOORS FOR VENTILATION AND ON THE OTHER PARTITION FOR TEXTURE AND TO PERMIT HANGING LIGHT SHELVES, ETC., ON COMMERCIAL BRACKETS.

CONSTRUCTION OF HEATER ENCLOSURE WILL DEPEND ON THE TYPE OF HEATING UNIT TO BE INSTALLED.

31

6. TWO-BEDROOM FRAME CABIN WITH SLEEPING LOFT

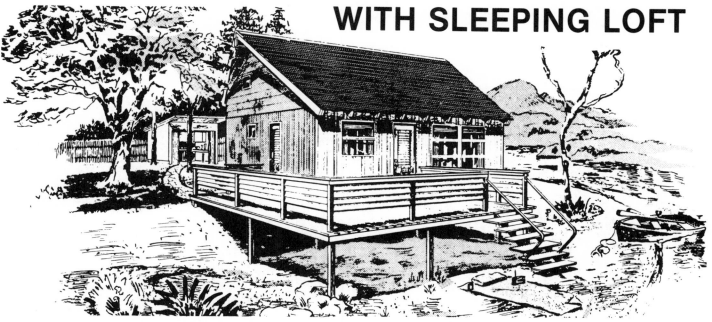

1 ST FLOOR . . 22' X 24'

LOFT . . . . 12' X 24'

BEDROOM

BATH

BEDROOM

KITCHEN
DINING

PRE-FAB. FIREPLACE

LIVING AREA

0   5   10
FEET

This one-and-a-half-story cabin has two bedrooms and a loft sleeping area. The loft is over the first floor bedrooms and has clearances of 7 feet at the ridge beam and 3 feet at the outside wall.

An open-type ceiling gives a feeling of spaciousness to the kitchen and living area and cuts construction costs. A prefabricated fireplace is suggested on the plan.

Pole framing helps to make construction easy for the less-experienced builder and eliminates the need for expensive masonry foundations. A wood-frame floor is used in the structure shown and is most suitable for a sloping site. A concrete floor would be more economical when the house is built on a well-drained, level site. A pole-supported deck is suggested for more indoor-outdoor relaxation space.

Rough-sawn native material is used wherever possible. The choice of interior finishing material is left to the builder. Slight changes in the wall framing could be made if insulation and interior finish are to be added.

DORMITORY

SECTION AT CENTER OF STRUCTURE

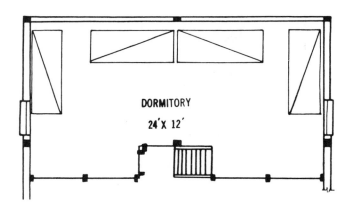

DORMITORY

24' X 12'

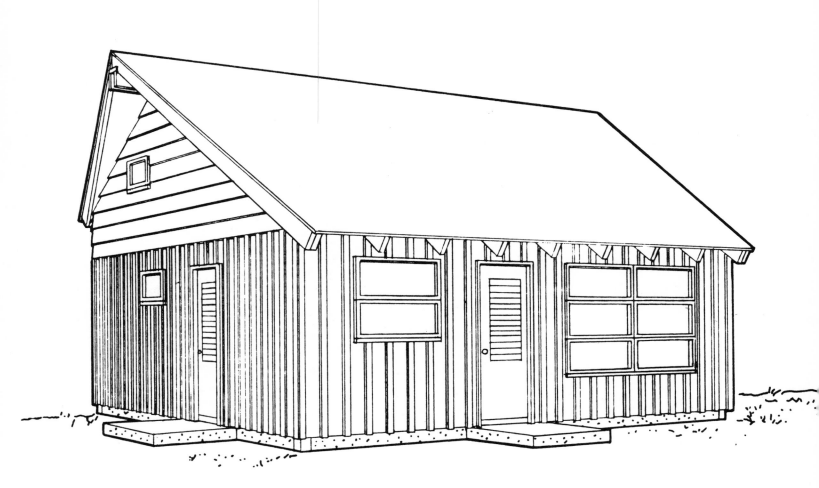

PERSPECTIVE

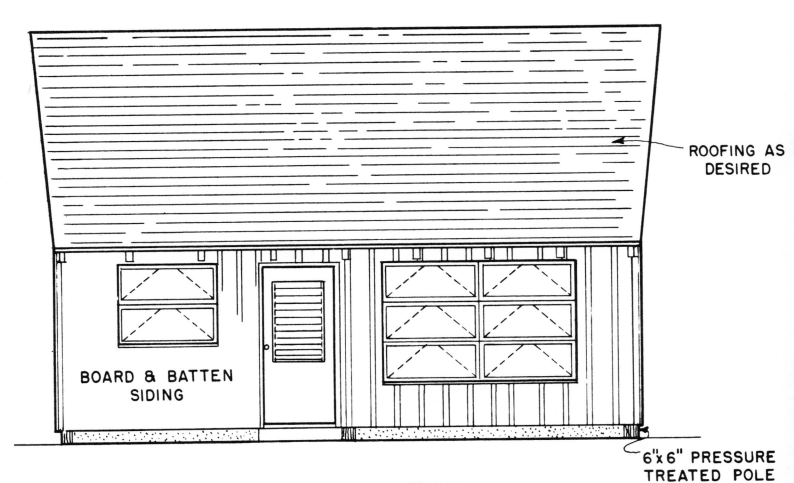

ROOFING AS
DESIRED

BOARD & BATTEN
SIDING

6"x 6" PRESSURE
TREATED POLE

FRONT ELEVATION

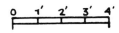

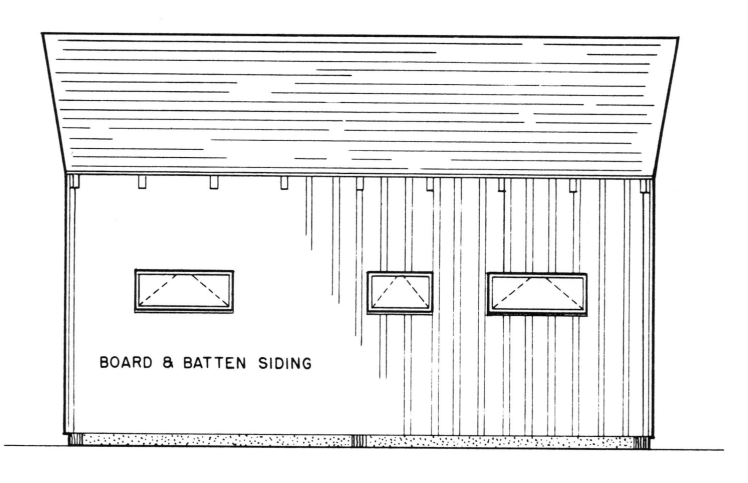

BOARD & BATTEN SIDING

REAR ELEVATION

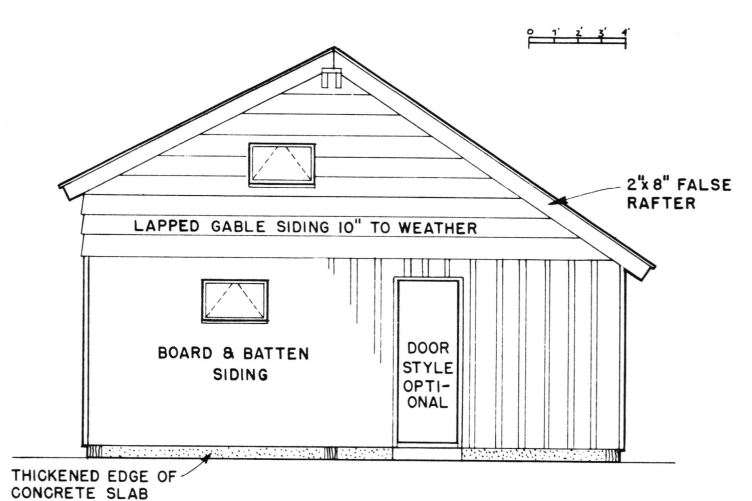

LAPPED GABLE SIDING 10" TO WEATHER

2"x 8" FALSE RAFTER

BOARD & BATTEN SIDING

DOOR STYLE OPTIONAL

THICKENED EDGE OF CONCRETE SLAB

SIDE ELEVATION

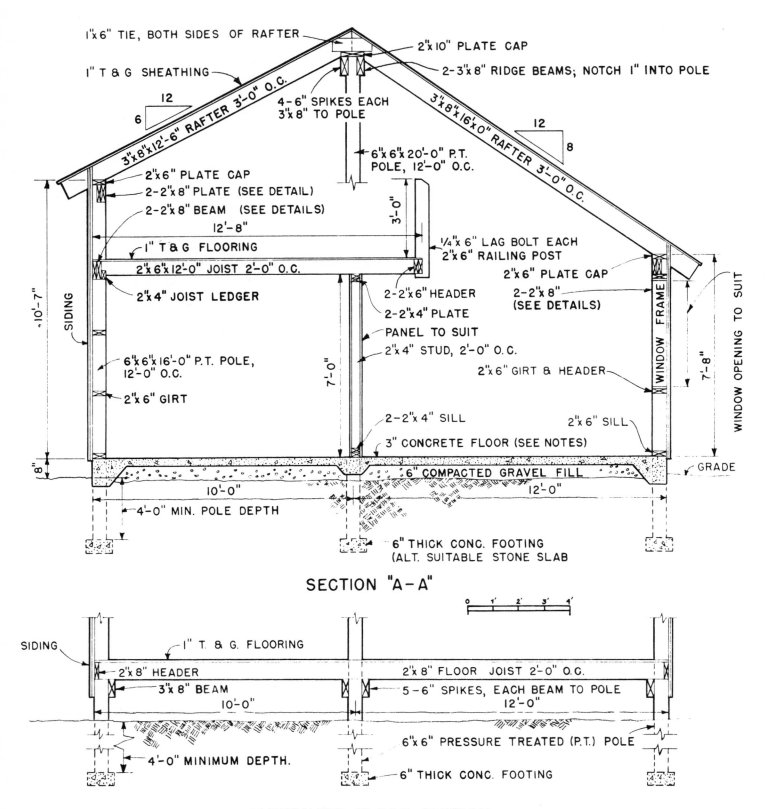

1"x6" TIE, BOTH SIDES OF RAFTER

2"x10" PLATE CAP

1" T & G SHEATHING

2-3"x8" RIDGE BEAMS; NOTCH 1" INTO POLE

3"x8"x12'-6" RAFTER 3'-0" O.C.

12
6

4-6" SPIKES EACH 3"x8" TO POLE

3"x8"x16'-0" RAFTER 3'-0" O.C.

12
8

6"x6"x20'-0" P.T. POLE, 12'-0" O.C.

2"x6" PLATE CAP

2-2"x8" PLATE (SEE DETAIL)

2-2"x8" BEAM (SEE DETAILS)

12'-8"

3'-0"

1" T & G FLOORING

1/4"x 6" LAG BOLT EACH 2"x6" RAILING POST

2"x6"x12'-0" JOIST 2'-0" O.C.

2"x6" PLATE CAP

2"x4" JOIST LEDGER

2-2"x6" HEADER

2-2"x8" (SEE DETAILS)

2-2"x4" PLATE

PANEL TO SUIT

6"x6"x16'-0" P.T. POLE, 12'-0" O.C.

2"x4" STUD, 2'-0" O.C.

2"x6" GIRT & HEADER

7'-0"

2"x6" GIRT

SIDING

10'-7"

WINDOW FRAME

7'-8"

WINDOW OPENING TO SUIT

2-2"x4" SILL

2"x6" SILL

3" CONCRETE FLOOR (SEE NOTES)

6" COMPACTED GRAVEL FILL

GRADE

8"

10'-0"

12'-0"

4'-0" MIN. POLE DEPTH

6" THICK CONC. FOOTING (ALT. SUITABLE STONE SLAB

SECTION "A-A"

SIDING

1" T. & G. FLOORING

0 1' 2' 3' 4'

2"x8" HEADER

2"x8" FLOOR JOIST 2'-0" O.C.

3"x8" BEAM

5-6" SPIKES, EACH BEAM TO POLE 12'-0"

10'-0"

6"x6" PRESSURE TREATED (P.T.) POLE

4'-0" MINIMUM DEPTH.

6" THICK CONC. FOOTING

ALTERNATE FLOOR SECTION

AWNING WINDOW SCHEDULE					
WINDOW	UNIT SIZE	NO. REQ'D	WINDOW	UNIT SIZE	NO. REQ'D
A	1'-8"x 2'-8"	1	G	1'-8"x 4'-1"	2
B	1'-8"x 4'-1"	1	H	1'-8"x 2'-8"	1
C	1'-8"x 2'-8"	1	I	1'-8"x 4'-1"	1
D	1'-8"x 2'-8"	1	J	1'-8"x 2'-8"	1
E	1'-8"x 2'-8"	1	K	1'-8"x 2'-8"	1
F	1'-8"x 4'-1"	6			

ALL AWNING WINDOW UNIT SIZES ARE APPROXIMATE.
OTHER WINDOW STYLES OR SIZES MAY BY SUBSTITUTED.

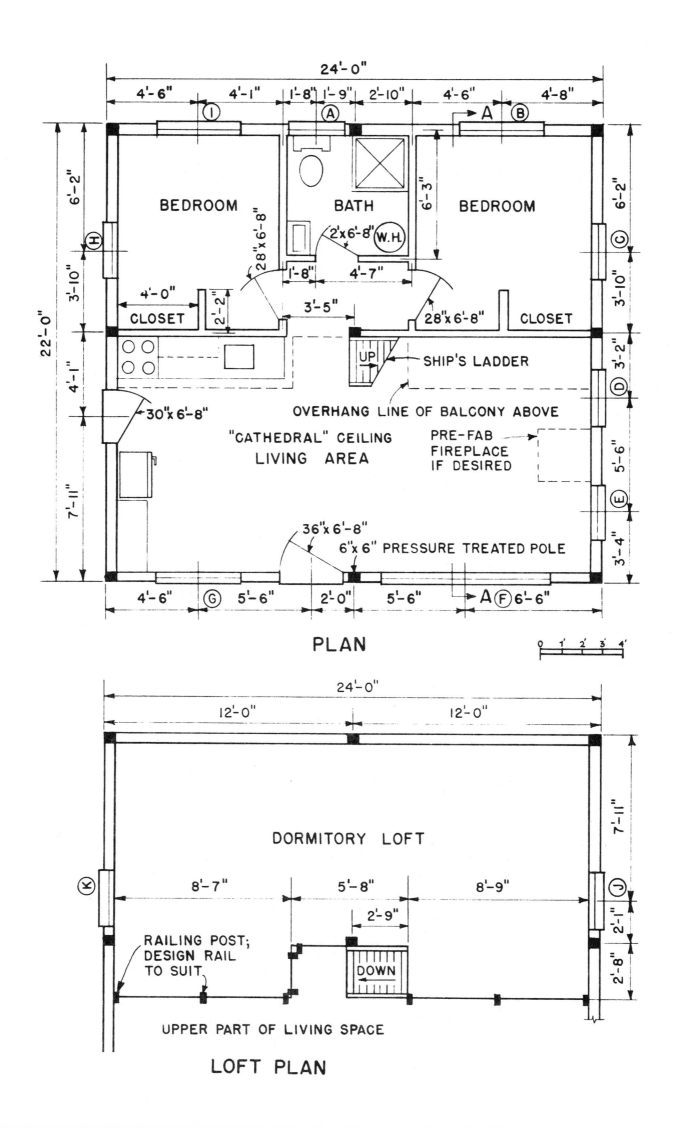

24'-0"

4'-6" | 4'-1" | 1'-8" | 1'-9" | 2'-10" | 4'-6" | 4'-8"

Ⓘ | Ⓐ | A Ⓑ

22'-0"

6'-2"

BEDROOM

28"x6'-8"

2'x6'-8" Ⓦ.Ⓗ.

BATH

6'-3"

BEDROOM

6'-2"

Ⓗ

3'-10"

4'-0"

CLOSET

2'-2"

1'-8"

4'-7"

3'-5"

28"x6'-8"

CLOSET

Ⓒ

3'-10"

4'-1"

UP

SHIP'S LADDER

30"x6'-8"

OVERHANG LINE OF BALCONY ABOVE

Ⓓ

3'-2"

7'-11"

"CATHEDRAL" CEILING
LIVING AREA

PRE-FAB
FIREPLACE
IF DESIRED

5'-6"

Ⓔ

36"x6'-8"

6"x 6" PRESSURE TREATED POLE

3'-4"

4'-6" | Ⓖ | 5'-6" | 2'-0" | 5'-6" | A Ⓕ 6'-6"

PLAN

0 1' 2' 3' 4'

24'-0"

12'-0" | 12'-0"

DORMITORY LOFT

7'-11"

Ⓚ

8'-7" | 5'-8" | 8'-9"

Ⓙ

2'-9"

2'-1"

RAILING POST;
DESIGN RAIL
TO SUIT

DOWN

2'-8"

UPPER PART OF LIVING SPACE

LOFT PLAN

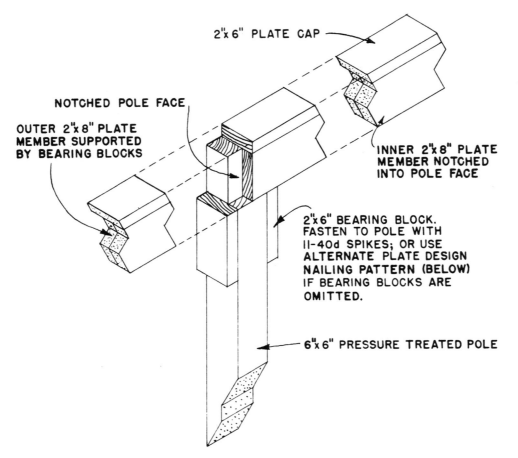

2"x 6" PLATE CAP

NOTCHED POLE FACE

OUTER 2"x 8" PLATE
MEMBER SUPPORTED
BY BEARING BLOCKS

INNER 2"x 8" PLATE
MEMBER NOTCHED
INTO POLE FACE

2"x 6" BEARING BLOCK.
FASTEN TO POLE WITH
11-40d SPIKES; OR USE
ALTERNATE PLATE DESIGN
NAILING PATTERN (BELOW)
IF BEARING BLOCKS ARE
OMITTED.

6"x 6" PRESSURE TREATED POLE

PLATE POLE DETAIL
NO SCALE

ALTERNATE PLATE DESIGN

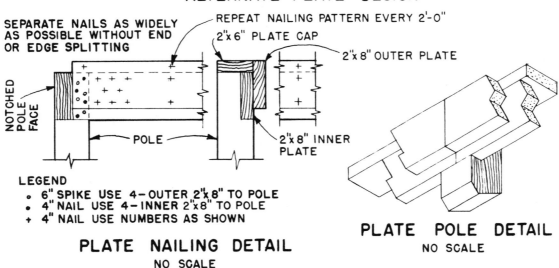

SEPARATE NAILS AS WIDELY
AS POSSIBLE WITHOUT END
OR EDGE SPLITTING

REPEAT NAILING PATTERN EVERY 2'-0"

2"x 6" PLATE CAP

2"x 8" OUTER PLATE

NOTCHED POLE FACE

POLE

2"x 8" INNER
PLATE

LEGEND
- o 6" SPIKE USE 4—OUTER 2"x 8" TO POLE
- • 4" NAIL USE 4—INNER 2"x 8" TO POLE
- + 4" NAIL USE NUMBERS AS SHOWN

PLATE NAILING DETAIL
NO SCALE

PLATE POLE DETAIL
NO SCALE

CONSTRUCTION NOTES

1. THIS DESIGN IS BASED ON ROUGH-SAWN EASTERN HEMLOCK.
2. DESIGN ROOF LOAD – 40 LBS. PER. SQ. FT.
3. DESIGN FLOOR LOAD (WOOD FRAME) 35 LBS. PER. SQ. FT.
4. CONCRETE SLAB FLOOR HAS THICKENED EDGE 12" DEEP, 8" WIDE ALONG BOTTOM EDGE; CONCRETE MIX: ¾" MAXIMUM AGGREGATE SIZE, 6½ SACKS OF CEMENT PER CUBIC YARD, AND 6 GAL. WATER CEMENT RATIO.
5. FOR CONCRETE SLABS ON OTHER THAN WELL DRAINED SOIL, WELL COMPACTED, USE 6"x 6"-NO. 10 WIRE REINFORCING MESH.
6. SPECIFIED POLE LENGTHS ARE FOR CONCRETE SLAB DESIGN ONLY. LONGER POLES ARE REQUIRED FOR WOOD FRAME FLOOR DESIGN; LENGTH OF POLE IS DEPENDENT ON SLOPE OF BUILDING SITE AND SETTING POLE IN GROUND TO MAX. DEPTH OR FIRM FOOTING.
7. CONVENTIONAL STUD FRAME CONSTRUCTION ON MASONRY FOUNDATION MAY BE SUBSTITUTED FOR POLE FRAME IF DESIRED.
8. INTERIOR AND EXTERIOR FINISH IS LEFT TO BUILDER'S DISCRETION, NO ATTEMPT WAS MADE TO PROVIDE MODULAR INTERIOR DIMENSIONS; SLIGHT CHANGES IN GIRT SPACING MAY BE DESIREABLE IF INTERIOR FINISHING IS DESIRED.

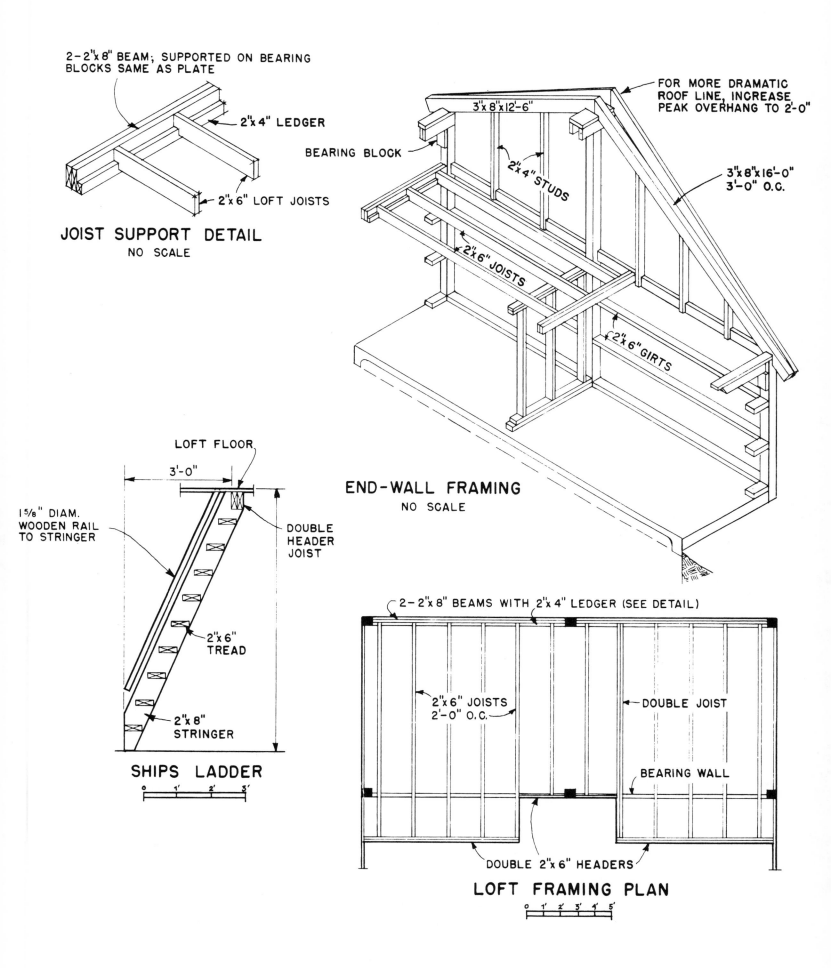

2-2"x 8" BEAM; SUPPORTED ON BEARING BLOCKS SAME AS PLATE

2"x 4" LEDGER

2"x 6" LOFT JOISTS

JOIST SUPPORT DETAIL
NO SCALE

FOR MORE DRAMATIC ROOF LINE, INCREASE PEAK OVERHANG TO 2'-0"

3"x 8"x12'-6"

BEARING BLOCK

2"x 4" STUDS

3"x 8"x16'-0" 3'-0" O.C.

2"x 6" JOISTS

2"x 6" GIRTS

END-WALL FRAMING
NO SCALE

LOFT FLOOR

3'-0"

1⁵⁄₈" DIAM. WOODEN RAIL TO STRINGER

DOUBLE HEADER JOIST

2"x 6" TREAD

2"x 8" STRINGER

SHIPS LADDER

0   1'   2'   3'

2-2"x 8" BEAMS WITH 2"x 4" LEDGER (SEE DETAIL)

2"x 6" JOISTS 2'-0" O.C.

DOUBLE JOIST

BEARING WALL

DOUBLE 2"x 6" HEADERS

LOFT FRAMING PLAN

0   1'   2'   3'   4'   5'

7. and 8. 24-FOOT and 36-FOOT A-FRAME VACATION HOMES

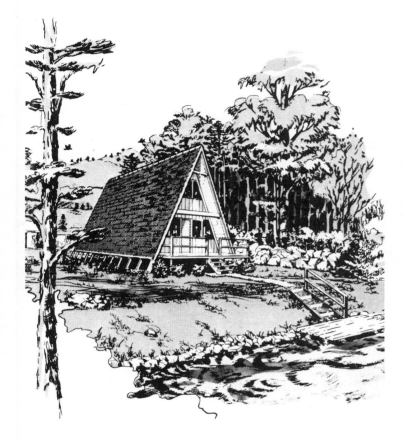

These two cabins are designed for recreational purposes in mountain areas or at a beach. They can be built by three or four people who have reasonable ability in the use of tools. Someone with a knowledge of concrete work may be required to place the footings. The frame itself should present no problems; nor should erection of the end walls, roof, and interior partitions. It is assumed that electricity will be available at the site to permit the use of power tools and to provide for lighting, heating, and cooking.

Each cabin is provided with a modern kitchen that contains a refrigerator, range, sink, and adequate cabinet space. Provision is made for a water heater under one corner of the floor cabinet arrangement. The bathroom contains a lavatory, toilet, and shower. A storage locker for linens is provided in the bathroom. The water supply would probably come from a well or spring; where the piping is exposed to the outside air it should be properly insulated and provided with drain valves so that all water can be drained from the system when the cabin is not occupied during winter weather.

See page 57 for additional information on construction of A-frame structures.

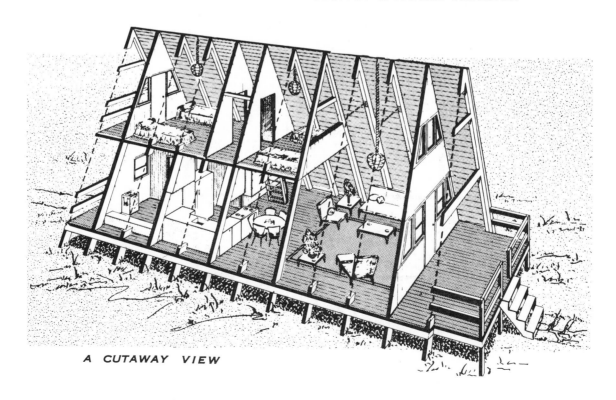

A CUTAWAY VIEW

The 36-foot-long cabin contains three bedrooms, one on the first floor and two on the second floor. The front bedroom on the second floor is a balcony that overlooks the two-story living room. If sleeping space for more than six persons is required, cots can be placed in the living room.

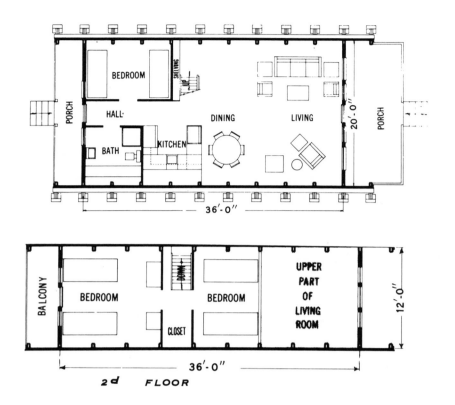

The 24-foot-long cabin contains two bedrooms, both on the second floor. The living-dining area is smaller than that in the 36-foot cabin. The living room is only one story high.

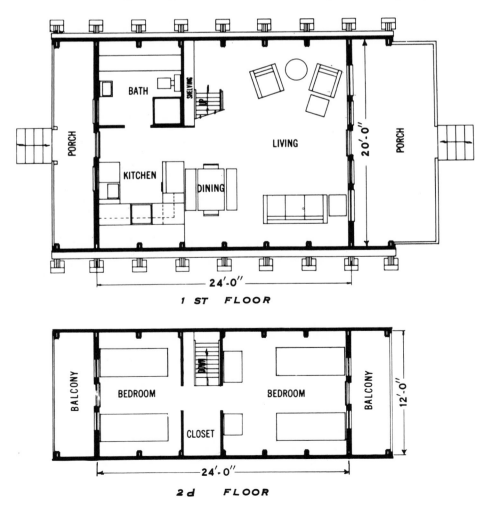

Other features in both cabins

Ventilation in both cabins is good; the windows at each end provide excellent circulation of air.

Storage shelving is indicated adjacent to the "ship's ladder" that leads to the second floor.

If a fireplace is desired, a prefabricated unit may be installed. Wood may be stored under the cabin for use during winter or for cooking.

The working drawings of the smaller cabin show that the size of the rear bedroom can be increased by extending the second floor to include the rear balcony. The second floor can also be extended at the front of the cabin if desired. If this is done, the door shown on the plan should be replaced by a double-hung window.

View of section

This section gives some ideas for constructing the A-frame. After the footings have been placed, the lower half of the frame may be erected and the rough flooring nailed in place at the first- and second-floor levels. The second floor can be used as a work platform while the upper half of the frame is put in place. The roof sheathing should then be put on, followed by the finished roofing. The end walls may then be framed and completed and, finally, the interior partitions.

For added protection in cold climates the space under the first floor and in the end walls should be insulated. Additional insulation may be installed on the underside of the roof sheathing between the frames if the climate requires.

SECTION
· VIEW FROM LIVING ROOM TOWARD THE REAR ·

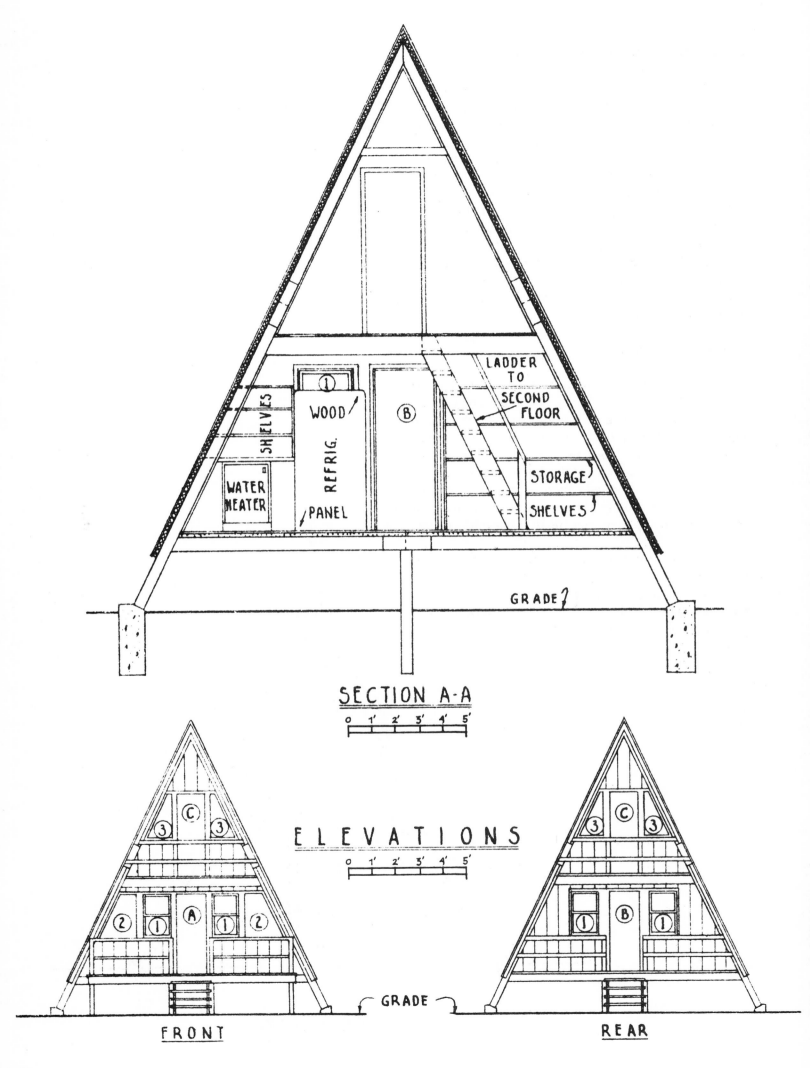

SECTION A-A

0 1' 2' 3' 4' 5'

ELEVATIONS

0 1' 2' 3' 4' 5'

FRONT

REAR

GRADE

44

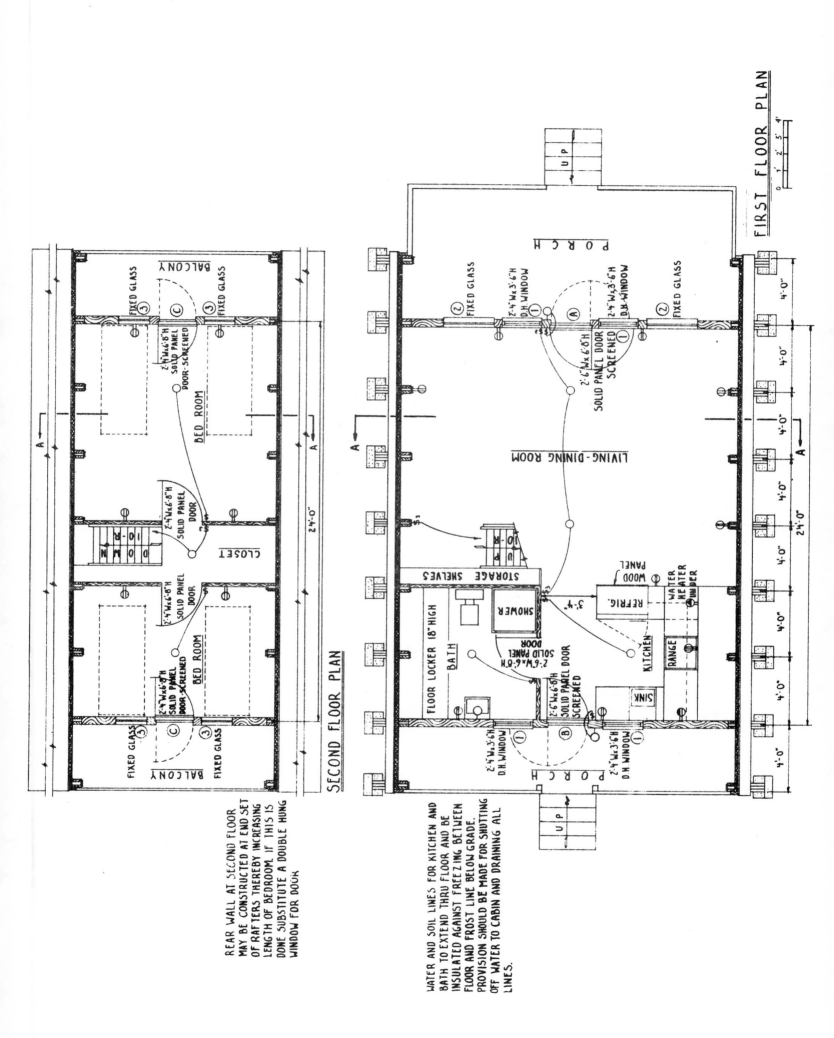

REAR WALL AT SECOND FLOOR MAY BE CONSTRUCTED AT END SET OF RAFTERS THEREBY INCREASING LENGTH OF BEDROOM. IF THIS IS DONE SUBSTITUTE A DOUBLE HUNG WINDOW FOR DOOR

SECOND FLOOR PLAN

WATER AND SOIL LINES FOR KITCHEN AND BATH TO EXTEND THRU FLOOR AND BE INSULATED AGAINST FREEZING BETWEEN FLOOR AND FROST LINE BELOW GRADE. PROVISION SHOULD BE MADE FOR SHUTTING OFF WATER TO CABIN AND DRAINING ALL LINES.

FIRST FLOOR PLAN

45

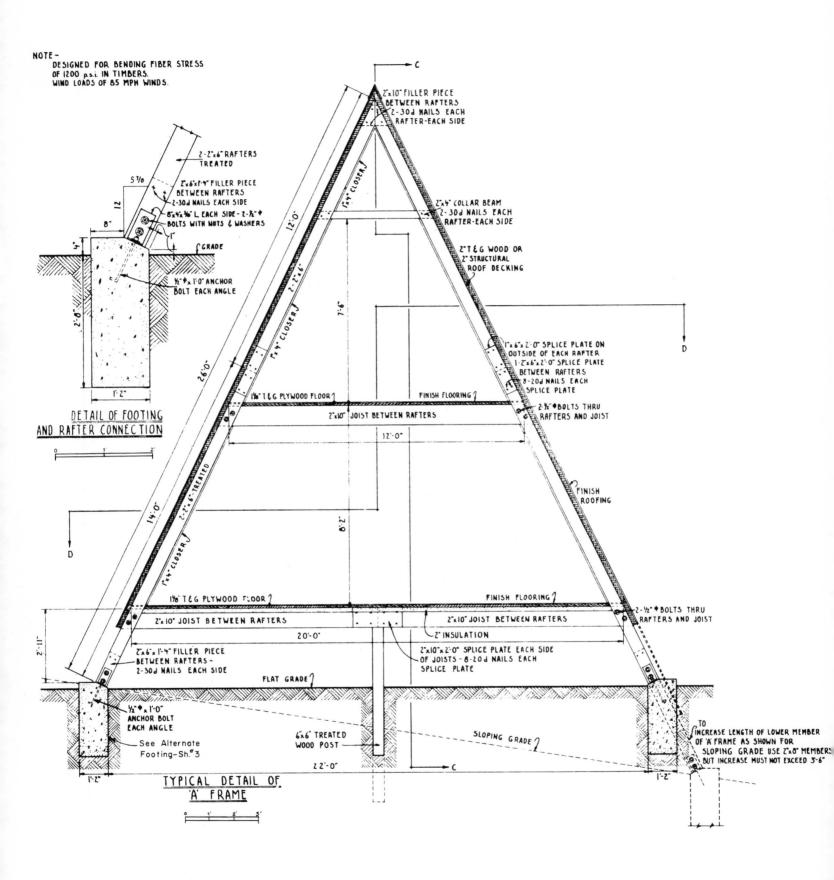

NOTE—
DESIGNED FOR BENDING FIBER STRESS
OF 1200 p.s.i. IN TIMBERS.
WIND LOADS OF 85 MPH WINDS.

2"x10" FILLER PIECE
BETWEEN RAFTERS
2-30d NAILS EACH
RAFTER-EACH SIDE

2-2"x6" RAFTERS
TREATED

2"x6"x1'-4" FILLER PIECE
BETWEEN RAFTERS
2-30d NAILS EACH SIDE
8"x4"x³⁄₈" L EACH SIDE-2-½" Ø
BOLTS WITH NUTS & WASHERS

2"x4" COLLAR BEAM
2-30d NAILS EACH
RAFTER-EACH SIDE

2"T&G WOOD OR
2" STRUCTURAL
ROOF DECKING

GRADE

½" Ø x 1'-0" ANCHOR
BOLT EACH ANGLE

1"x6"x2'-0" SPLICE PLATE ON
OUTSIDE OF EACH RAFTER
1-2"x6"x2'-0" SPLICE PLATE
BETWEEN RAFTERS
8-20d NAILS EACH
SPLICE PLATE

DETAIL OF FOOTING
AND RAFTER CONNECTION

1⅛" T&G PLYWOOD FLOOR

FINISH FLOORING

2"x10" JOIST BETWEEN RAFTERS

2-½" Ø BOLTS THRU
RAFTERS AND JOIST

12'-0"

FINISH
ROOFING

1⅛" T&G PLYWOOD FLOOR

FINISH FLOORING

2"x10" JOIST BETWEEN RAFTERS

2"x10" JOIST BETWEEN RAFTERS

2-½" Ø BOLTS THRU
RAFTERS AND JOIST

20'-0"

2" INSULATION

2"x6"x1'-4" FILLER PIECE
BETWEEN RAFTERS-
2-30d NAILS EACH SIDE

2"x10"x2'-0" SPLICE PLATE EACH SIDE
OF JOISTS-8-20d NAILS EACH
SPLICE PLATE

FLAT GRADE

½" Ø x 1'-0"
ANCHOR BOLT
EACH ANGLE

See Alternate
Footing-Sh.#3

6"x6" TREATED
WOOD POST

SLOPING GRADE

TO
INCREASE LENGTH OF LOWER MEMBER
OF 'A' FRAME AS SHOWN FOR
SLOPING GRADE USE 2"x8" MEMBERS
BUT INCREASE MUST NOT EXCEED 3'-6"

22'-0"

TYPICAL DETAIL OF
'A' FRAME

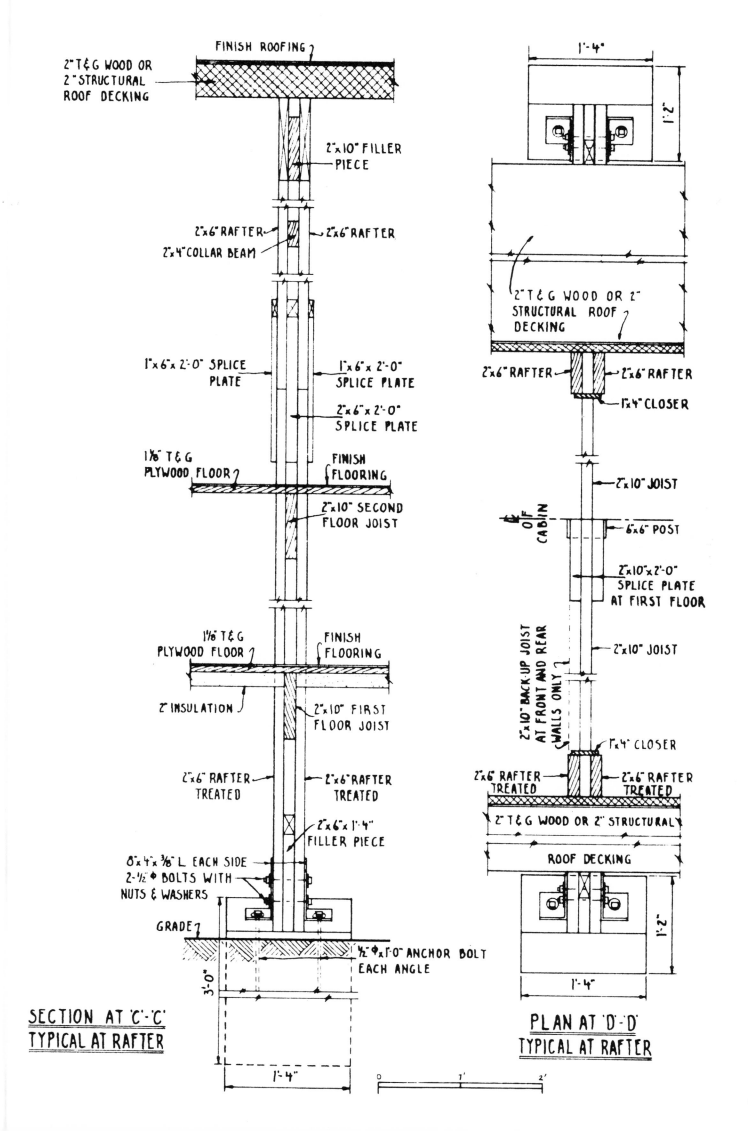

FINISH ROOFING

2" T&G WOOD OR 2" STRUCTURAL ROOF DECKING

2"x10" FILLER PIECE

2"x6" RAFTER

2"x6" RAFTER

2"x4" COLLAR BEAM

1"x6"x2'-0" SPLICE PLATE

1"x6"x2'-0" SPLICE PLATE

2"x6"x2'-0" SPLICE PLATE

1⅛" T&G PLYWOOD FLOOR

FINISH FLOORING

2"x10" SECOND FLOOR JOIST

1⅛" T&G PLYWOOD FLOOR

FINISH FLOORING

2" INSULATION

2"x10" FIRST FLOOR JOIST

2"x6" RAFTER TREATED

2"x6" RAFTER TREATED

2"x6"x1'-4" FILLER PIECE

8"x4"x⅜" L EACH SIDE
2-½" Φ BOLTS WITH NUTS & WASHERS

GRADE

½"Φ x 1'-0" ANCHOR BOLT EACH ANGLE

3'-0"

1'-4"

SECTION AT 'C'-'C'
TYPICAL AT RAFTER

1'-4"

1'-2"

2" T&G WOOD OR 2" STRUCTURAL ROOF DECKING

2"x6" RAFTER

2"x6" RAFTER

1"x4" CLOSER

2"x10" JOIST

6"x6" POST

2"x10"x2'-0" SPLICE PLATE AT FIRST FLOOR

2"x10" JOIST

2"x10" BACK-UP JOIST AT FRONT AND REAR (WALLS ONLY)

℄ OF CABIN

1"x4" CLOSER

2"x6" RAFTER TREATED

2"x6" RAFTER TREATED

2" T&G WOOD OR 2" STRUCTURAL

ROOF DECKING

1'-2"

1'-4"

PLAN AT 'D'-'D'
TYPICAL AT RAFTER

0   1'   2'

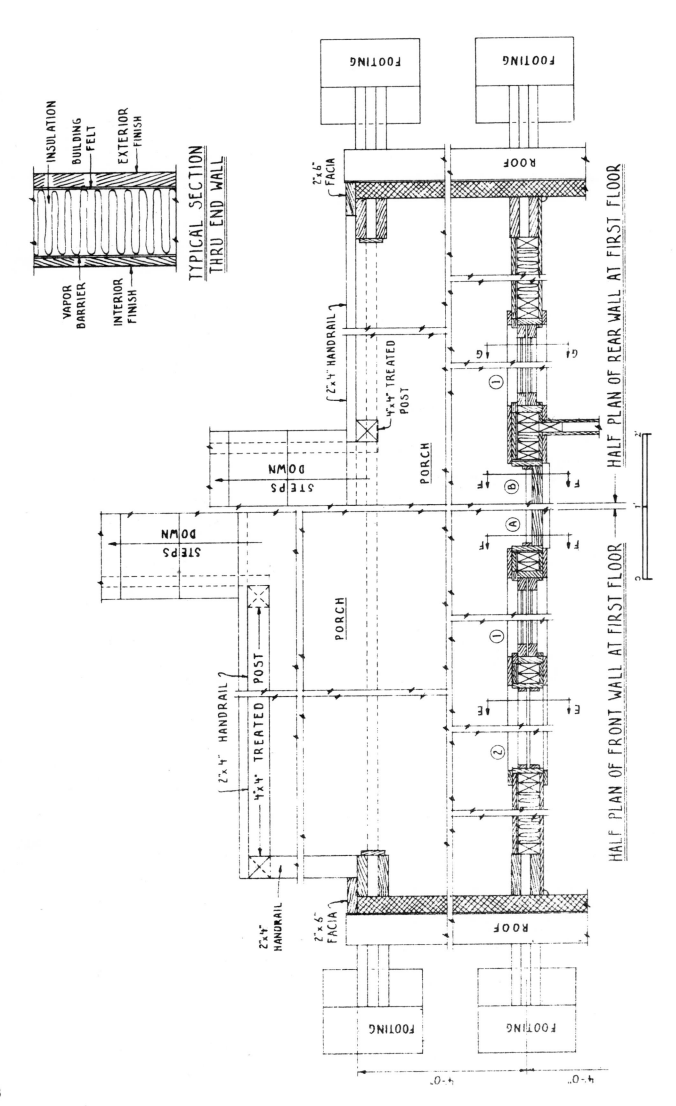

INSULATION
BUILDING FELT
EXTERIOR FINISH

VAPOR BARRIER
INTERIOR FINISH

TYPICAL SECTION
THRU END WALL

FOOTING

FOOTING

ROOF

2"x6" FACIA

HALF PLAN OF REAR WALL AT FIRST FLOOR

2"x4" HANDRAIL

4"x4" TREATED POST

PORCH

STEPS DOWN

G

G

①

B

F

F

A

F

F

①

E

E

②

HALF PLAN OF FRONT WALL AT FIRST FLOOR

STEPS DOWN

PORCH

2"x4" HANDRAIL

4"x4" TREATED POST

2"x4" HANDRAIL

2"x6" FACIA

ROOF

FOOTING

FOOTING

4'-0"

4'-0"

48

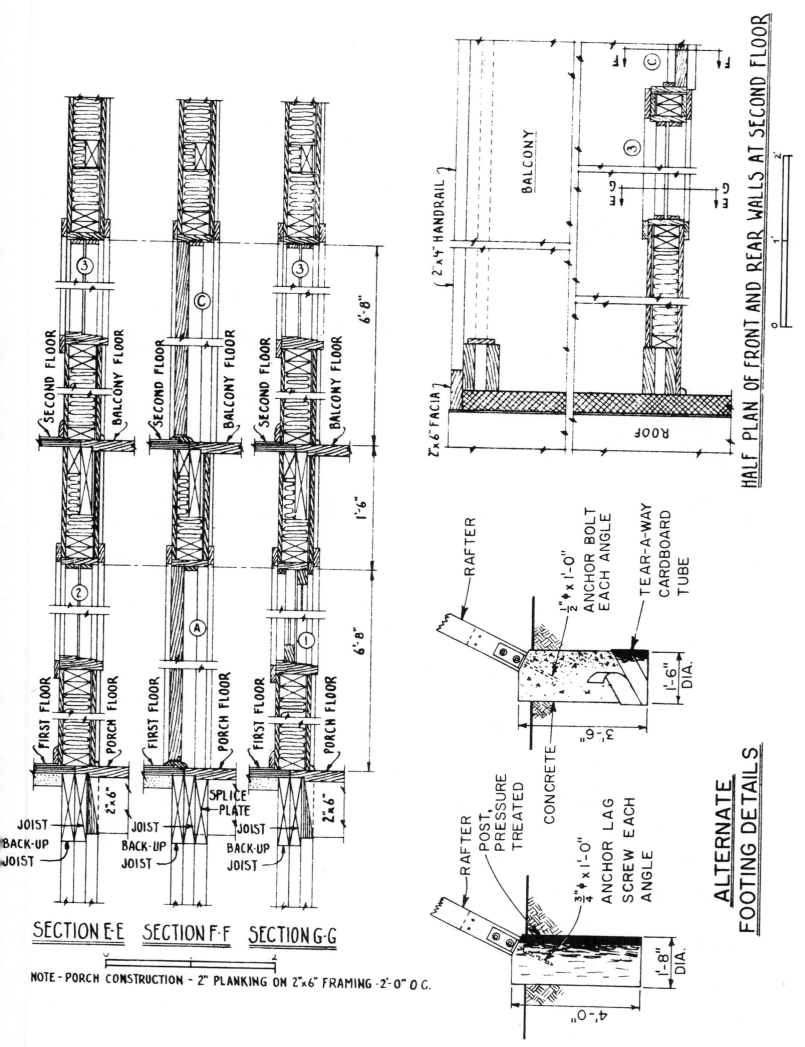

SECTION E-E   SECTION F-F   SECTION G-G

NOTE - PORCH CONSTRUCTION - 2" PLANKING ON 2"x6" FRAMING - 2'-0" O.C.

SECOND FLOOR
BALCONY FLOOR
6'-8"
1'-6"
6'-8"
FIRST FLOOR
PORCH FLOOR

JOIST
BACK-UP JOIST
2"x6"
SPLICE PLATE

2"x4" HANDRAIL
2"x6" FACIA
BALCONY
ROOF

HALF PLAN OF FRONT AND REAR WALLS AT SECOND FLOOR

RAFTER
½"φ x 1'-0" ANCHOR BOLT EACH ANGLE
TEAR-A-WAY CARDBOARD TUBE
1'-6" DIA.
3'-6"
CONCRETE

RAFTER
POST, PRESSURE TREATED
¾"φ x 1'-0" ANCHOR LAG SCREW EACH ANGLE
1'-8" DIA.
4'-0"

ALTERNATE FOOTING DETAILS

49

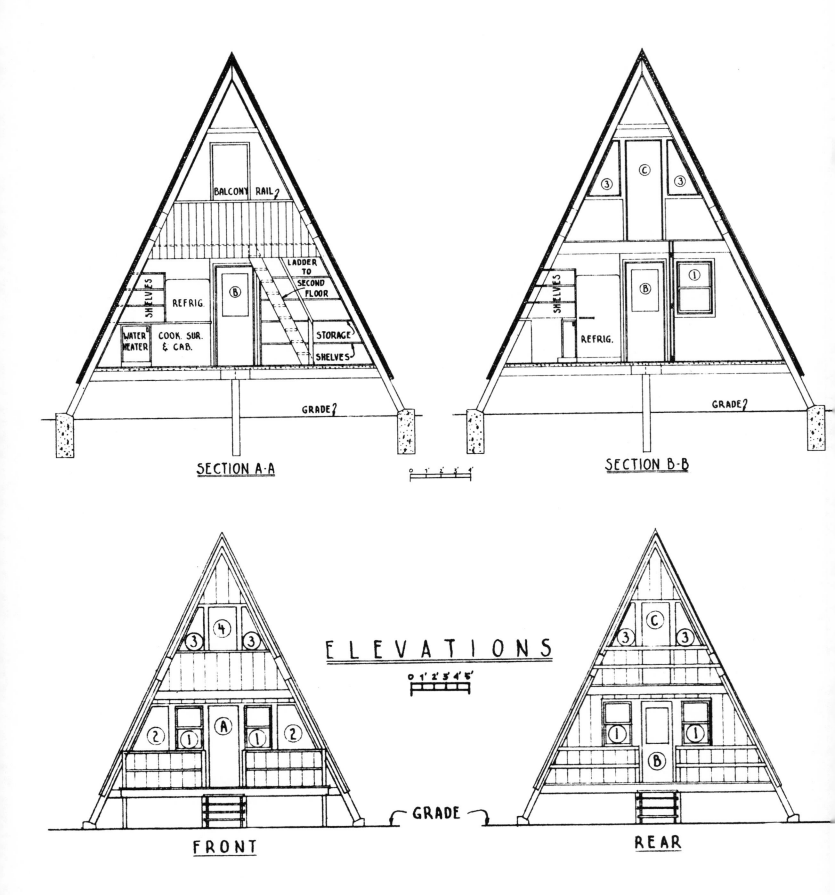

BALCONY RAIL

SHELVES
REFRIG.
WATER HEATER
COOK. SUR. & CAB.

LADDER TO SECOND FLOOR

STORAGE
SHELVES

GRADE

SECTION A-A

SHELVES
REFRIG.

GRADE

SECTION B-B

ELEVATIONS

FRONT

REAR

GRADE

50

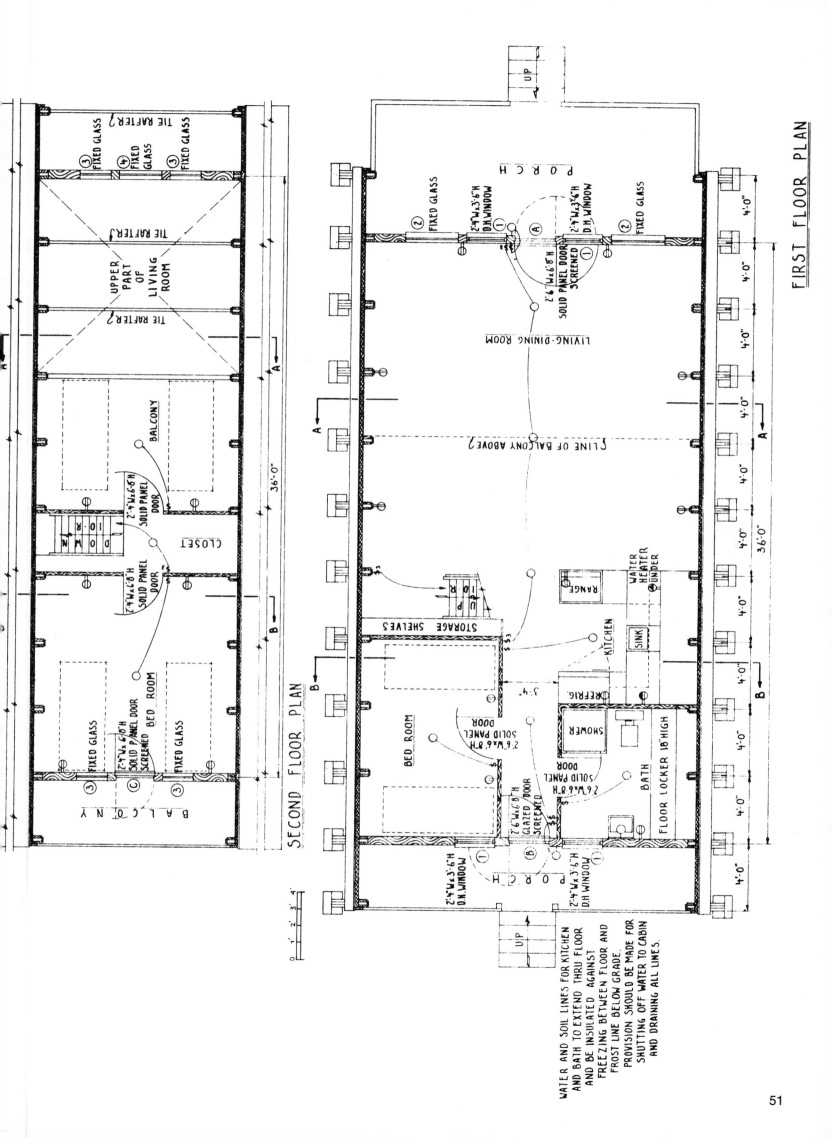

SECOND FLOOR PLAN

TIE RAFTER
FIXED GLASS ③
FIXED GLASS ④
FIXED GLASS ③
TIE RAFTER
UPPER PART OF LIVING ROOM
TIE RAFTER
BALCONY
2'-4"W x 6'-6" H SOLID PANEL DOOR
D O O R
2'-4"W x 6'-6" H SOLID PANEL DOOR
CLOSET
BED ROOM
2'-4"W x 6'-6" H SOLID PANEL DOOR SCREENED
FIXED GLASS ③
FIXED GLASS ③
Ⓒ
B A L C O N Y
36'-0"

FIRST FLOOR PLAN

UP
P O R C H
FIXED GLASS ②
2'-4"W x 3'-6" H D.H. WINDOW ①
Ⓐ
2'-6"W x 6'-9" H SOLID PANEL DOOR SCREENED
2'-4"W x 3'-6" H D.H. WINDOW ①
FIXED GLASS ②
LIVING-DINING ROOM
Ⓛ LINE OF BALCONY ABOVE
STORAGE SHELVES
UP
RANGE
WATER HEATER UNDER
KITCHEN
SINK
REFRIG.
BED ROOM
2'-6"W x 6'-8" H SOLID PANEL DOOR
3'-4"
SHOWER
2'-6"W x 6'-8" H SOLID PANEL DOOR
BATH
FLOOR LOCKER 18" HIGH
2'-6"W x 6'-9" H GLAZED DOOR SCREENED
Ⓑ
2'-4"W x 3'-6" H D.H. WINDOW ①
P O R C H
2'-4"W x 3'-6" H D.H. WINDOW ①
UP
36'-0"

4'-0" (×9)

WATER AND SOIL LINES FOR KITCHEN AND BATH TO EXTEND THRU FLOOR AND BE INSULATED AGAINST FREEZING BETWEEN FLOOR AND FROST LINE BELOW GRADE. PROVISION SHOULD BE MADE FOR SHUTTING OFF WATER TO CABIN AND DRAINING ALL LINES.

0 1' 2' 3' 4'

51

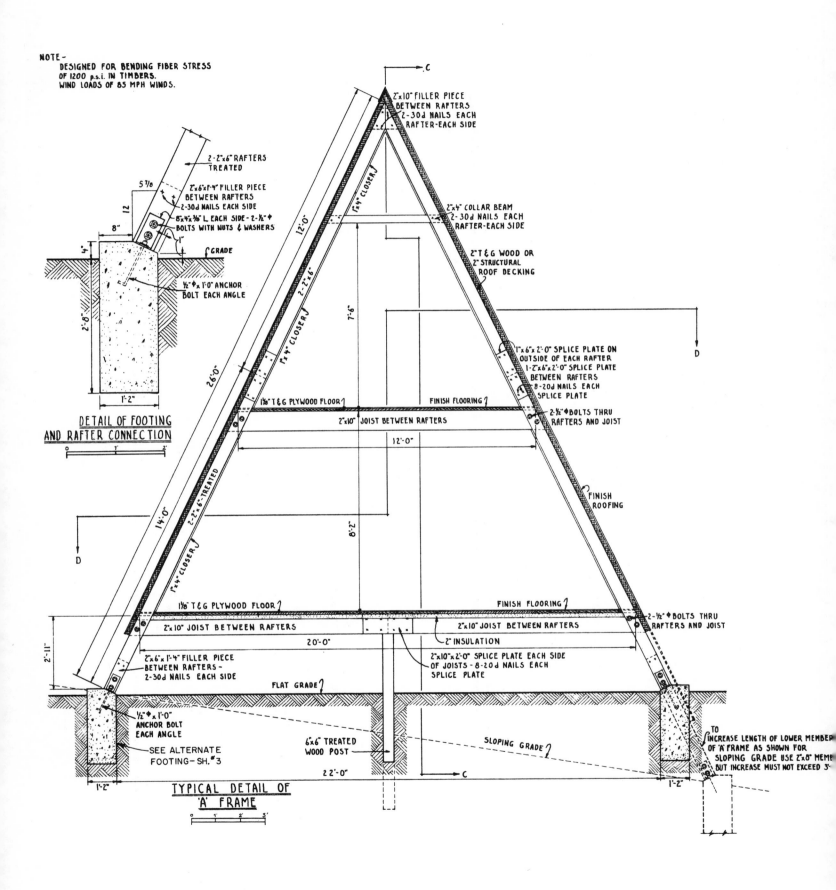

NOTE-
DESIGNED FOR BENDING FIBER STRESS
OF 1200 p.s.i. IN TIMBERS.
WIND LOADS OF 85 MPH WINDS.

2"x6" RAFTERS TREATED

2"x6"x1'-4" FILLER PIECE
BETWEEN RAFTERS
2-30d NAILS EACH SIDE

5⅞

12

8"

8"x4"x⅜" L EACH SIDE-2-½"⌀
BOLTS WITH NUTS & WASHERS

4"

1"

GRADE

2'-8"

½"⌀x1'-0" ANCHOR
BOLT EACH ANGLE

1'-2"

DETAIL OF FOOTING
AND RAFTER CONNECTION

0   1   2

2"x10" FILLER PIECE
BETWEEN RAFTERS
2-30d NAILS EACH
RAFTER-EACH SIDE

C

1"x4" CLOSER

12'-0"

2-2"x6"

2"x4" COLLAR BEAM
2-30d NAILS EACH
RAFTER-EACH SIDE

2"T&G WOOD OR
2" STRUCTURAL
ROOF DECKING

1"x4" CLOSER

7'-6"

26'-0"

D

1"x6"x2'-0" SPLICE PLATE ON
OUTSIDE OF EACH RAFTER
1-2"x6"x2'-0" SPLICE PLATE
BETWEEN RAFTERS
8-20d NAILS EACH
SPLICE PLATE

1⅛" T&G PLYWOOD FLOOR

FINISH FLOORING

2"x10" JOIST BETWEEN RAFTERS

12'-0"

2-½"⌀BOLTS THRU
RAFTERS AND JOIST

14'-0"

2-2"x6"-TREATED

8'-2"

FINISH
ROOFING

D

1"x4" CLOSER

2'-11"

1⅛" T&G PLYWOOD FLOOR

FINISH FLOORING

2"x10" JOIST BETWEEN RAFTERS

20'-0"

2"x10" JOIST BETWEEN RAFTERS

2-½"⌀ BOLTS THRU
RAFTERS AND JOIST

2" INSULATION

2"x6"x1'-4" FILLER PIECE
BETWEEN RAFTERS-
2-30d NAILS EACH SIDE

FLAT GRADE

2"x10"x2'-0" SPLICE PLATE EACH SIDE
OF JOISTS-8-20d NAILS EACH
SPLICE PLATE

½"⌀x1'-0"
ANCHOR BOLT
EACH ANGLE

SEE ALTERNATE
FOOTING-SH. #3

6"x6" TREATED
WOOD POST

SLOPING GRADE

22'-0"

C

1'-2"

1'-2"

TO
INCREASE LENGTH OF LOWER MEMBER
OF 'A' FRAME AS SHOWN FOR
SLOPING GRADE USE 2"x8" MEMBER
BUT INCREASE MUST NOT EXCEED 3'

TYPICAL DETAIL OF
'A' FRAME

0   1   2   3

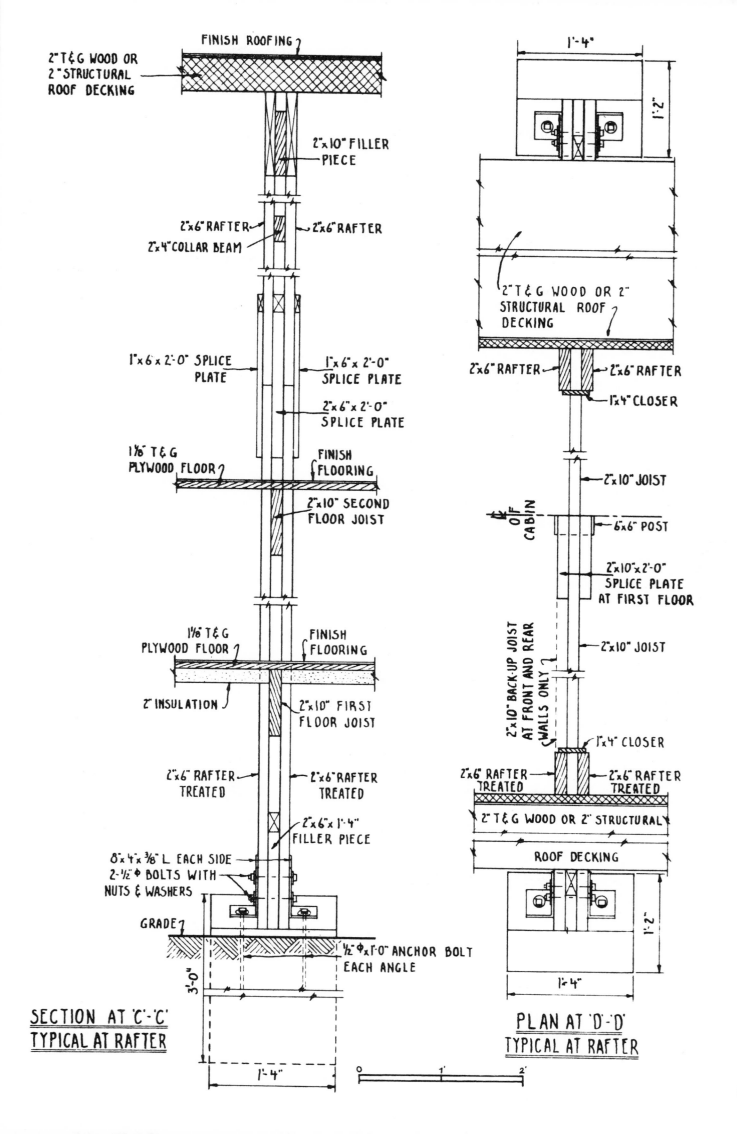

FINISH ROOFING

2" T&G WOOD OR
2" STRUCTURAL
ROOF DECKING

2"x10" FILLER
PIECE

2"x6" RAFTER   2"x6" RAFTER
2"x4" COLLAR BEAM

1"x 6"x 2'-0" SPLICE
PLATE

1"x 6"x 2'-0"
SPLICE PLATE

2"x 6"x 2'-0"
SPLICE PLATE

1⅛" T&G
PLYWOOD FLOOR   FINISH
                      FLOORING

2"x10" SECOND
FLOOR JOIST

1⅛" T&G
PLYWOOD FLOOR   FINISH
                      FLOORING

2" INSULATION

2"x10" FIRST
FLOOR JOIST

2"x6" RAFTER   2"x6" RAFTER
TREATED   TREATED

2"x6"x 1'-4"
FILLER PIECE

8"x 4"x ⅜" L EACH SIDE
2-½" ⏀ BOLTS WITH
NUTS & WASHERS

GRADE

½" ⏀ x 1'-0" ANCHOR BOLT
EACH ANGLE

3'-0"

1'-4"

SECTION AT 'C'-'C'
TYPICAL AT RAFTER

0   1'   2'

1'-4"

1'-2"

2" T&G WOOD OR 2"
STRUCTURAL ROOF
DECKING

2"x6" RAFTER   2"x6" RAFTER

1"x4" CLOSER

2"x10" JOIST

₵ OF CABIN   6x6" POST

2"x10"x2'-0"
SPLICE PLATE
AT FIRST FLOOR

2"x10" BACK-UP JOIST
AT FRONT AND REAR
WALLS ONLY

2"x10" JOIST

1"x4" CLOSER

2"x6" RAFTER   2"x6" RAFTER
TREATED   TREATED

2" T&G WOOD OR 2" STRUCTURAL

ROOF DECKING

1'-2"

1'-4"

PLAN AT 'D'-'D'
TYPICAL AT RAFTER

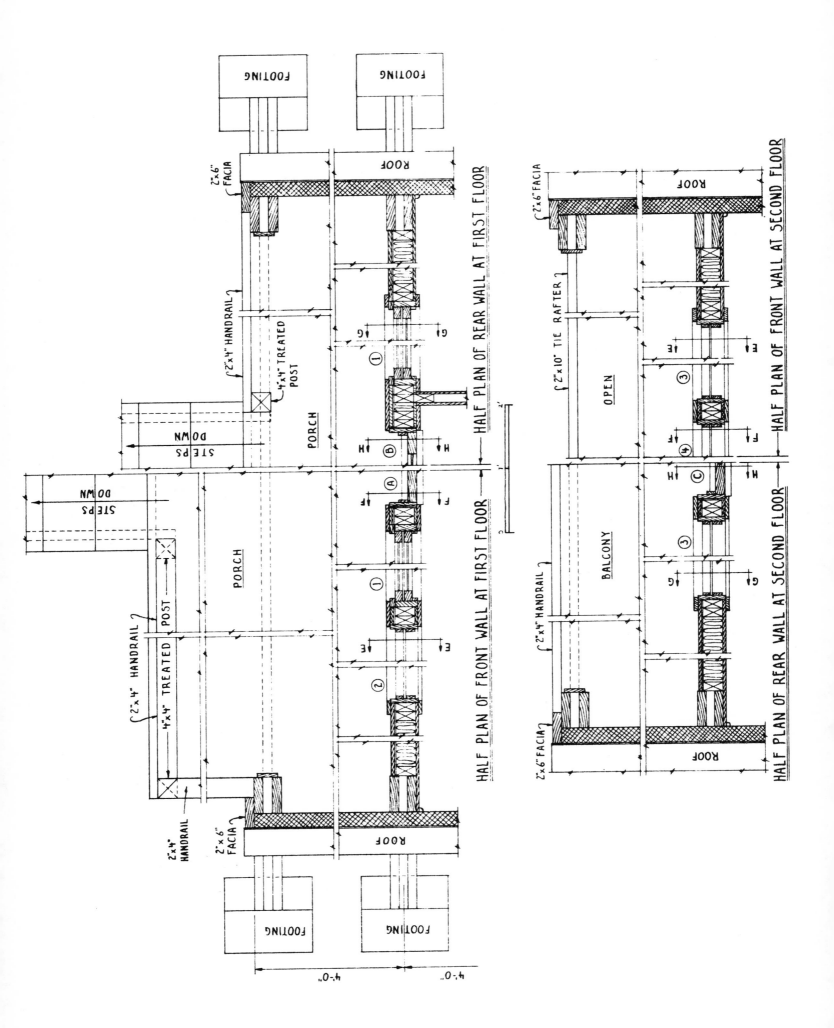

2"×6" FACIA

2"×4" HANDRAIL

4"×4" TREATED POST

STEPS DOWN

PORCH

HALF PLAN OF REAR WALL AT FIRST FLOOR

ROOF

FOOTING

FOOTING

2"×4" HANDRAIL

4"×4" TREATED POST

STEPS DOWN

PORCH

2"×4" HANDRAIL

2"×6" FACIA

ROOF

FOOTING

FOOTING

4'-0"

4'-0"

HALF PLAN OF FRONT WALL AT FIRST FLOOR

2"×6" FACIA

2"×10" TIE RAFTER

OPEN

HALF PLAN OF FRONT WALL AT SECOND FLOOR

ROOF

2"×4" HANDRAIL

BALCONY

2"×6" FACIA

ROOF

HALF PLAN OF REAR WALL AT SECOND FLOOR

54

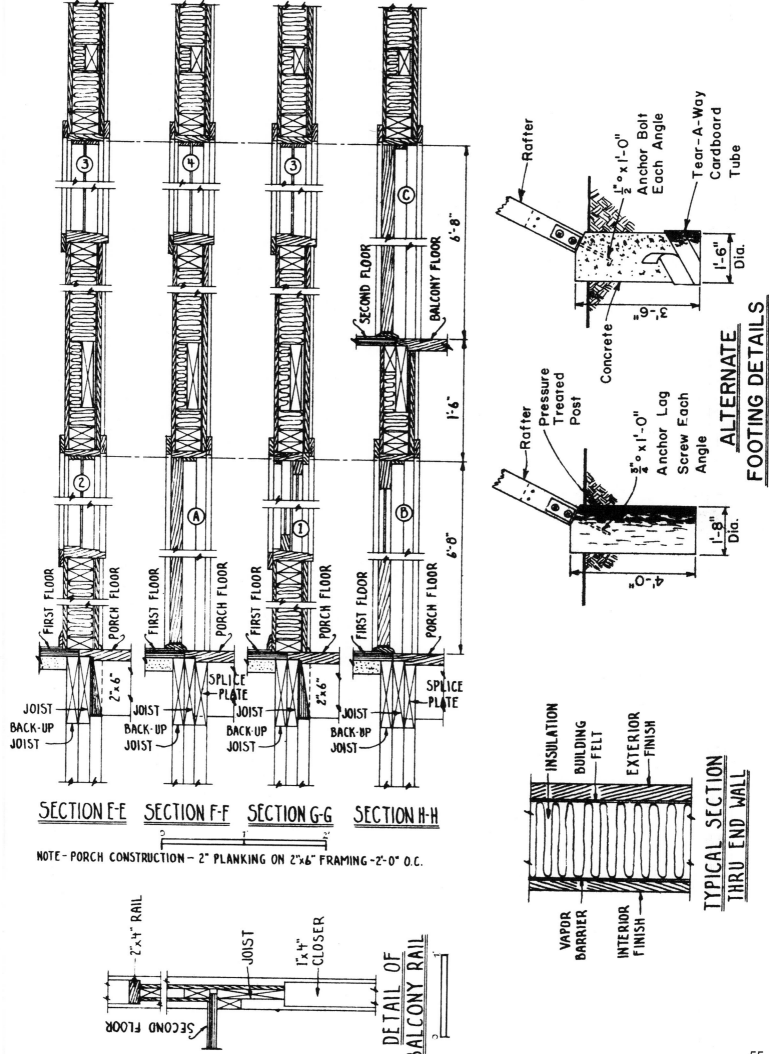

SECTION E-E SECTION F-F SECTION G-G SECTION H-H

NOTE-PORCH CONSTRUCTION-2" PLANKING ON 2"x6" FRAMING-2'-0" O.C.

DETAIL OF
BALCONY RAIL

ALTERNATE
FOOTING DETAILS

TYPICAL SECTION
THRU END WALL

55

9. ALL-PURPOSE 24-FOOT × 24-FOOT A-FRAME CABIN

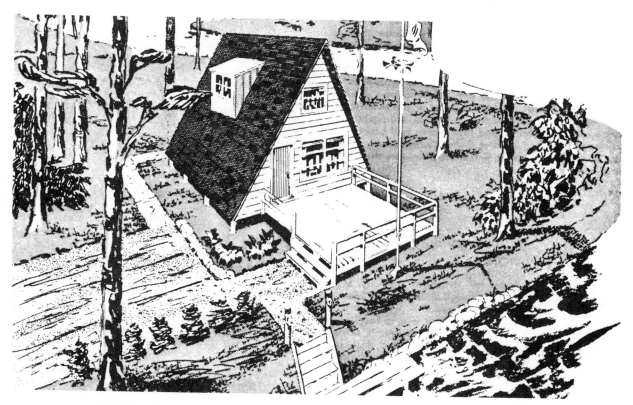

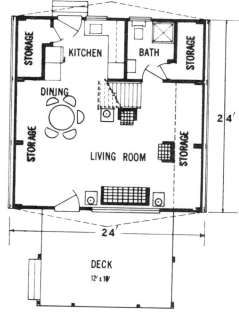

This 24- by 24-foot A-frame cabin, a recreational second home that is popular throughout the United States, has been built in mountain areas, at the shore from Maine to Florida, and across the country. Like the traditional cabins, this A-frame cabin provides quite comfortable living space for a family of four or five. Sleeping space for weekend visitors can be provided easily by rearranging the furniture in the large bedroom on the second floor.

The first floor of the cabin contains a living-dining room, a compact kitchen, a bathroom with shower, and adequate storage space. The living-dining room runs the full width of the building, with storage space on each side.

The locale and climatic conditions are major factors for the builder to consider when deciding if a heating system and insulation are needed.

The kitchen at the rear of the cabin contains space for a sink, a refrigerator, a range, and base and wall cabinets. A "ship's ladder" stairway leads to the second floor, and a dormer-type window extension in the roof adds light and ventilation to this area.

With some knowledge of carpentry and the ability to use ordinary hand tools, three or four men should have no serious problems building this cabin. Care should be taken in locating and setting the pressure-treated posts. The A-frames should be assembled flat on the ground, raised into position, and braced until the flooring is put in place. The roof sheathing should be placed, the ends cut to the shape of the overhang, then the roofing applied. The end walls and partitions may easily be installed and the kitchen and bathroom fixtures placed. Redwood or cypress lumber siding will take on a weathered finish and eliminate the need for periodic painting.

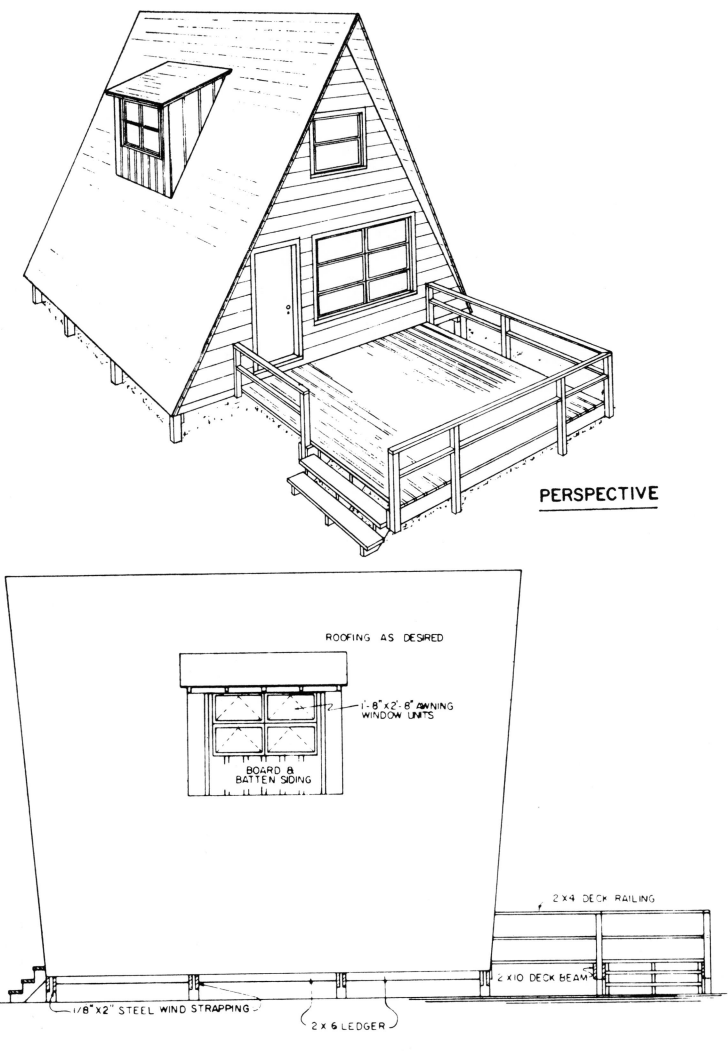

PERSPECTIVE

ROOFING AS DESIRED

1'-8" X 2'-8" AWNING WINDOW UNITS

BOARD & BATTEN SIDING

2 X 4 DECK RAILING

2 X 10 DECK BEAM

1/8" X 2" STEEL WIND STRAPPING

2 X 6 LEDGER

58

SIDE ELEVATION

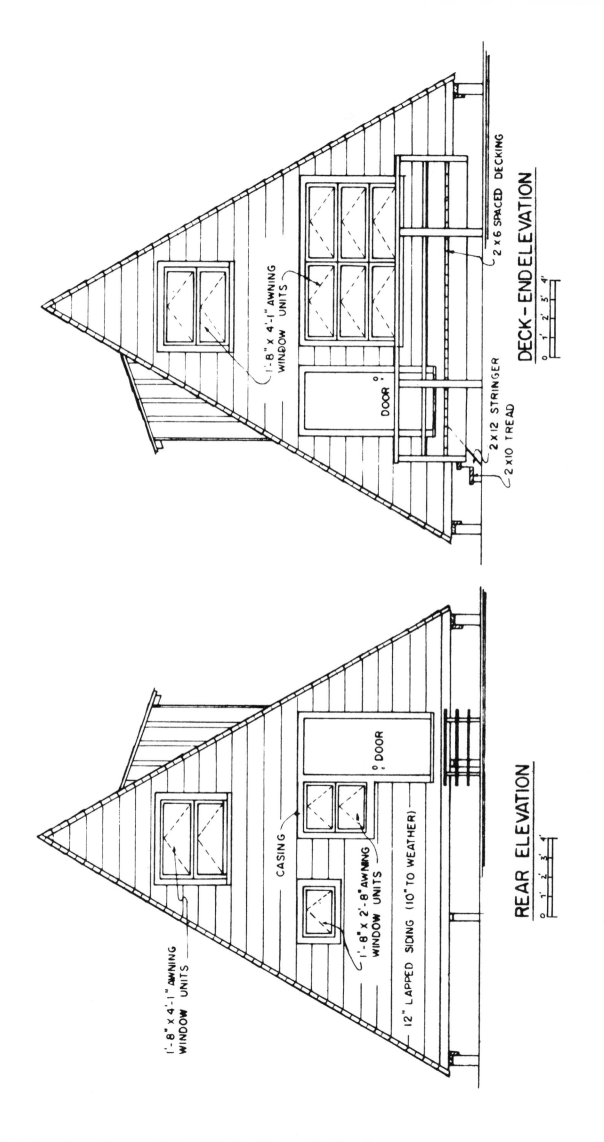

DECK-END ELEVATION

2 x 6 SPACED DECKING

1'-8" x 4'-1" AWNING WINDOW UNITS

DOOR

2 x 12 STRINGER

2 x 10 TREAD

0' 1' 2' 3' 4'

REAR ELEVATION

1'-8" x 4'-1" AWNING WINDOW UNITS

CASING

DOOR

1'-8" x 2'-8" AWNING WINDOW UNITS

12" LAPPED SIDING (10" TO WEATHER)

0' 1' 2' 3' 4'

59

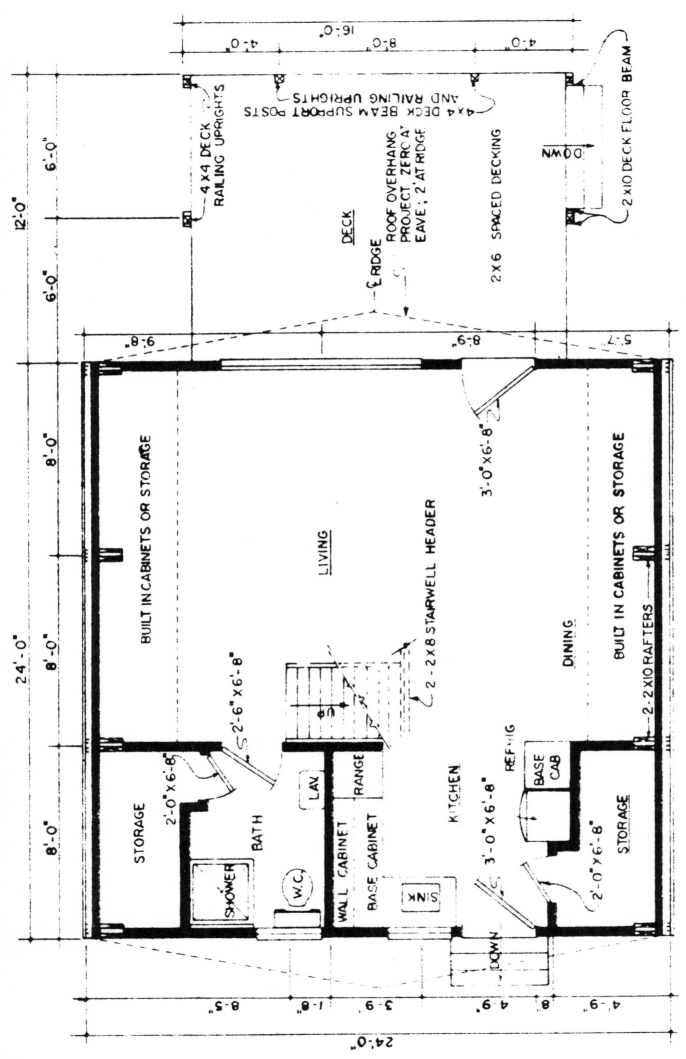

FLOOR PLAN

0 1 2 3 4

60

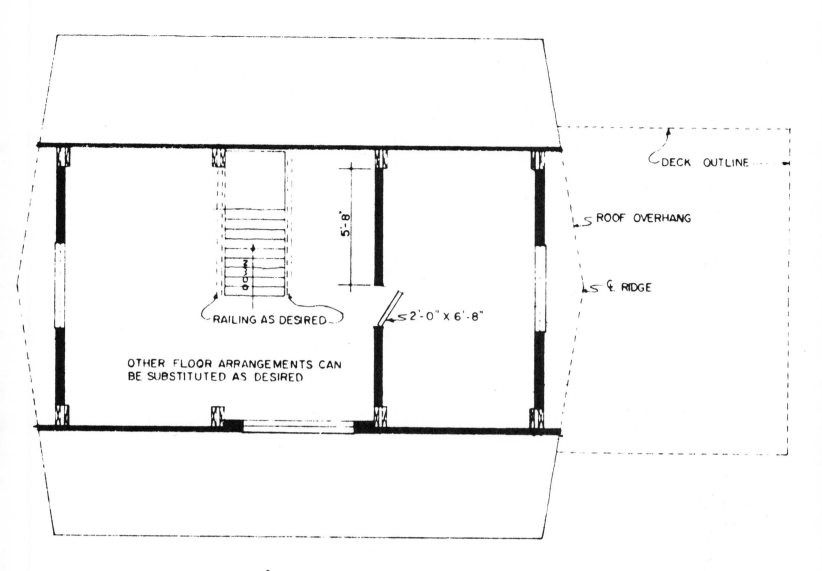

5'-8"

RAILING AS DESIRED

OTHER FLOOR ARRANGEMENTS CAN
BE SUBSTITUTED AS DESIRED

≤2'-0" X 6'-8"

DECK OUTLINE

ROOF OVERHANG

℄ RIDGE

2nd FLOOR PLAN

0   1'   2'   3'   4'

CONSTRUCTION NOTES:

Use rough lumber for all structural framing. Lap
rough, 1-inch boards for end-wall siding. Other materials or methods may be substituted.

Rafters and floor beams are 24-feet long to facilitate construction of the A-frame on the ground.
If some saving in intial cost is necessary, add the deck
in the front later. Interior finish is left to builder's
choice.

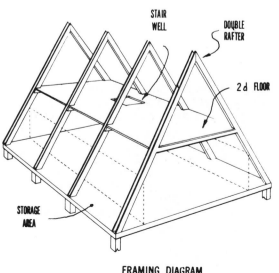

STAIR
WELL

DOUBLE
RAFTER

2d FLOOR

STORAGE
AREA

FRAMING DIAGRAM

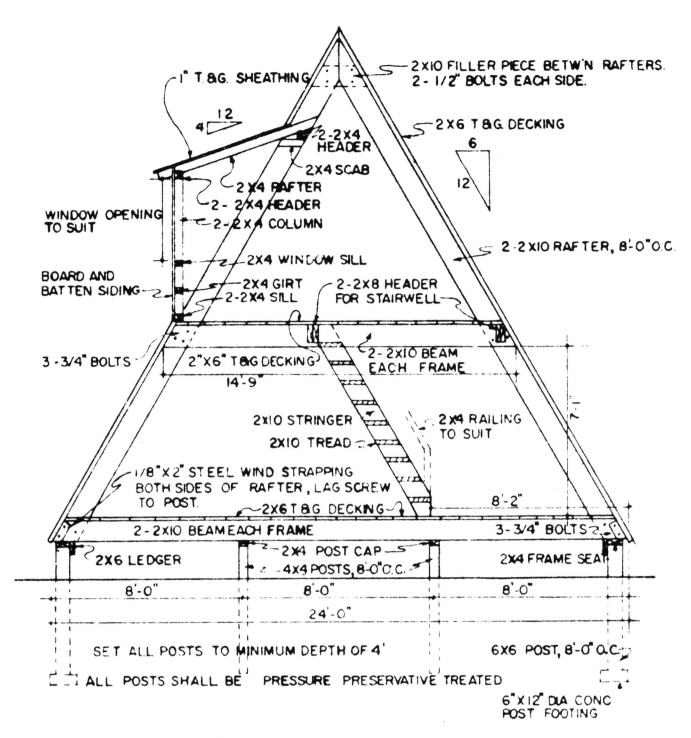

CROSS SECTION

0 1' 2 3 4'

NOTES:

1. DESIGN FLOOR LOAD = 30 PSF
2. DESIGN FIBER STRESS IN BENDING = 1200 PSI
3. FLOOR MEMBER DEFLECTION LIMIT = ℓ /360
4. FLOOR - DECKING JOINTS SHALL BE STAGGERED AS MUCH AS POSSIBLE
5. RAFTERS AND FLOOR BEAMS ARE INTENDED TO BE 24' LONG IN ORDER TO FACILITATE CONSTRUCTION OF THE "A" FRAMES ON THE GROUND. IF SPLICES ARE NECESSARY, LOCATE RAFTER JOINTS ABOVE 2ND FLOOR LEVEL AND FLOOR - BEAM JOINTS (STAGGER JOINTS IN TWO FLOOR BEAMS) ABOVE THE INTERIOR SUPPORT POSTS

6. ALL STRUCTURAL FRAMING SHALL BE ROUGH LUMBER
7. LAPPED ROUGH 1" BOARDS (NOMINAL SIZE) IS SUGGESTED FOR END-WALL SIDING OTHER MATERIALS OR METHODS MAY BE SUBSTITUTED IF DESIRED
8. ALL AWNING WINDOWS UNIT SIZE ARE APPROXIMATE. OTHER WINDOW SIZES AND / OR STYLES MAY BE SUBSTITUTED AS DESIRED.
9. INTERIOR FINISH IS LEFT TO BUILDER'S DISCRETION.

10. FIVE-ROOM LOG CABIN

This cabin is designed principally for camping but would make a fairly comfortable house for a small family. A basement could be provided, with the entrance down a stairway from the back porch. Loft space could be reached from an open stair in the living room.

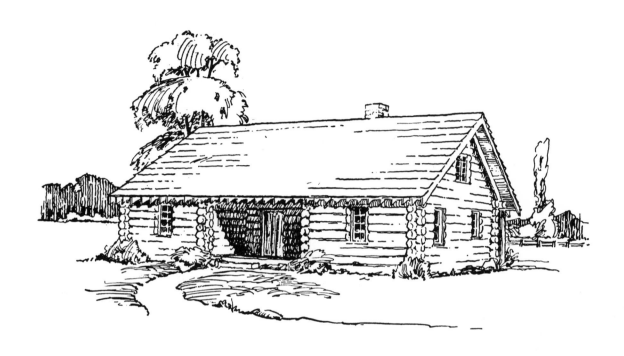

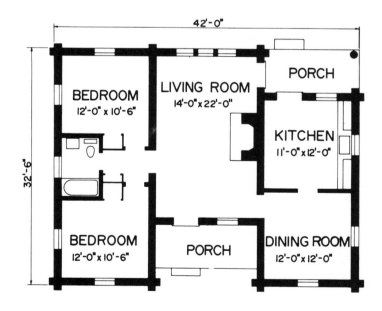

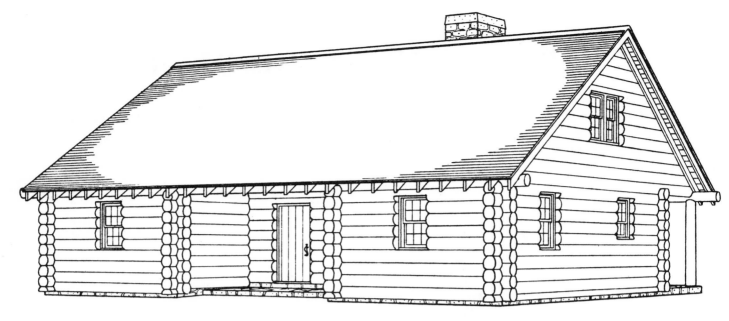

PERSPECTIVE

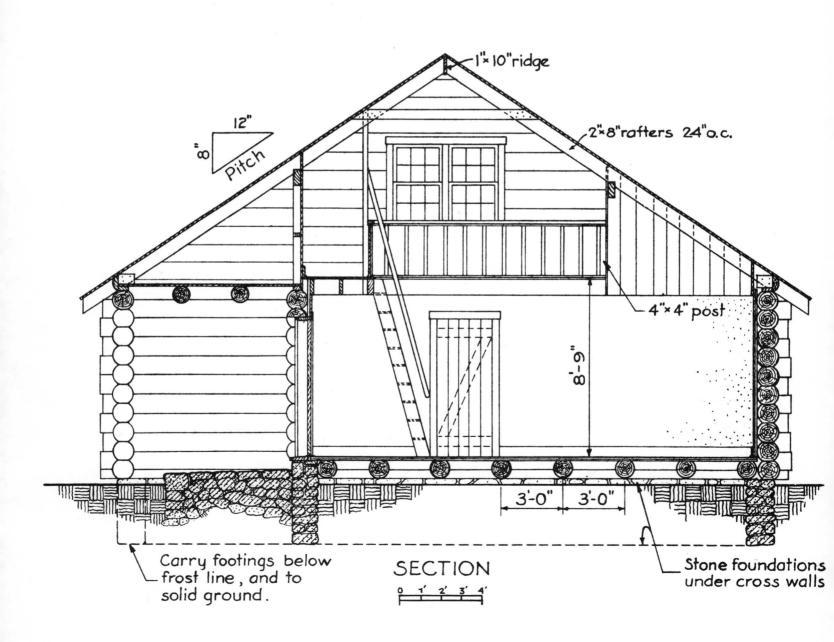

1"× 10" ridge

12"
8"
Pitch

2"× 8" rafters 24" o.c.

4"× 4" post

8'-9"

3'-0"   3'-0"

Carry footings below
frost line, and to
solid ground.

SECTION

0 1' 2' 3' 4'

Stone foundations
under cross walls

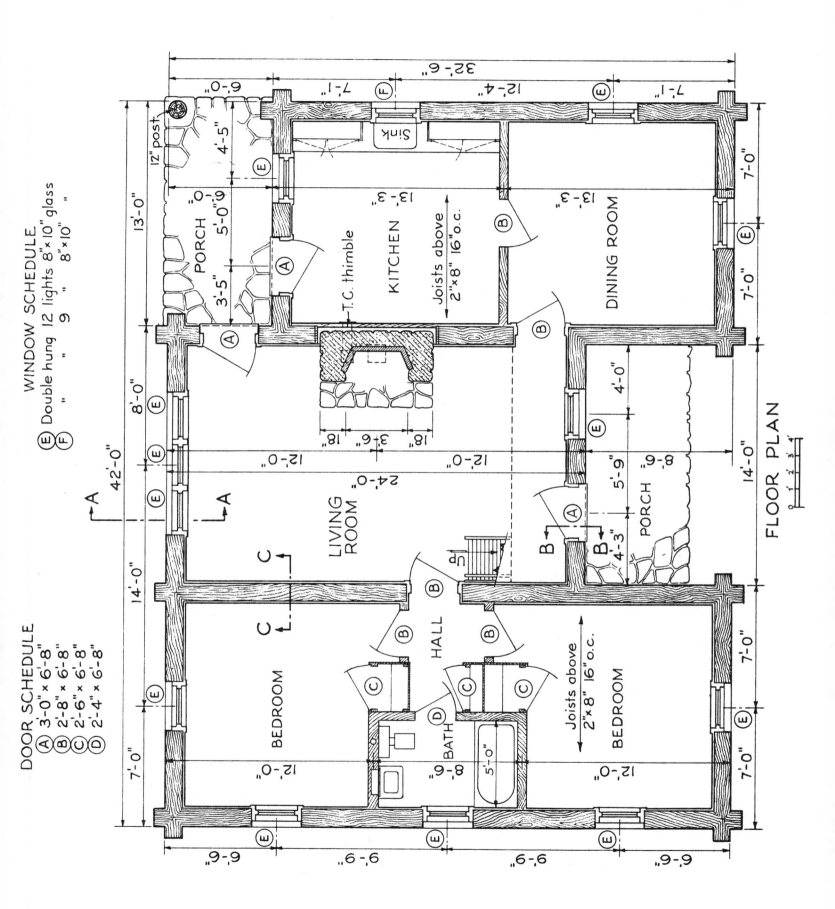

WINDOW SCHEDULE
Ⓔ Double hung 12 lights 8"×10" glass
Ⓕ " 9 " 8"×10" "

DOOR SCHEDULE
Ⓐ 3'-0" × 6'-8"
Ⓑ 2'-8" × 6'-8"
Ⓒ 2'-6" × 6'-8"
Ⓓ 2'-4" × 6'-8"

FLOOR PLAN

PORCH

KITCHEN
Joists above
2"×8" 16" o.c.

Sink

T.C. thimble

DINING ROOM

LIVING ROOM

PORCH

BEDROOM

HALL

BATH

BEDROOM
Joists above
2"×8" 16" o.c.

UP

65

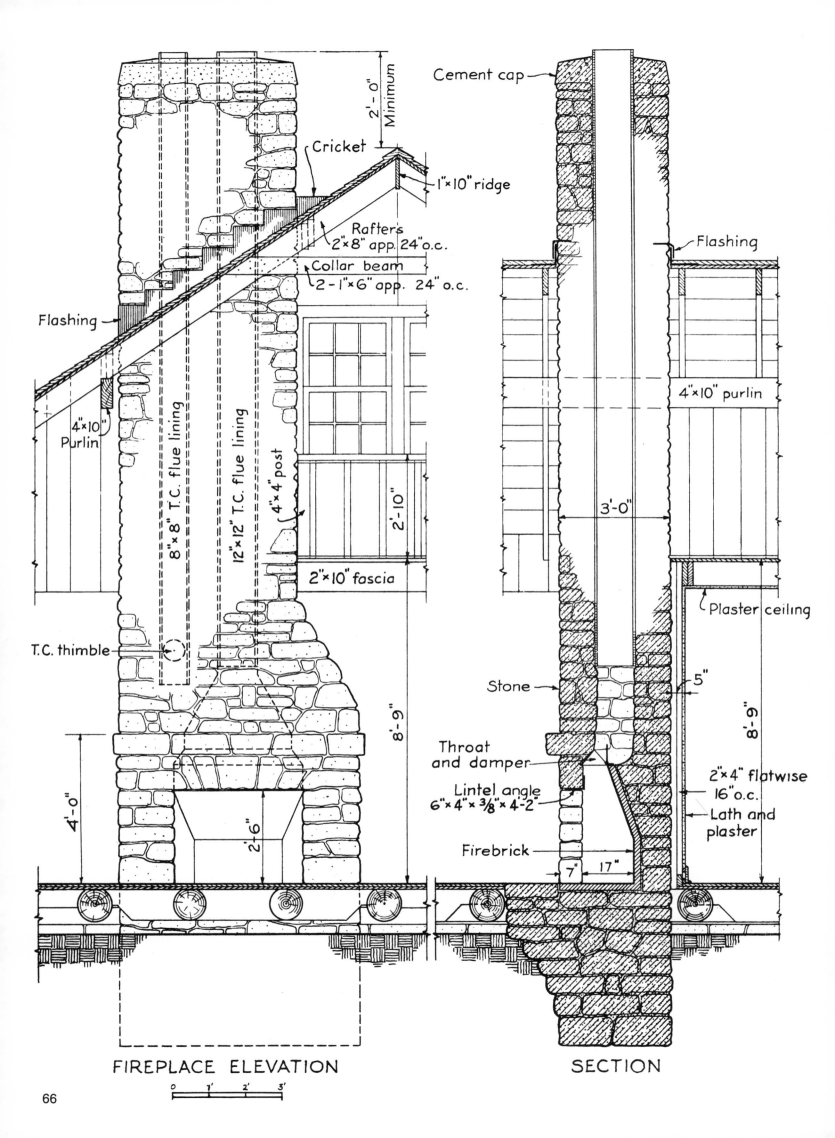

Cement cap

2'-0" Minimum

Cricket

1"×10" ridge

Rafters 2"×8" app. 24" o.c.

Collar beam 2-1"×6" app. 24" o.c.

Flashing

Flashing

4"×10" Purlin

4"×10" purlin

8"×8" T.C. flue lining

12"×12" T.C. flue lining

4"×4" post

2'-10"

2"×10" fascia

3'-0"

Plaster ceiling

T.C. thimble

Stone

5"

8'-9"

8'-9"

Throat and damper

2"×4" flatwise 16" o.c.

Lintel angle 6"×4"×³⁄₈"×4-2"

Lath and plaster

4'-0"

2'-6"

Firebrick

7"   17"

FIREPLACE ELEVATION

0   1'   2'   3'

SECTION

66

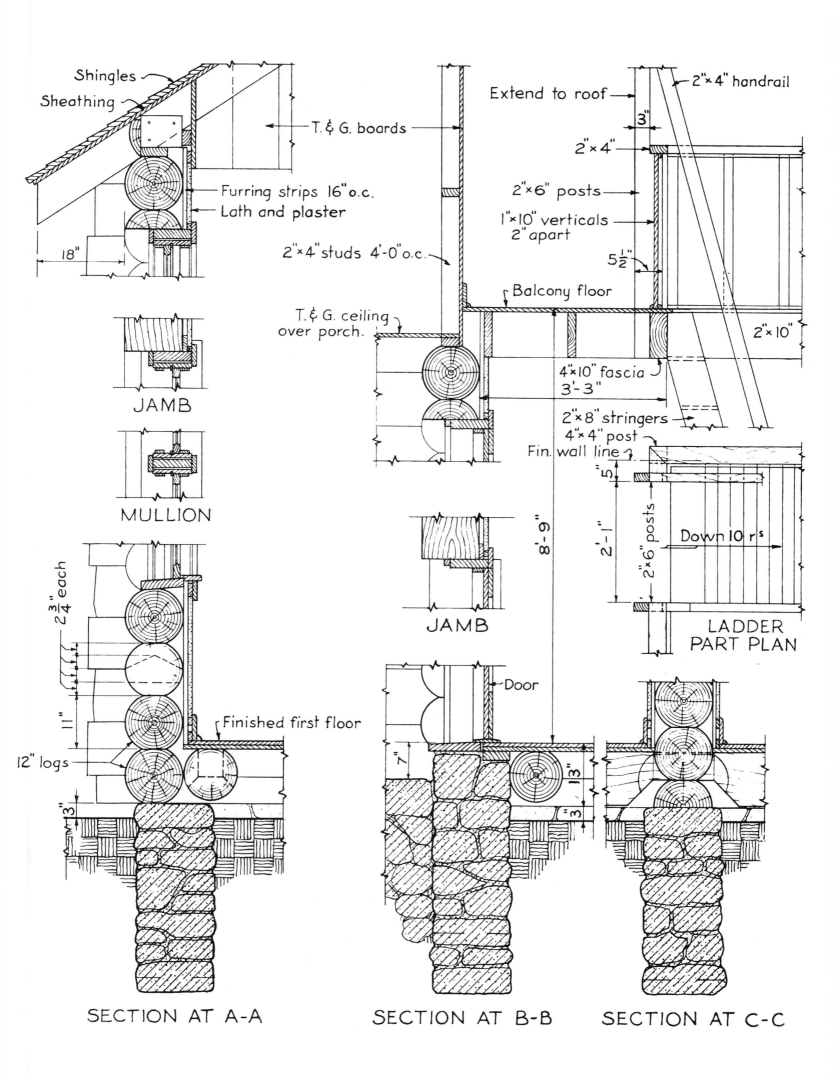

Shingles

Sheathing

T. & G. boards

Furring strips 16" o.c.

Lath and plaster

18"

JAMB

MULLION

Extend to roof

2"×4" handrail

3"

2"×4"

2"×6" posts

1"×10" verticals 2" apart

5½"

2"×4" studs 4'-0" o.c.

Balcony floor

T. & G. ceiling over porch.

4"×10" fascia

3'-3"

2"×8" stringers

4"×4" post

Fin. wall line

2"×10"

LADDER PART PLAN

Down 10 r's

2"×6" posts

5"

2'-1"

JAMB

Door

8'-9"

2¾" each

11"

12" logs

Finished first floor

3"

SECTION AT A-A

7"

13"

3"

SECTION AT B-B

SECTION AT C-C

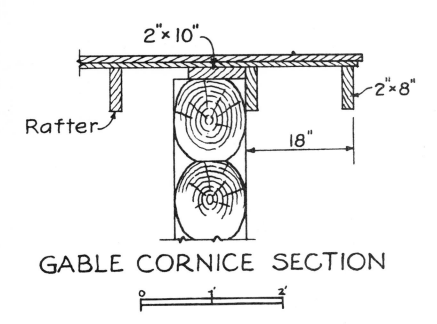

GABLE CORNICE SECTION

2"×10"

Rafter

2"×8"

18"

0   1   2'

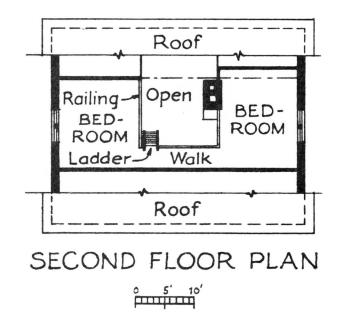

SECOND FLOOR PLAN

Roof

Railing Open

BED-ROOM

BED-ROOM

Ladder Walk

Roof

0   5'   10'

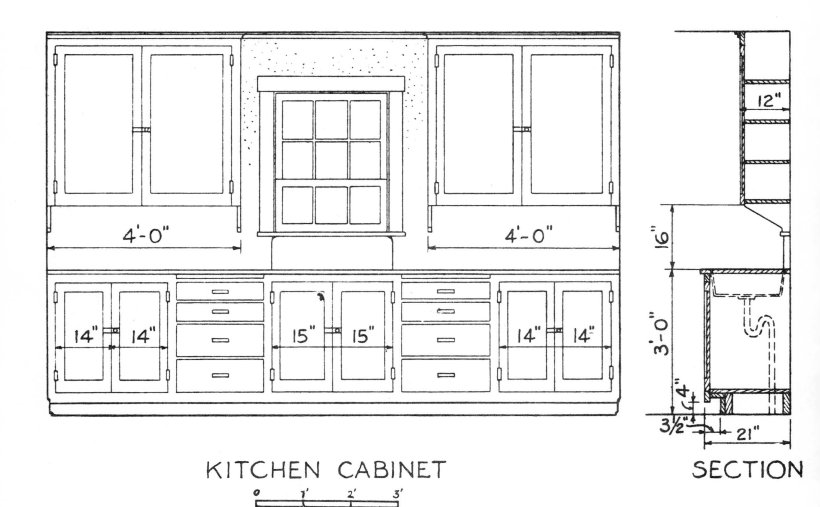

KITCHEN CABINET

4'-0"

4'-0"

14" 14"

15" 15"

14" 14"

0   1'   2'   3'

SECTION

12"

16"

3'-0"

4"

3½"

21"

11. THREE-ROOM LOG CABIN

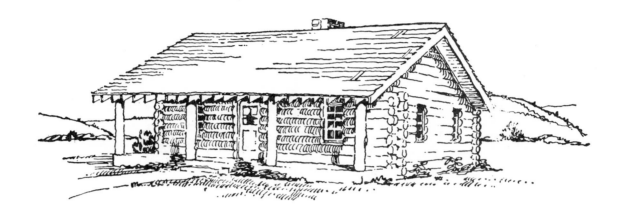

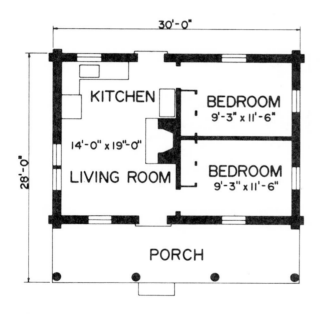

This cabin would be especially appropriate for a camp in the woods or on the lakeshore. The back of the fireplace in the living room gives heat to the bedrooms. The large porch is especially desirable if the house is to be used as a summer home. Porch posts of peeled logs are appropriate for this cabin.

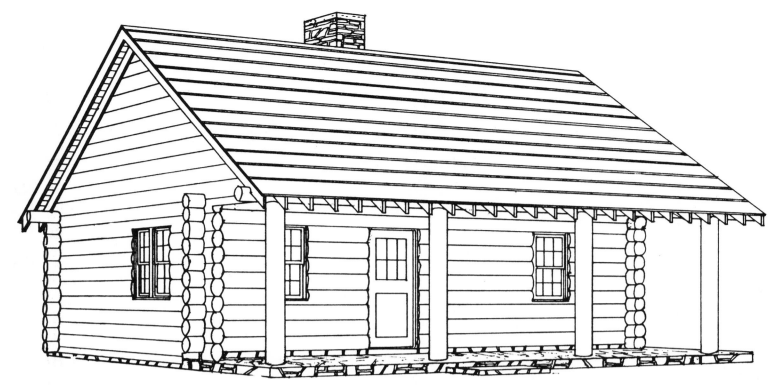

PERSPECTIVE

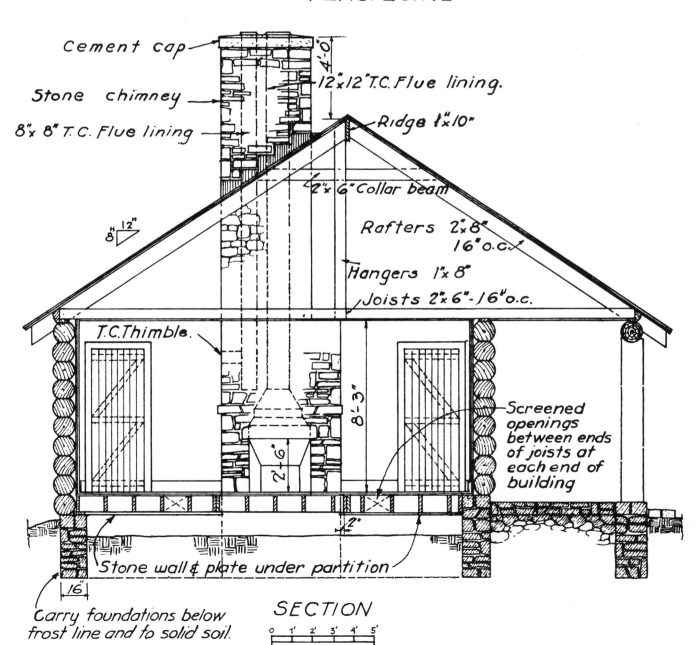

Cement cap

Stone chimney

8"x 8" T.C. Flue lining

4'-0"

12"x12" T.C. Flue lining.

Ridge 1"x10"

2"x 6" Collar beam

8" 12"

Rafters 2"x8" 16" o.c.

Hangers 1"x 8"

Joists 2"x 6"-16" o.c.

T.C. Thimble.

8'-3"

2'-6"

Screened openings between ends of joists at each end of building

Stone wall & plate under partition

2'

16"

Carry foundations below frost line and to solid soil.

SECTION

0 1' 2' 3' 4' 5'

70

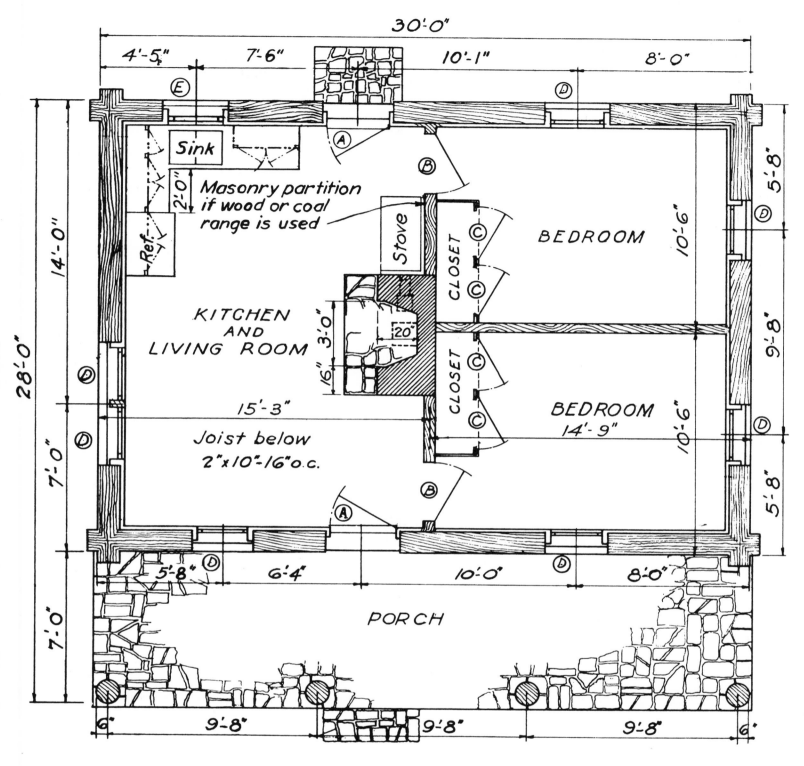

Sink

Masonry partition
if wood or coal
range is used

Ref.

Stove

KITCHEN
AND
LIVING ROOM

CLOSET

CLOSET

BEDROOM

BEDROOM
14'-9"

Joist below
2"x10"-16" o.c.

PORCH

30'-0"

4'-5" 7'-6" 10'-1" 8'-0"

14'-0"

28'-0"

7'-0"

7'-0"

5'-8"

9'-8"

10'-6"

10'-6"

5'-8"

9'-8"

15'-3"

2'-0"

3'-0"

6"

20"

6" 5'-8" 6'-4" 10'-0" 8'-0"

6" 9'-8" 9'-8" 9'-8" 6"

PLAN

0 1' 2' 3' 4' 5'

DOOR SCHEDULE
A. 3'-0" x 6'-8"   Glazed.
B. 2'-8" x 6'-8"   Wood batten
C. 2'-4" x 6'-8"   "   "

WINDOW SCHEDULE
D - Double hung 12 lights 8"x10" glass.
E -   "   "   9 "   8"x10" "

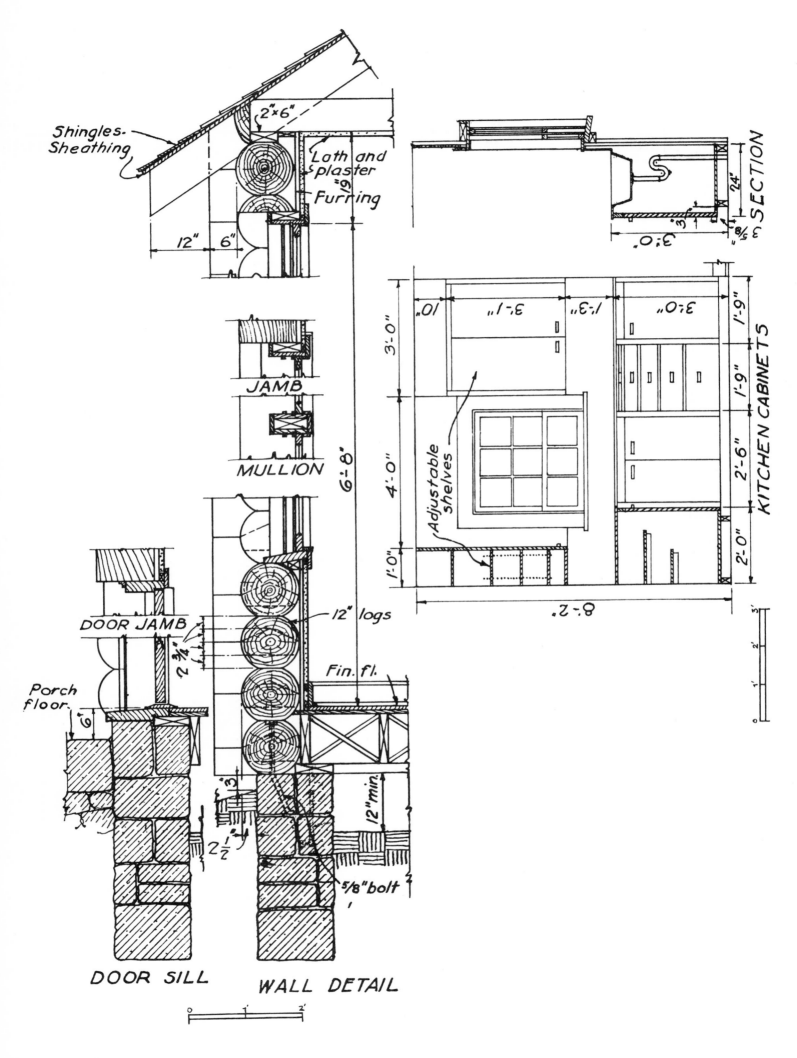

Shingles. Sheathing

2"x6"

Lath and plaster

"⁵⁄₈" Furring

12" 6"

SECTION

24"

3'-0"

3"

"⁵⁄₈"

JAMB

MULLION

6'-8"

3'-0"

10"

3'-1"

1'-3"

3'-0"

1'-9"

Adjustable shelves

4'-0"

1'-9"

2'-6"

KITCHEN CABINETS

DOOR JAMB

2 ¾"

12" logs

1'-0"

2'-0"

Porch floor.

6'

Fin. fl.

8'-2"

3"

12" min.

2 ½"

5/8" bolt

0 1 2 3'

DOOR SILL   WALL DETAIL

0   1   2'

12. FIVE-ROOM LOG CABIN

In a well-wooded region, this rustic log cabin would be suitable for a small family starting farm life. Or, it might be used as a tenant house or a summer cottage. The grouping of doors and windows reduces the work that usually goes into log construction and provides good cross ventilation. The single, main-bearing partition and other partitions are easily framed. A circulator heater, large living-room fireplace, and the wood or coal kitchen range furnish heat.

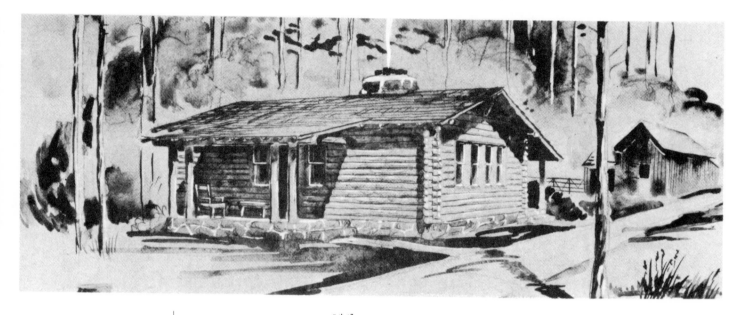

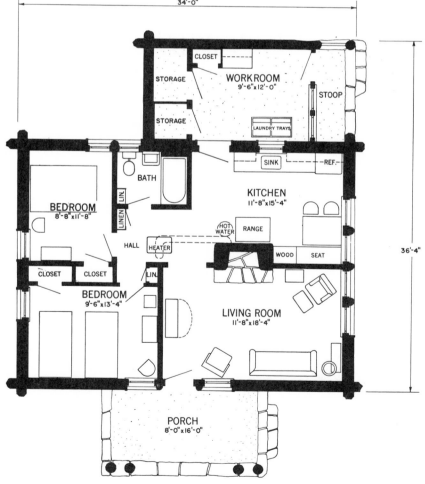

FLOOR PLAN

PERSPECTIVE

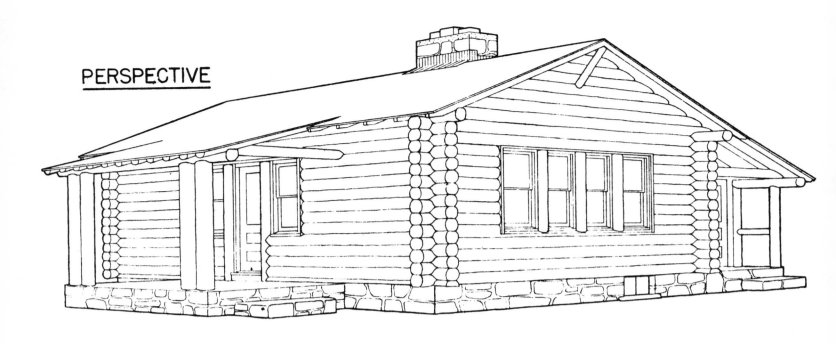

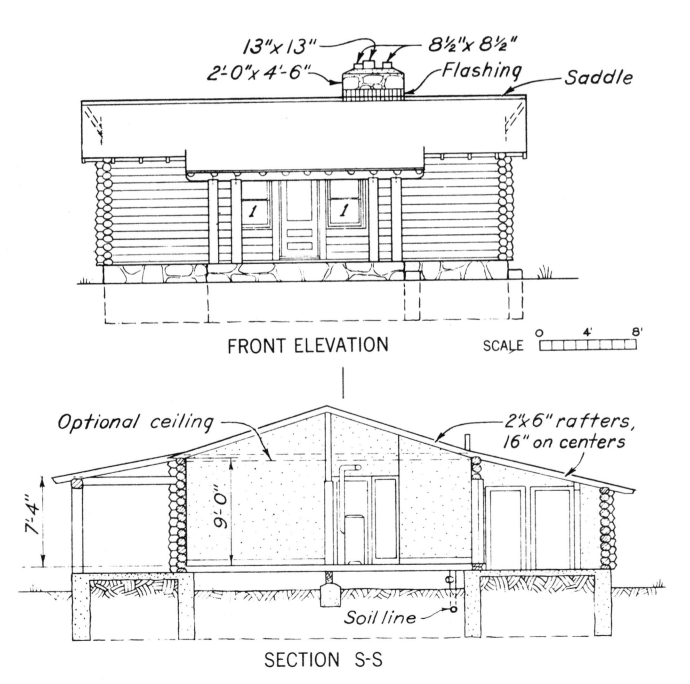

13"x 13"

8½"x 8½"

2'-0"x 4'-6"

Flashing

Saddle

1   1

FRONT ELEVATION

SCALE   0   4'   8'

Optional ceiling

2"x 6" rafters,
16" on centers

7'-4"

9'-0"

Soil line

SECTION S-S

74

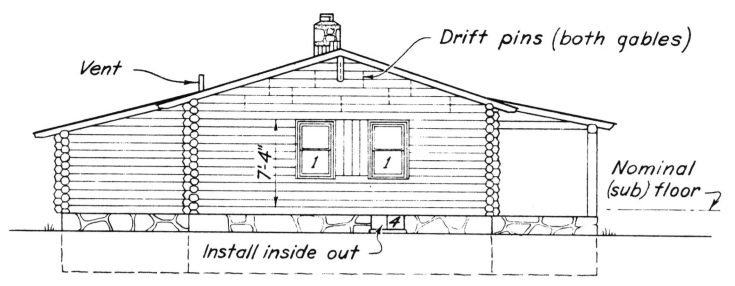

Vent

Drift pins (both gables)

7'-4"

Nominal (sub) floor

Install inside out

4

LEFT ELEVATION, BED ROOM

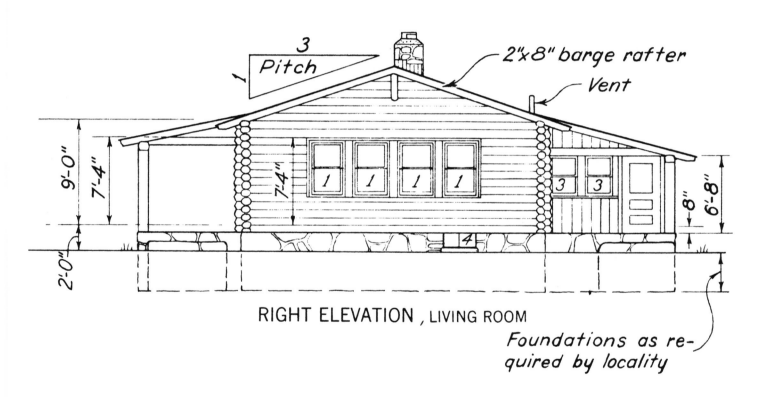

3
1 Pitch

2"x8" barge rafter

Vent

9'-0"

7'-4"

7'-4"

1 1 1 1

3 3

8"

6'-8"

2'-0"

4

RIGHT ELEVATION, LIVING ROOM

Foundations as required by locality

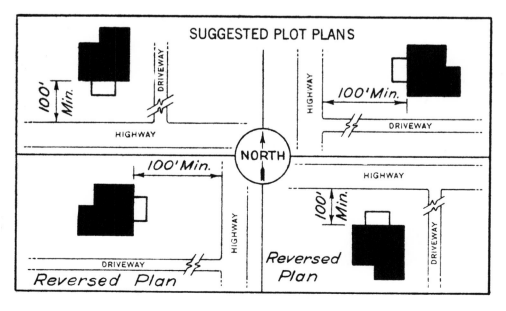

SUGGESTED PLOT PLANS

100' Min.

DRIVEWAY

HIGHWAY

HIGHWAY

100' Min.

DRIVEWAY

NORTH

100' Min.

DRIVEWAY

HIGHWAY

HIGHWAY

Reversed Plan

100' Min.

DRIVEWAY

Reversed Plan

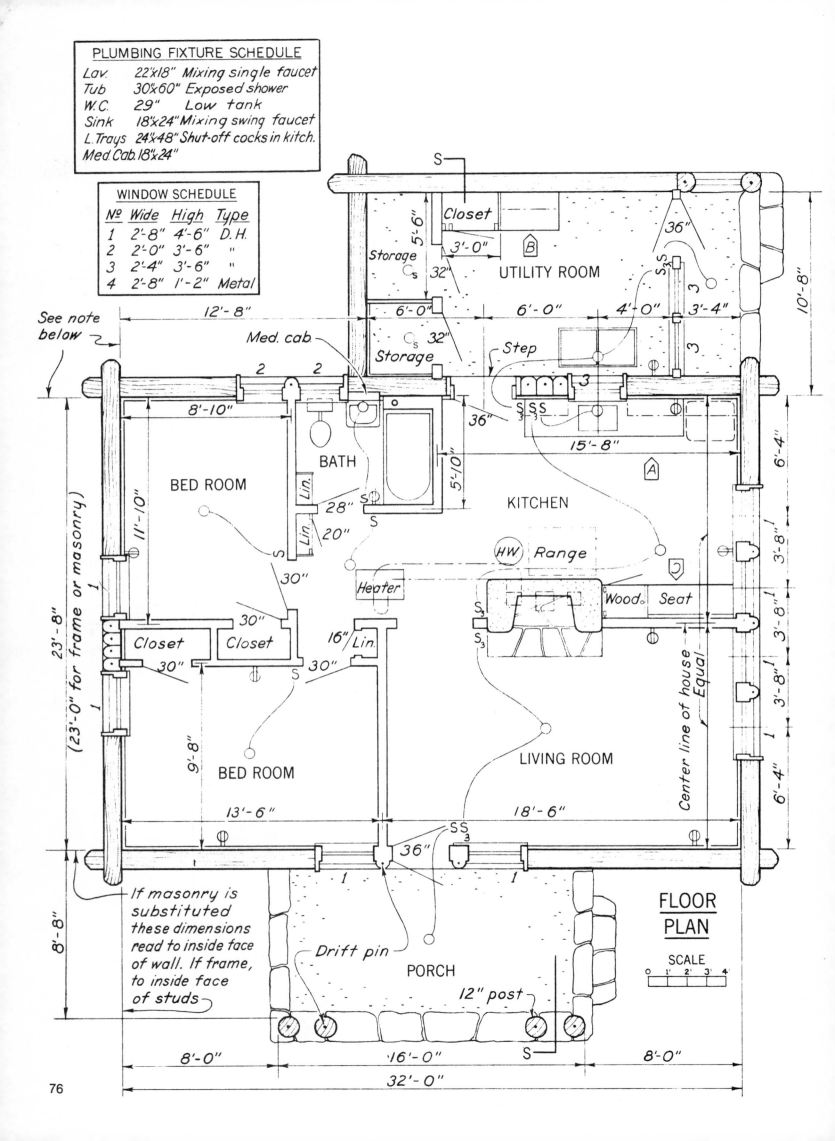

PLUMBING FIXTURE SCHEDULE

Lav.   22"x18" Mixing single faucet
Tub   30"x60" Exposed shower
W.C.   29"   Low tank
Sink   18"x24" Mixing swing faucet
L.Trays 24"x48" Shut-off cocks in kitch.
Med.Cab. 18"x24"

WINDOW SCHEDULE

№	Wide	High	Type
1	2'-8"	4'-6"	D.H.
2	2'-0"	3'-6"	"
3	2'-4"	3'-6"	"
4	2'-8"	1'-2"	Metal

See note below

Closet

Storage

UTILITY ROOM

5'-6"

3'-0"

B

32"

Storage

32"

6'-0"

6'-0"

4'-0"

3'-4"

10'-8"

36"

S₃ S

3

3

Med. cab.

2   2

8'-10"

Step

36"

S S S
3 3

15'-8"

6'-4"

A

BATH

BED ROOM

11'-10"

5'-10"

KITCHEN

28"

Lin.

20"

S

S

30"

30"

HW   Range

Heater

Wood   Seat

3'-8"

3'-8"

3'-8"

3'-8"

S₃

S₃

Closet   Closet

30"

30"

16" Lin.

30"

Center line of house

Equal

23'-8"

(23'-0" for frame or masonry)

1

1

BED ROOM

9'-8"

13'-6"

LIVING ROOM

18'-6"

6'-4"

1

If masonry is substituted these dimensions read to inside face of wall. If frame, to inside face of studs

S S
3

36"

1   1

FLOOR PLAN

SCALE

0   1'   2'   3'   4'

8'-8"

Drift pin

PORCH

12" post

S

8'-0"

16'-0"

8'-0"

32'-0"

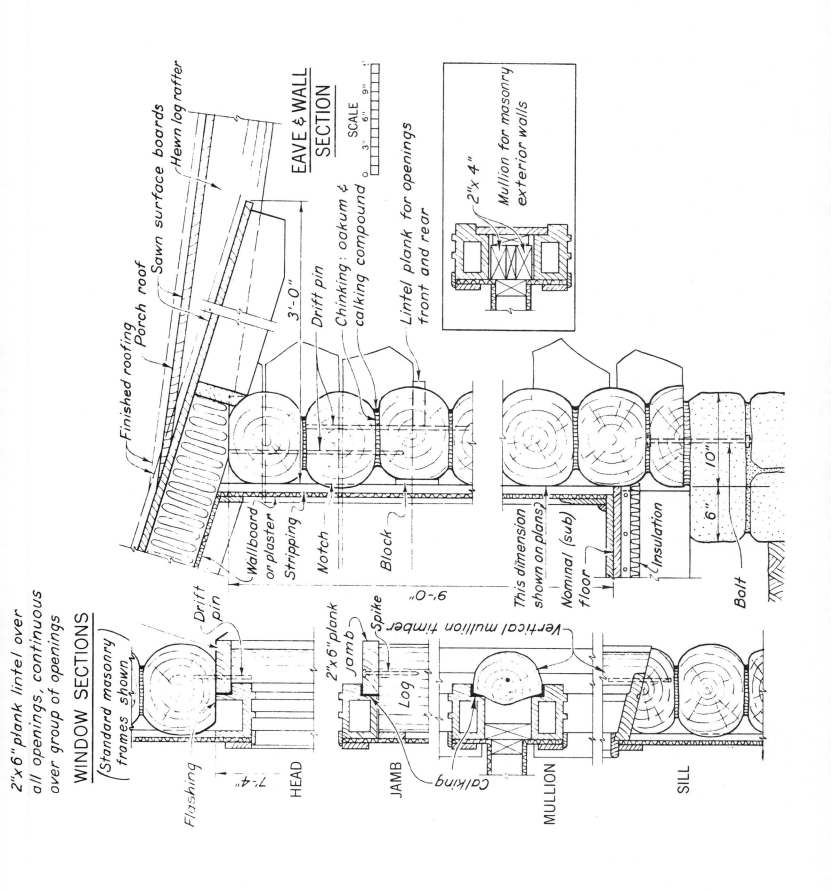

2"x 6" plank lintel over all openings, continuous over group of openings

WINDOW SECTIONS
(Standard masonry frames shown)

Flashing

Drift pin

HEAD

7'-4"

2"x 6" plank jamb

Log

JAMB

Spike

Calking

Vertical mullion timber

MULLION

SILL

EAVE & WALL SECTION

SCALE
0   3"   6"   9"   1'

Finished roofing
Porch roof
Sawn surface boards
Hewn log rafter

3'-0"

Drift pin

Chinking: oakum & calking compound

Lintel plank for openings front and rear

Wallboard or plaster
Stripping
Notch
Block

9'-0"

This dimension shown on plans

Nominal (sub) floor

Insulation

Bolt

10"

6"

2"x 4"
Mullion for masonry exterior walls

77

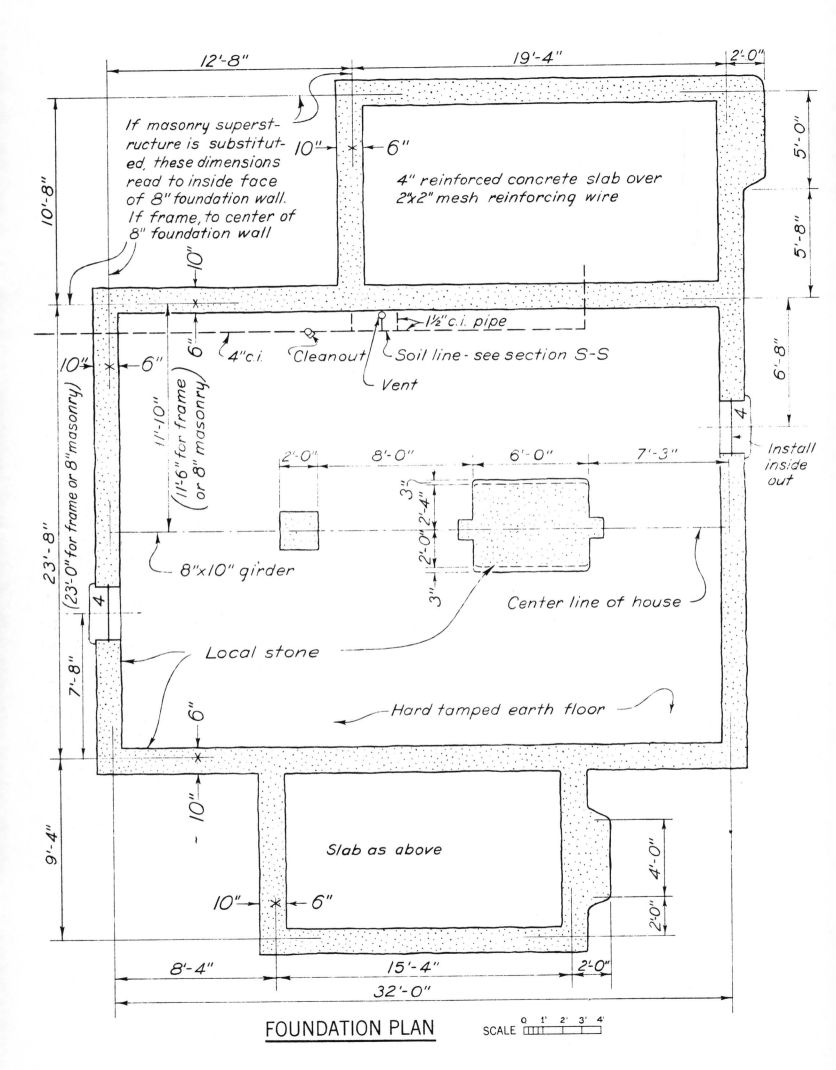

12'-8" 19'-4" 2'-0"

10'-8"

If masonry superstructure is substituted, these dimensions read to inside face of 8" foundation wall. If frame, to center of 8" foundation wall

10" 6"

5'-0"

5'-8"

4" reinforced concrete slab over 2"x2" mesh reinforcing wire

10"

6"

6'-8"

1½" c.i. pipe

4" c.i. Cleanout Soil line - see section S-S

Vent

10" 6"

Install inside out

4

23'-8"

(23'-0" for frame or 8" masonry)

11'-10"

(11'-6" for frame or 8" masonry)

2'-0" 8'-0" 6'-0" 7'-3"

3"

2'-4"

2'-0"

2'-0"

3"

8"x10" girder

Center line of house

4

Local stone

7'-8"

6"

Hard tamped earth floor

- 10"

9'-4"

Slab as above

4'-0"

10" 6"

2'-0"

8'-4" 15'-4" 2'-0"

32'-0"

FOUNDATION PLAN

SCALE 0 1' 2' 3' 4'

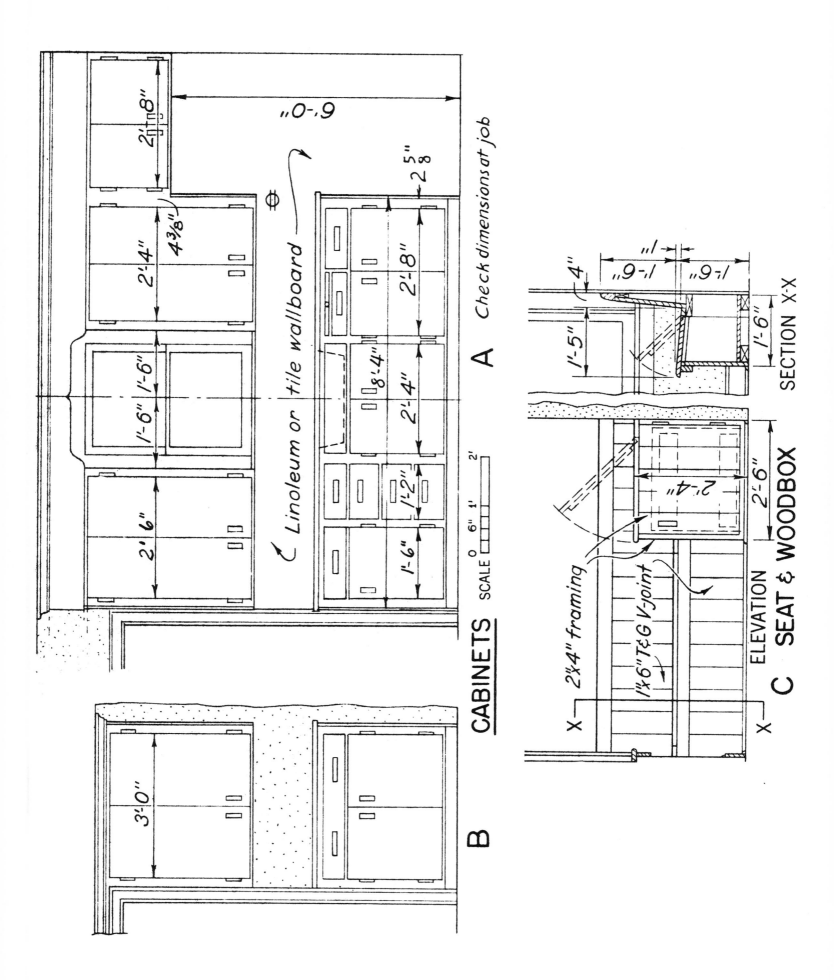

A Check dimensions at job

CABINETS SCALE 0 6" 1' 2'

B

C SEAT & WOODBOX
ELEVATION
SECTION X-X

79

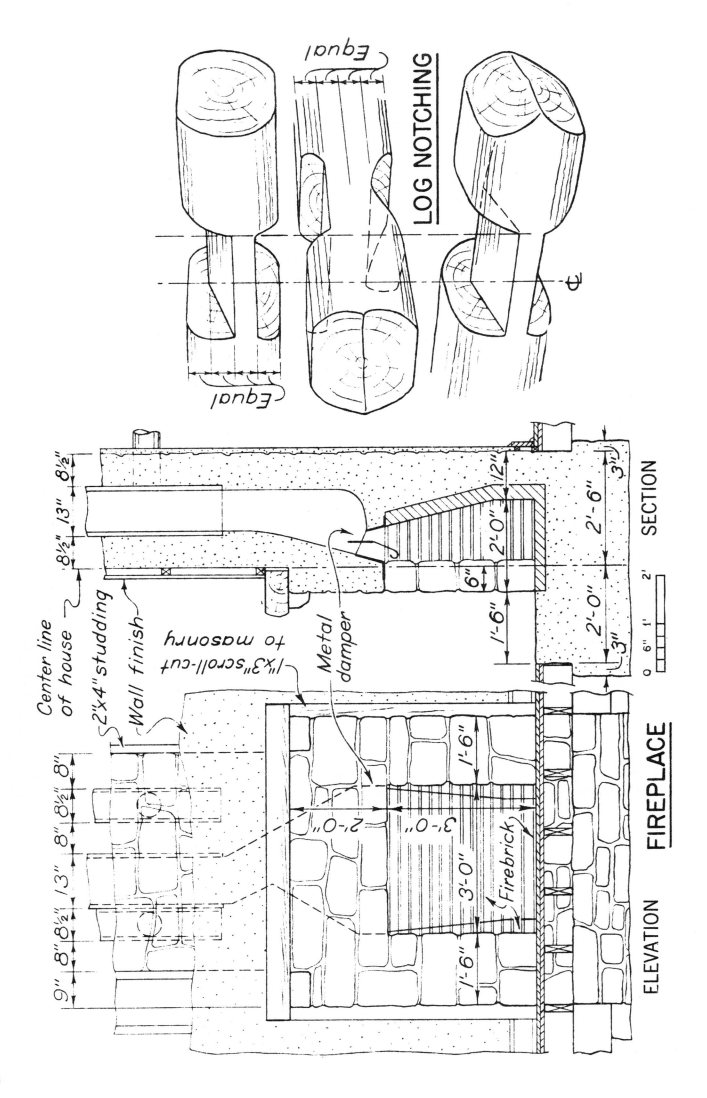

LOG NOTCHING

Equal

Equal

SECTION

8½" 13" 8½"

8½"

2'-0"

2'-0"

3"

2'-0"

3"

1'-6"

6"

12"

0 6" 1' 2'

FIREPLACE

Center line of house

2"x4" studding

Wall finish

1"x3" scroll-cut to masonry

Metal damper

Firebrick

9" 8" 8½" 13" 8" 8½" 8"

2'-0"

3'-0"

3'-0"

1'-6"

1'-6"

ELEVATION

13. ONE-BEDROOM POLE-FRAME CABIN

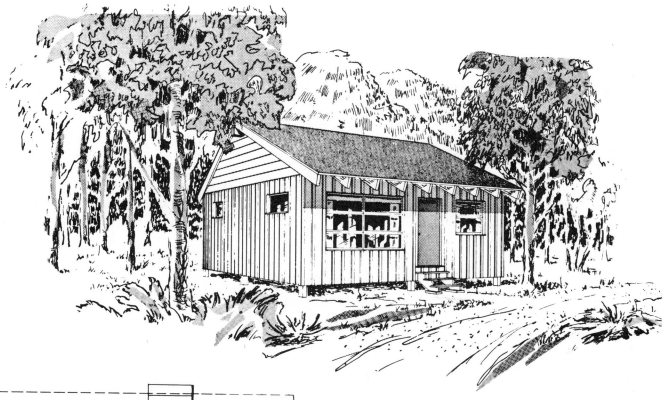

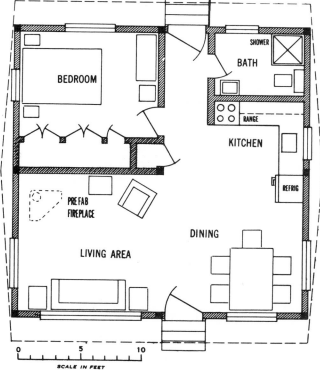

SCALE IN FEET

This 24-foot x 24-foot one-bedroom structure, simply designed for comfort and economy, can be used as a vacation retreat or campsite. It features low-cost pole-frame construction, design simplicity, and flexibility of arrangement.

The use of poles permits rapid erection, minimum site preparation, and decreased foundation expenses. The poles also serve as the wall framework to which other members are fastened. The life expectancy of a pole-frame structure, with the commercial preservative-treating processes in use today, can be as long as 75 years. The structure can be made very attractive both inside and out, depending on materials available, taste, and cost.

Rough-sawn native lumber is used in the board-and-batten siding. Several kinds of material are available for use as coverings.

Location and type of windows are flexible.

With kitchen and bath as suggested, the interior is efficiently arranged for pleasant living. A prefabricated fireplace could be installed.

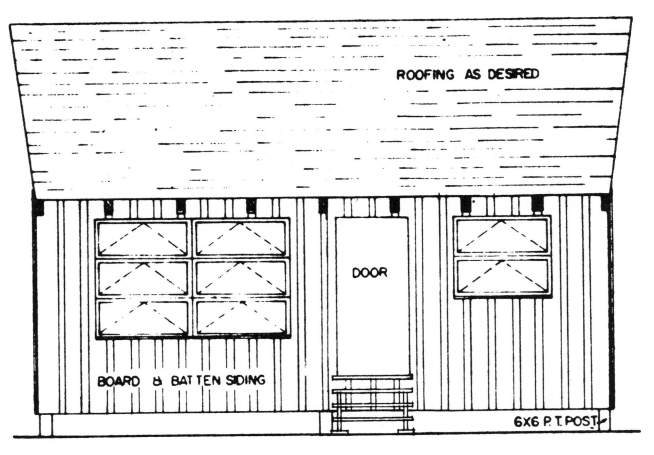

ROOFING AS DESIRED

DOOR

BOARD & BATTEN SIDING

6X6 P.T. POST

FRONT ELEVATION

0 1' 2' 3' 4'

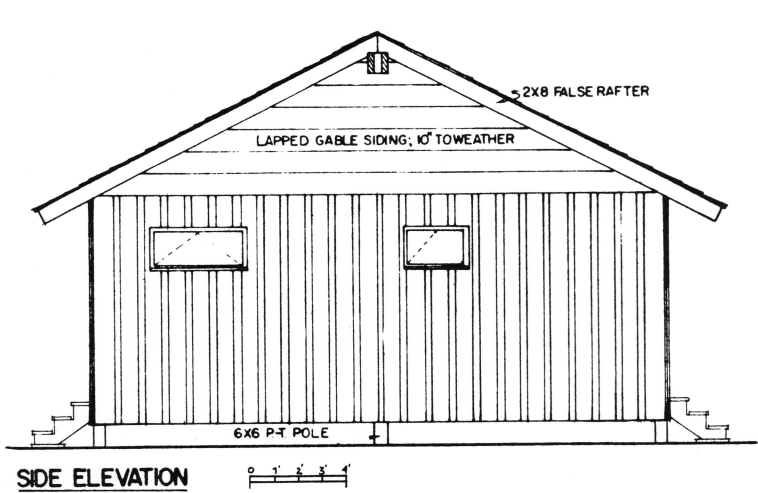

2X8 FALSE RAFTER

LAPPED GABLE SIDING; 10" TO WEATHER

6X6 P.T. POLE

SIDE ELEVATION

0 1' 2' 3' 4'

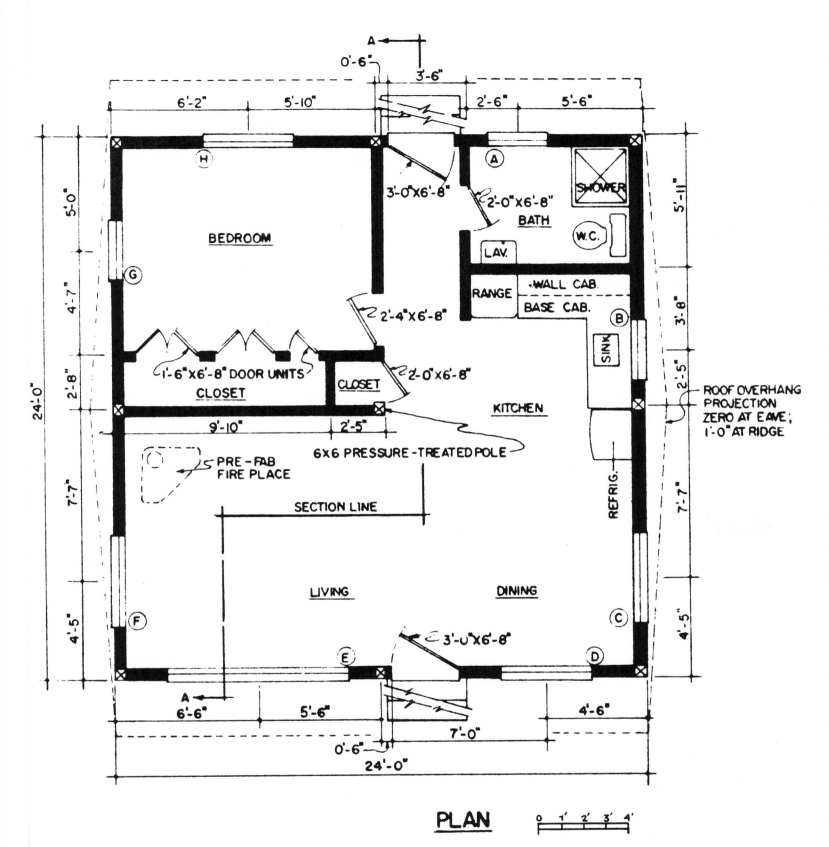

PLAN

0 1' 2' 3' 4'

ROOF OVERHANG
PROJECTION
ZERO AT EAVE;
1'-0" AT RIDGE

6x6 PRESSURE-TREATED POLE

SECTION LINE

PRE-FAB
FIRE PLACE

1'-6"X6'-8" DOOR UNITS

BEDROOM

CLOSET

CLOSET

KITCHEN

BATH

SHOWER

W.C.

LAV.

RANGE

*WALL CAB.

BASE CAB.

SINK

REFRIG.

LIVING

DINING

2'-4"X6'-8"

2'-0"X6'-8"

3'-0"X6'-8"

2'-0"X6'-8"

3'-0"X6'-8"

WINDOW SCHEDULE

WINDOW	UNIT SIZE	NO. OF UNITS
A	1'-8"X2'-8"	1
B	1'-8"X2'-8"	1
C	1'-8"X4'-1"	1
D	1'-8"X4'-1"	2
E	1'-8"X4'-1"	6
F	1'-8"X4'-1"	1
G	1'-8"X2'-8"	1
H	1'-8"X4'-1"	1

*ALL AWNING WINDOW UNITS SIZES
ARE APPROXIMATE. OTHER WINDOW
SIZES AND/OR STYLES MAY BE
SUBSTITUTED AS DESIRED.

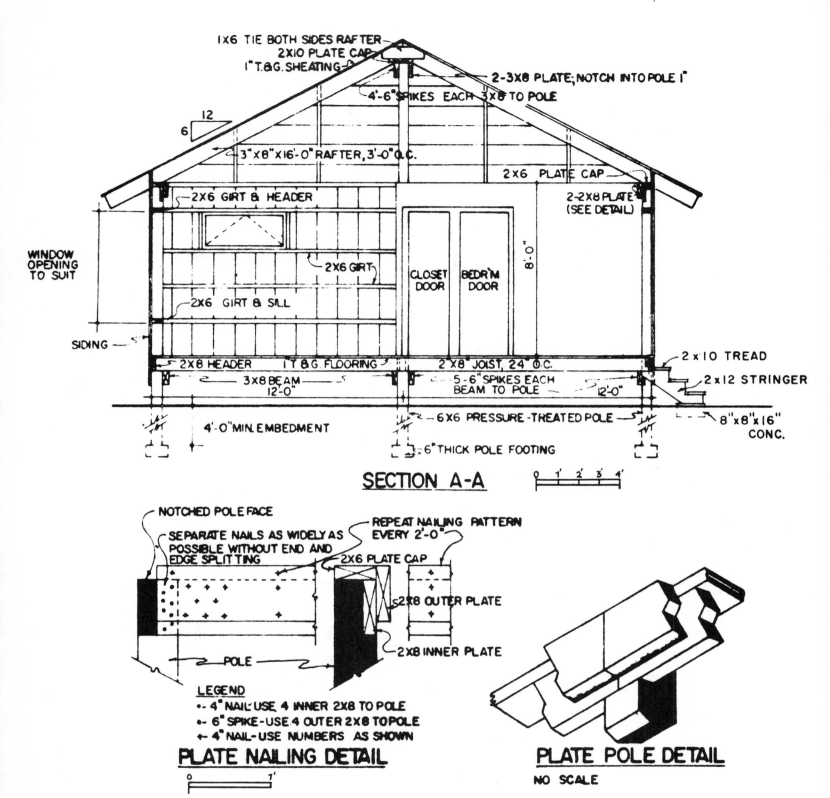

1X6 TIE BOTH SIDES RAFTER
2X10 PLATE CAP
1" T.& G. SHEATING

2-3X8 PLATE; NOTCH INTO POLE 1"
4'-6" SPIKES EACH 3X8 TO POLE

12
6

3"X8"X16'-0" RAFTER, 3'-0" O.C.

2X6 PLATE CAP

2-2X8 PLATE (SEE DETAIL)

2X6 GIRT & HEADER

2X6 GIRT

CLOSET DOOR

BEDR'M DOOR

8'-0"

WINDOW OPENING TO SUIT

2X6 GIRT & SILL

SIDING

2X8 HEADER

1" T.& G. FLOORING

2X8 JOIST, 24" O.C.

2 x 10 TREAD

2 x 12 STRINGER

3X8 BEAM 12'-0"

5-6" SPIKES EACH BEAM TO POLE

12'-0"

4'-0" MIN. EMBEDMENT

6X6 PRESSURE-TREATED POLE

6" THICK POLE FOOTING

8"X8"X16" CONC.

SECTION A-A

0 1 2 3 4'

NOTCHED POLE FACE

SEPARATE NAILS AS WIDELY AS POSSIBLE WITHOUT END AND EDGE SPLITTING

REPEAT NAILING PATTERN EVERY 2'-0"

2X6 PLATE CAP

2X8 OUTER PLATE

2X8 INNER PLATE

POLE

LEGEND
- • - 4" NAIL-USE 4 INNER 2X8 TO POLE
- ● - 6" SPIKE-USE 4 OUTER 2X8 TO POLE
- ✛ - 4" NAIL-USE NUMBERS AS SHOWN

PLATE NAILING DETAIL

0   1'

PLATE POLE DETAIL
NO SCALE

NOTES:
1. DESIGN BASED ON ROUGH-SAWN EASTERN HEMLOCK.

2. DESIGN ROOF LOAD - 40 PSF

3. DESIGN FLOOR LOAD - 35 PSF.

4. ALL FRAMING NAILS SHOULD BE OF HARDENED THREADED TYPE.

5. FLOOR- AND ROOF-DECKING JOINTS SHOULD BE WELL STAGGERED.

6. ROUGH 1" BOARDS ARE SUGGESTED FOR SIDING.

7. INTERIOR FINISH IS LEFT TO BUILDER'S DISCRETION.

14. ONE-ROOM POLE-FRAME CABIN

This structure was designed for builders having limited finances, time, and construction skills. Besides being used as campsite living quarters, it can be an auxiliary structure for such other uses as a concession stand or a storage shelter.

The use of pole framing is in keeping with the objectives of design simplicity, low cost, and flexibility of arrangement. Pole framing is not necessarily unattractive from either the exterior or the interior. Several kinds of covering materials can be used, depending on cost, desired appearance, and availability. This plan suggests using rough-sawn board-and-batten siding with 10- to 12-inch-wide boards and 2- to 3-inch-wide battens over cracks between the boards. Such siding is economical, attractive, and easily applied.

Though a wood-framed floor structure on a level site is shown here, this type of construction is also adaptable to a sloping site. A concrete floor slab could be substituted on a well-drained, level site.

The window treatment is quite flexible as to type and location.

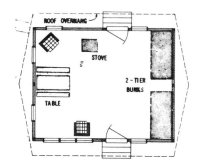

THE FLOOR PLAN IS 16 FEET BY 20 FEET WITH SIDE-WALL POLES SPACED 10 FEET ON CENTER. THE STRUCTURE CAN BE EXTENDED TO 30 FEET THEREBY ALLOWING ONE END TO BE PARTITIONED INTO SLEEPING AREAS.

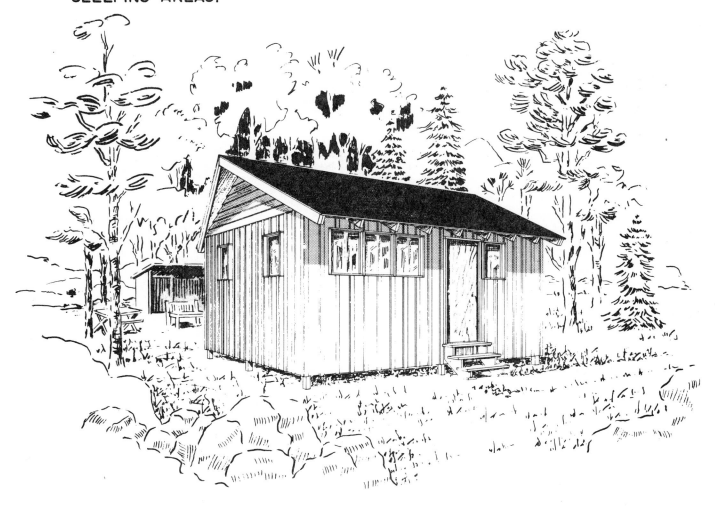

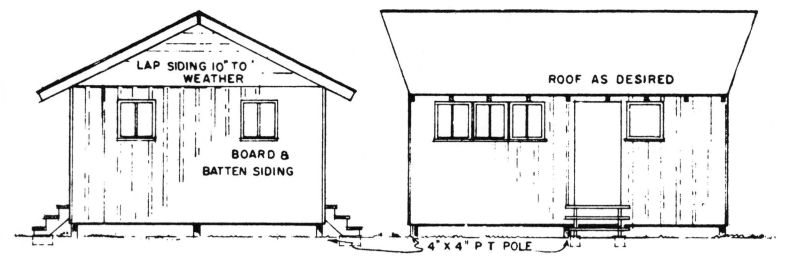

LAP SIDING 10" TO
WEATHER

BOARD 8
BATTEN SIDING

ROOF AS DESIRED

4" X 4" P T POLE

END ELEVATION

FRONT ELEVATION

0 1' 2' 3' 4' 5'

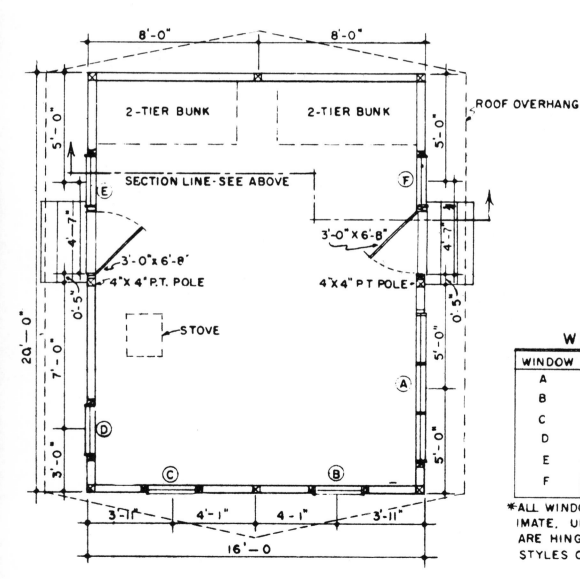

8'-0"   8'-0"

5'-0"

2-TIER BUNK   2-TIER BUNK

5'-0"

ROOF OVERHANG

E

SECTION LINE - SEE ABOVE

F

4'-7"

3'-0" X 6'-8'

3'-0" x 6'-8'

4'-7"

4" X 4" P.T. POLE

4"X 4" PT POLE

0'-5"

0'-5"

20'-0"

7'-0"

STOVE

5'-0"

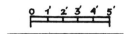
A

5'-0"

D

3'-0"

C   B

3'-1"   4'-1"   4-1"   3'-11"

16'-0"

PLAN

0 1' 2' 3' 4' 5'

WINDOW SCHEDULE

WINDOW	UNIT SIZE*	NO. OF UNITS
A	28" x 28"	3
B		1
C		1
D		1
E		1
F		1

*ALL WINDOW UNIT SIZES ARE APPROX-
IMATE, UNITS ARE INSWINGING &
ARE HINGED AT THE TOP OTHER
STYLES OR SIZES MAY BE SUBSTITUTED

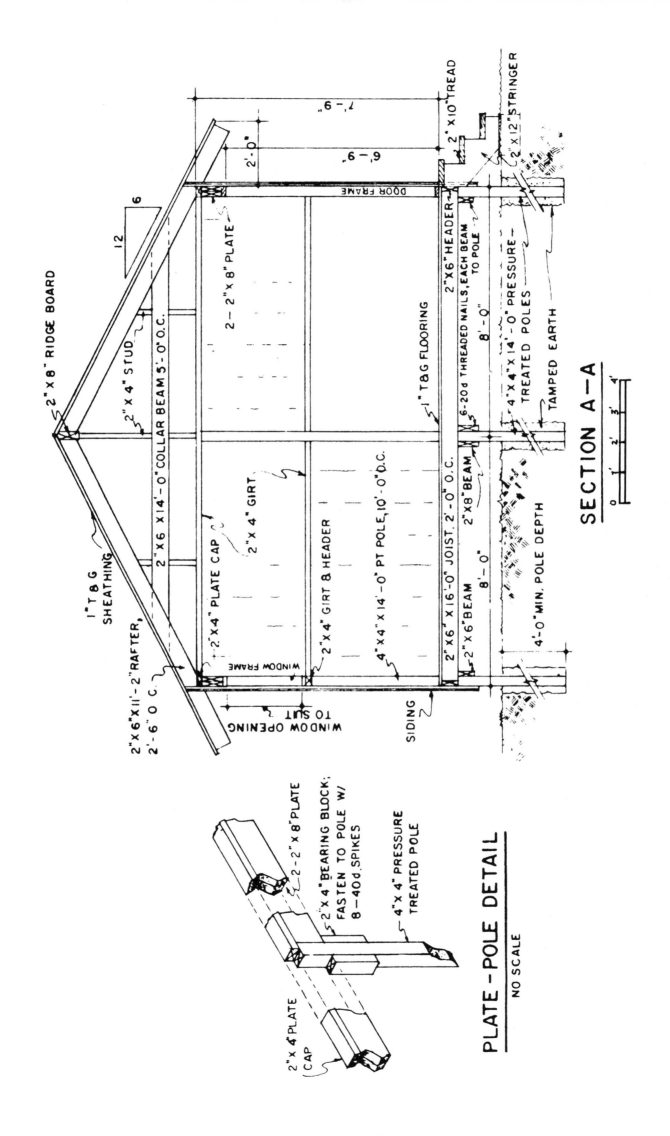

2"x8" RIDGE BOARD

1" T&G SHEATHING

2"x6"x11'-2" RAFTER, 2'-6" O.C.

2"x4" STUD

2"x6"x14'-0" COLLAR BEAM 5'-0" O.C.

2-2"x8" PLATE

12
6

7'-9"
2'-0"
6'-9"

DOOR FRAME

2"x6" HEADER
6-20d THREADED NAILS, EACH BEAM TO POLE
8'-0"
4"x4"x14'-0" PRESSURE TREATED POLES
TAMPED EARTH

2"x10" TREAD
2"x12" STRINGER

SECTION A-A

0 1 2 3 4

2"x4" PLATE CAP

2"x4" GIRT

2"x4" GIRT & HEADER

4"x4"x14'-0" PT POLE, 10'-0" O.C.

WINDOW FRAME

WINDOW OPENING TO SUIT

SIDING

1" T&G FLOORING

2"x6"x16'-0" JOIST, 2'-0" O.C.

2"x8" BEAM
2"x6" BEAM
8'-0"

4'-0" MIN. POLE DEPTH

2-2"x8" PLATE

2"x4" BEARING BLOCK; FASTEN TO POLE W/ 8-40d SPIKES

4"x4" PRESSURE TREATED POLE

2"x4" PLATE CAP

PLATE-POLE DETAIL

NO SCALE

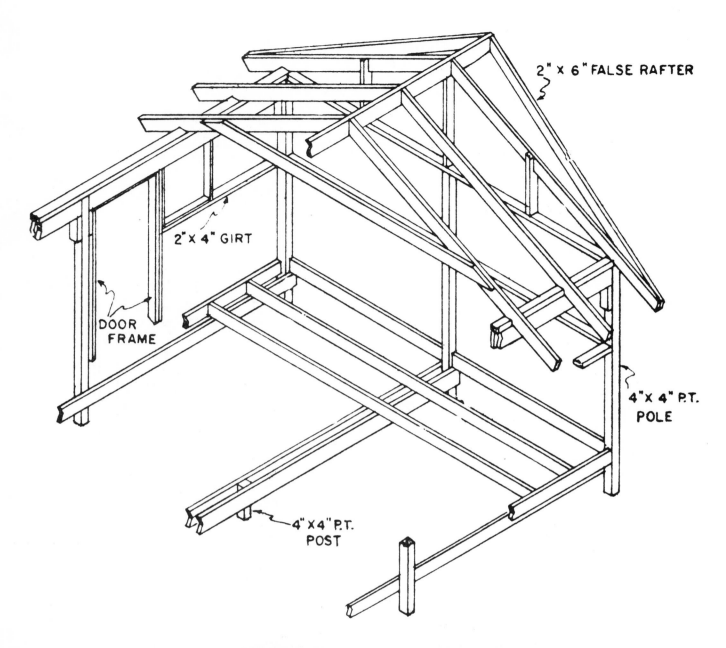

2" X 6" FALSE RAFTER

2" X 4" GIRT

DOOR
FRAME

4" X 4" P.T.
POLE

4" X 4" P.T.
POST

FRAMING PERSPECTIVE

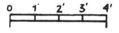

0   1'   2'   3'   4'

CONSTRUCTION NOTES

1......THIS DESIGN IS BASED ON THE USE OF ROUGH-SAWN EASTERN HEMLOCK
2 ..DESIGN ROOF LOAD 40 LBS. PER. SQ. FT.
3 DESIGN FLOOR LOAD 40 LBS PER SQ. FT.
4 ..LENGTHS OF POLES ARE DEPENDENT ON SLOPE OF BUILDING SITE
5 ...ALL FRAMING NAILS SHOULD BE HARDENED AND THREADED.
6......ALL WOOD IN CONTACT WITH EARTH SHOULD BE PRESSURE TREATED
         WITH A PRESERVATIVE.
7 ..ROUGH-SAWN BOARD & BATTEN SIDING WITH 10" TO 12" WIDE BOARDS &
         2" TO 3" WIDE BATTENS ON THE BETWEEN-BOARD CRACKS IS ATTRACTIVE.
         OTHER SIDING MATERIALS MAY BE USED IF DESIRED.
8 .. INTERIOR FINISH IS LEFT TO THE BUILDERS DISCRETION.

15. TWO-BEDROOM FRAME VACATION HOME

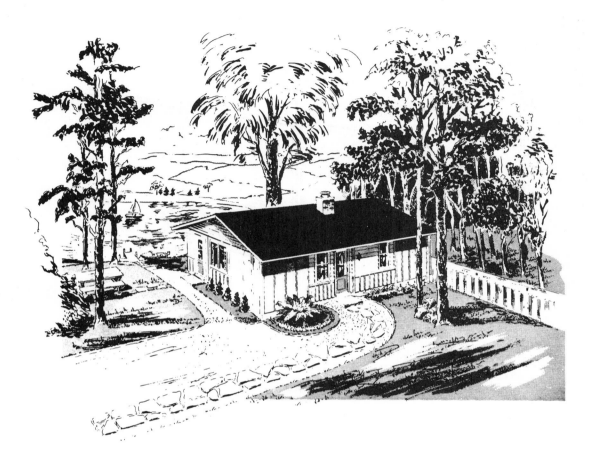

Comfort, convenience, safety, and economy were designed into this house by agricultural engineers at Beltsville, Md. The heating system uniformly distributes heat from any type of heater—wood, coal, gas, or oil-fired. The standards of convenience and sanitation that are found in the most expensive home are maintained in this low-cost house. The framing timber is used efficiently so that cost of material is reduced without loss of the framing strength. Wall panels, trusses, and floor systems were load-tested to prove the strength.

The outstanding features of this house are the post-and-girt construction and a free-floating floor that promotes central heating without ductwork—that is, perimeter distribution of warmed air. Besides these improvements in construction methods, the house plan embodies the usual cost-saving features —multiple use of space, minimum traffic lanes, and omission of unnecessary trim or doors.

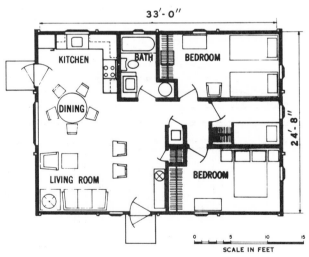

See page 95 for additional information on post-and-girt construction and this structure's heating system.

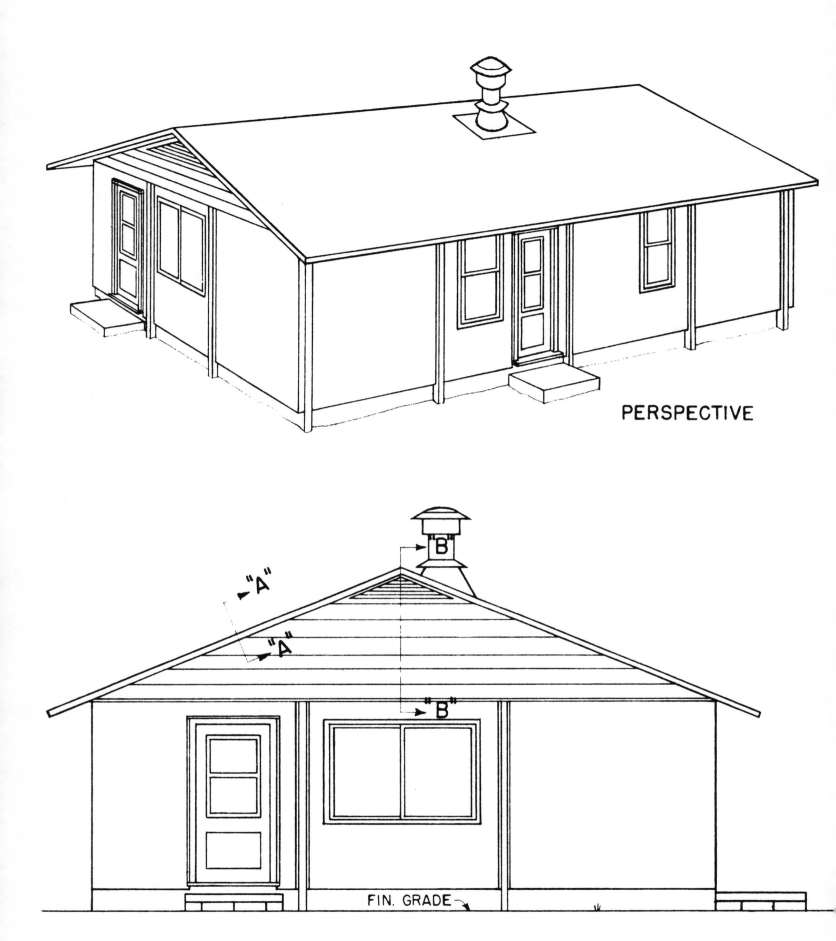

PERSPECTIVE

"A"

"A"

"B"

"B"

FIN. GRADE

LEFT END ELEVATION
SCALE: 1/4"= 1'-0"

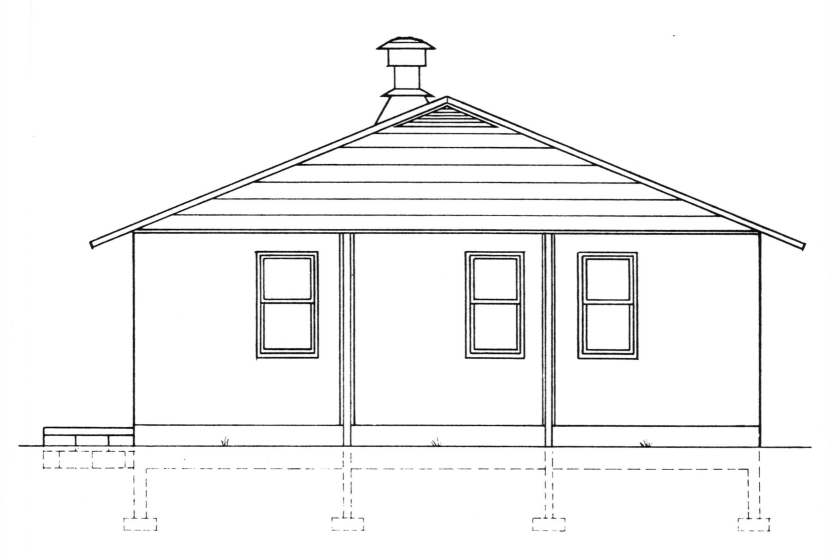

RIGHT END ELEVATION
SCALE: ¼"= 1'-0"

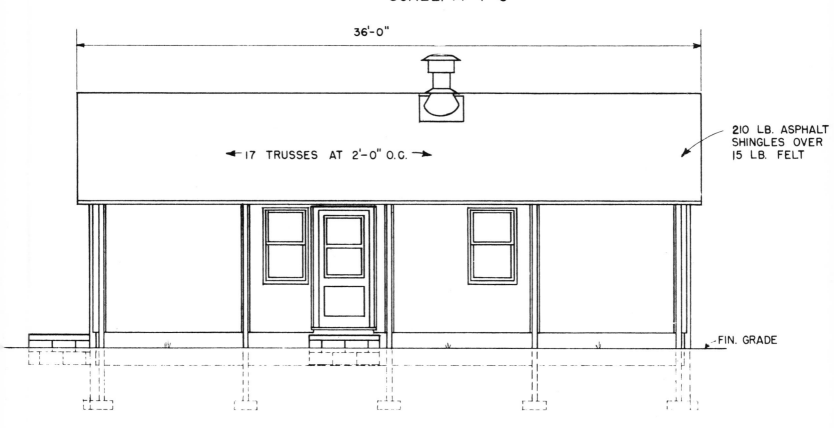

36'-0"

← 17 TRUSSES AT 2'-0" O.C. →

210 LB. ASPHALT
SHINGLES OVER
15 LB. FELT

FIN. GRADE

FRONT ELEVATION

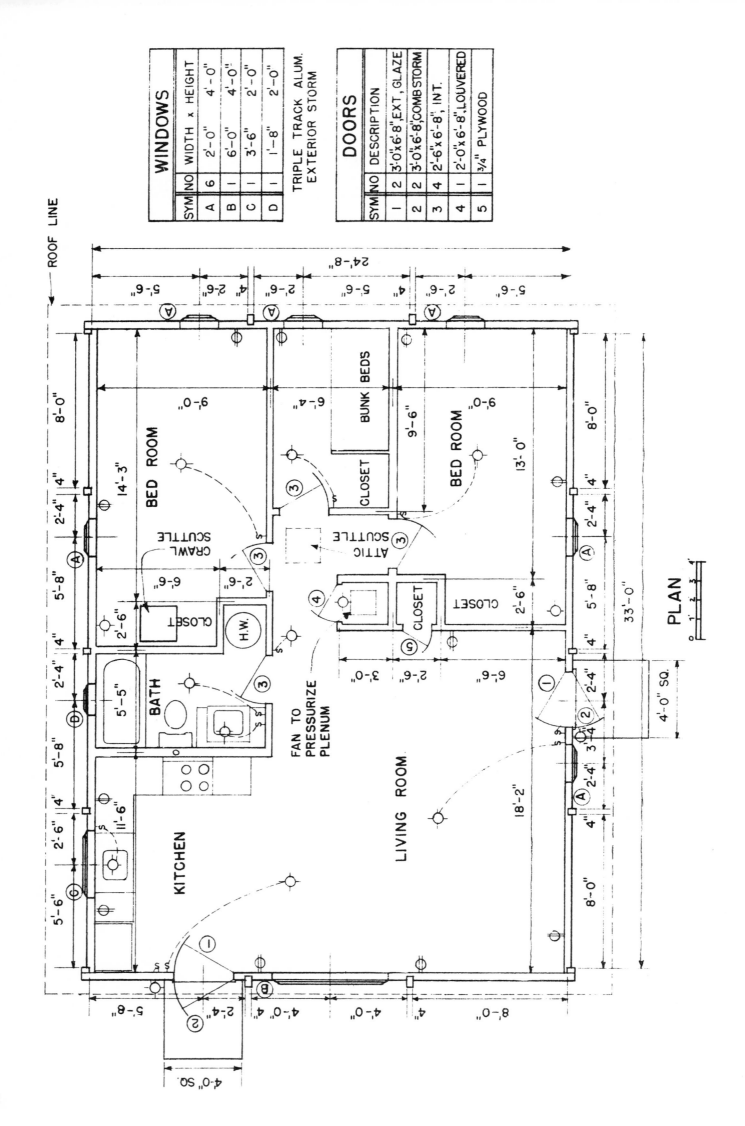

WINDOWS

SYM	NO	WIDTH x HEIGHT	
A	6	2'-0"	4'-0"
B	1	6'-0"	4'-0"
C	1	3'-6"	2'-0"
D	1	1'-8"	2'-0"

TRIPLE TRACK ALUM. EXTERIOR STORM

DOORS

SYM	NO	DESCRIPTION
1	2	3'-0"x6'-8",EXT, GLAZE
2	2	3'-0"x6'-8",COMB STORM
3	4	2'-6"x6'-8", INT.
4	1	2'-0"x6'-8",LOUVERED
5	1	3/4" PLYWOOD

ROOF LINE

BED ROOM

BUNK BEDS

CLOSET

BED ROOM

CRAWL SCUTTLE

ATTIC SCUTTLE

CLOSET

CLOSET

H.W.

BATH

FAN TO PRESSURIZE PLENUM

LIVING ROOM

KITCHEN

PLAN

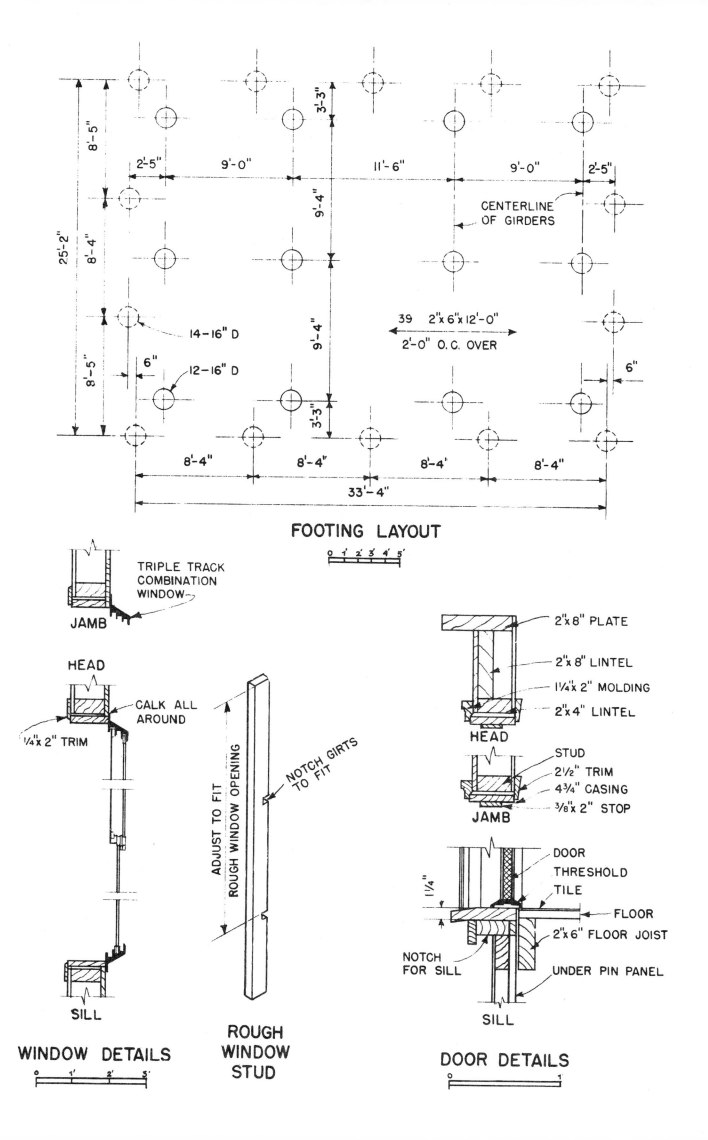

FOOTING LAYOUT

25'-2"
8'-5"
8'-4"
8'-5"

2'-5" 9'-0" 11'-6" 9'-0" 2'-5"

3'-3"

9'-4"

CENTERLINE OF GIRDERS

14–16" D

12–16" D

6"

9'-4"

39 2"x 6"x 12'-0"
2'-0" O.C. OVER

6"

3'-3"

8'-4" 8'-4" 8'-4' 8'-4"

33'-4"

0 1 2 3 4 5'

TRIPLE TRACK
COMBINATION
WINDOW

JAMB

HEAD

CALK ALL
AROUND

1/4"x 2" TRIM

ADJUST TO FIT
ROUGH WINDOW OPENING

NOTCH GIRTS
TO FIT

SILL

WINDOW DETAILS

0 1 2 3

**ROUGH
WINDOW
STUD**

2"x 8" PLATE

2"x 8" LINTEL

1 1/4"x 2" MOLDING

2"x 4" LINTEL

HEAD

STUD

2 1/2" TRIM

4 3/4" CASING

3/8"x 2" STOP

JAMB

DOOR
THRESHOLD
TILE

1 1/4"

FLOOR

2"x 6" FLOOR JOIST

NOTCH
FOR SILL

UNDER PIN PANEL

SILL

DOOR DETAILS

0 1

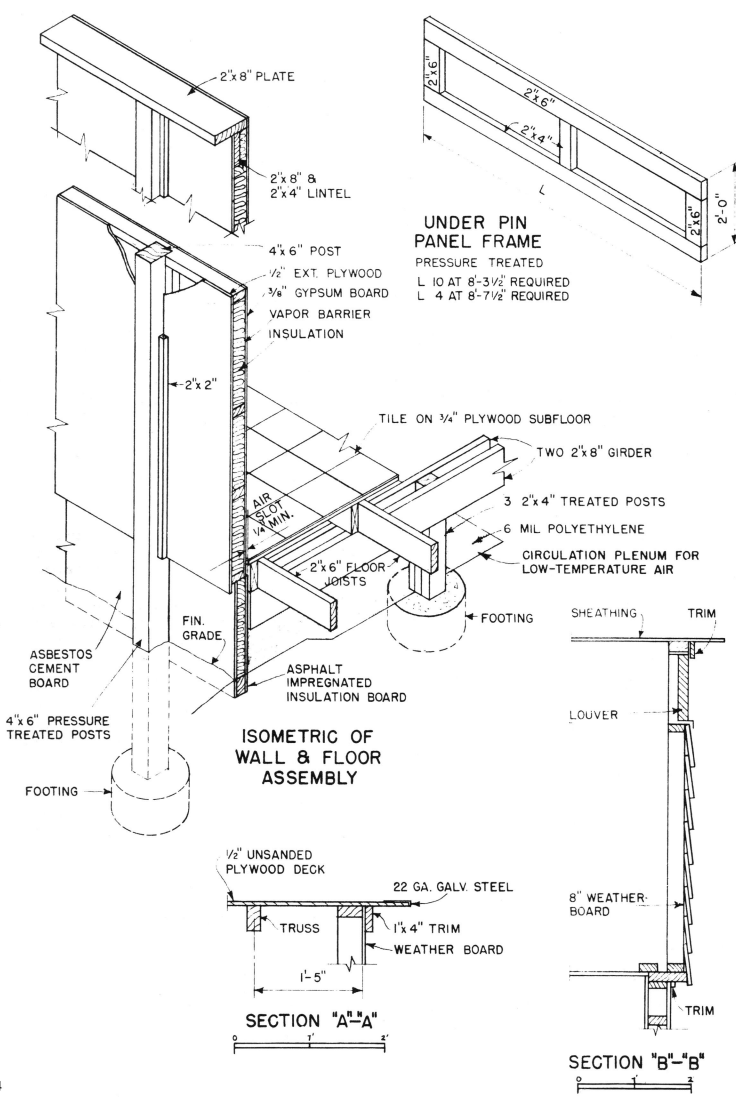

2"x 8" PLATE

2"x 8" &
2"x 4" LINTEL

4"x 6" POST

½" EXT. PLYWOOD
⅜" GYPSUM BOARD
VAPOR BARRIER
INSULATION

2"x 2"

ASBESTOS
CEMENT
BOARD

4"x 6" PRESSURE
TREATED POSTS

FOOTING

FIN.
GRADE

AIR
SLOT
¼" MIN.

2"x 6" FLOOR
JOISTS

ASPHALT
IMPREGNATED
INSULATION BOARD

ISOMETRIC OF
WALL & FLOOR
ASSEMBLY

UNDER PIN
PANEL FRAME
PRESSURE TREATED
L 10 AT 8'-3½" REQUIRED
L 4 AT 8'-7½" REQUIRED

2"x 6"
2"x 6"
2"x 4"
2"x 6"
2'-0"

TILE ON ¾" PLYWOOD SUBFLOOR

TWO 2"x 8" GIRDER

3 2"x 4" TREATED POSTS

6 MIL POLYETHYLENE

CIRCULATION PLENUM FOR
LOW-TEMPERATURE AIR

FOOTING

½" UNSANDED
PLYWOOD DECK

22 GA. GALV. STEEL

TRUSS

1"x 4" TRIM

WEATHER BOARD

1'-5"

SECTION "A"-"A"

0   1'   2'

SHEATHING   TRIM

LOUVER

8" WEATHER-
BOARD

TRIM

SECTION "B"-"B"

0   1'   2'

94

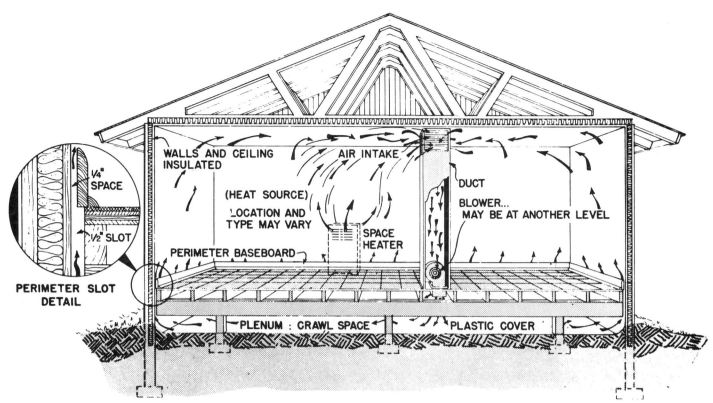

Detail labels:
- ¼" SPACE
- ½" SLOT
- PERIMETER SLOT DETAIL
- WALLS AND CEILING INSULATED
- (HEAT SOURCE) LOCATION AND TYPE MAY VARY
- PERIMETER BASEBOARD
- AIR INTAKE
- SPACE HEATER
- DUCT
- BLOWER... MAY BE AT ANOTHER LEVEL
- PLENUM : CRAWL SPACE
- PLASTIC COVER

AIR DIFFUSION SYSTEM USING UNDER-FLOOR PLENUM WITH PERIMETER SLOT

Post-and-girt construction

Pressure treated 4- x 6-inch posts, set 8 feet 4 inches on center, serve as foundation members; as the columnar support for the airtight, insulated, skirt wall around the crawl space and as the columnar supports for the curtain-wall sides and roof. The built-up plate and lintel system is continuous around the entire periphery of the house. No further lintels are needed over the doors and windows. The full 8-inch-wide top plate member and the 8-inch-deep lintel form an excellent foundation for fastening the roof trusses. A building with this continuous tie from the foundation through the trusses is more resistant to wind damage than a building with conventional platform framing.

Horizontal nail ties, 2 feet on center, are notched onto the posts for precision spacing and alignment —a help in speedy erection. The curtain-wall sides are continuous on the interior, but are placed between the posts on the exterior. The skirt wall beneath the floor is a little over 2 inches thick and is installed on the inside of the posts. Because of its continuity, the skirt can easily be made airtight. No ventilators are installed in the crawl space of this house.

Continuous cantilevered joists and girders support the floor and carry the interior loads independently of the exterior loads and shrinkage. This improve-ment in construction technique prevents doors and windows from being pulled out of line and sticking. In conventional construction, floor settlement creates problems in the walls. With post-and-girt construction, the floor can be installed after the roof and walls are placed, and interior partitions can be installed after the floor and ceiling are in place.

Superior heating at low cost

The perimeter-slot heating system used in this house provides draft-free comfort and a uniform temperature. A fan draws warm air from a centrally located intake near the ceiling and delivers it into the crawl space beneath the floor. Since air pressure in the crawl space is a little higher than that inside the house, air flows through the ¼-inch-wide slot around the entire periphery of the house This air warms the floor and walls, and the result is draft-free uniform temperatures in the house.

The uniformity is somewhat better when the air is heated with a down-draft type of hot air furnace than when it is heated with a space heater in one corner of the living room. However, tests of the heating systems show that while both of the above systems are superior to the perimeter loop type, the perimeter-slot heating system gives the best heat distribution at lower cost than the other systems.

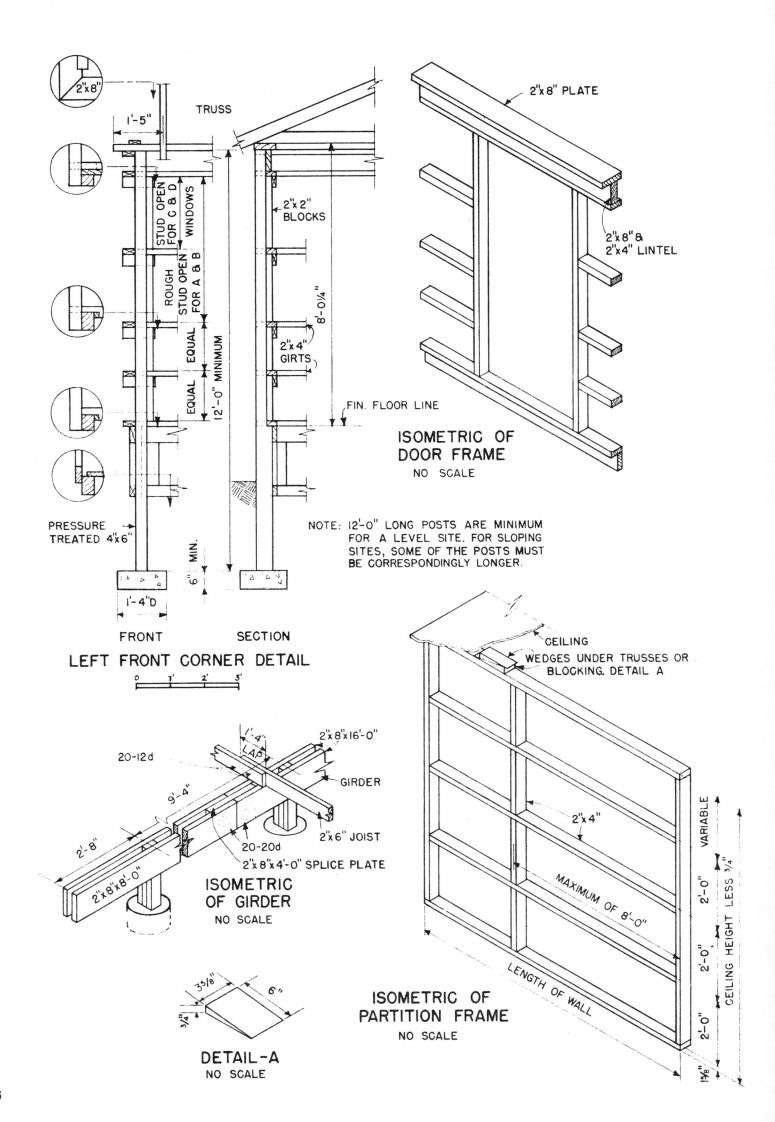

2"x8"

1'-5"

TRUSS

STUD OPEN FOR C & D WINDOWS

ROUGH

STUD OPEN FOR A & B

EQUAL

EQUAL

EQUAL

12'-0" MINIMUM

2"x2" BLOCKS

8'-0¼"

2"x4" GIRTS

FIN. FLOOR LINE

PRESSURE TREATED 4"x6"

6" MIN.

1'-4"D

FRONT   SECTION

LEFT FRONT CORNER DETAIL

0   1'   2'   3'

2"x8" PLATE

2"x8" & 2"x4" LINTEL

ISOMETRIC OF DOOR FRAME
NO SCALE

NOTE: 12'-0" LONG POSTS ARE MINIMUM FOR A LEVEL SITE. FOR SLOPING SITES, SOME OF THE POSTS MUST BE CORRESPONDINGLY LONGER.

20-12d

1'-4" LAP

2"x8"x16'-0"

GIRDER

9'-4"

2'-8"

2"x8"x8'-0"

20-20d

2"x6" JOIST

2"x8"x4'-0" SPLICE PLATE

ISOMETRIC OF GIRDER
NO SCALE

3⅝"

6"

¾"

DETAIL-A
NO SCALE

CEILING

WEDGES UNDER TRUSSES OR BLOCKING. DETAIL A

2"x4"

MAXIMUM OF 8'-0"

VARIABLE

2'-0" ¾"

2'-0"

2'-0"

1⅝"

CEILING HEIGHT LESS ¾"

LENGTH OF WALL

ISOMETRIC OF PARTITION FRAME
NO SCALE

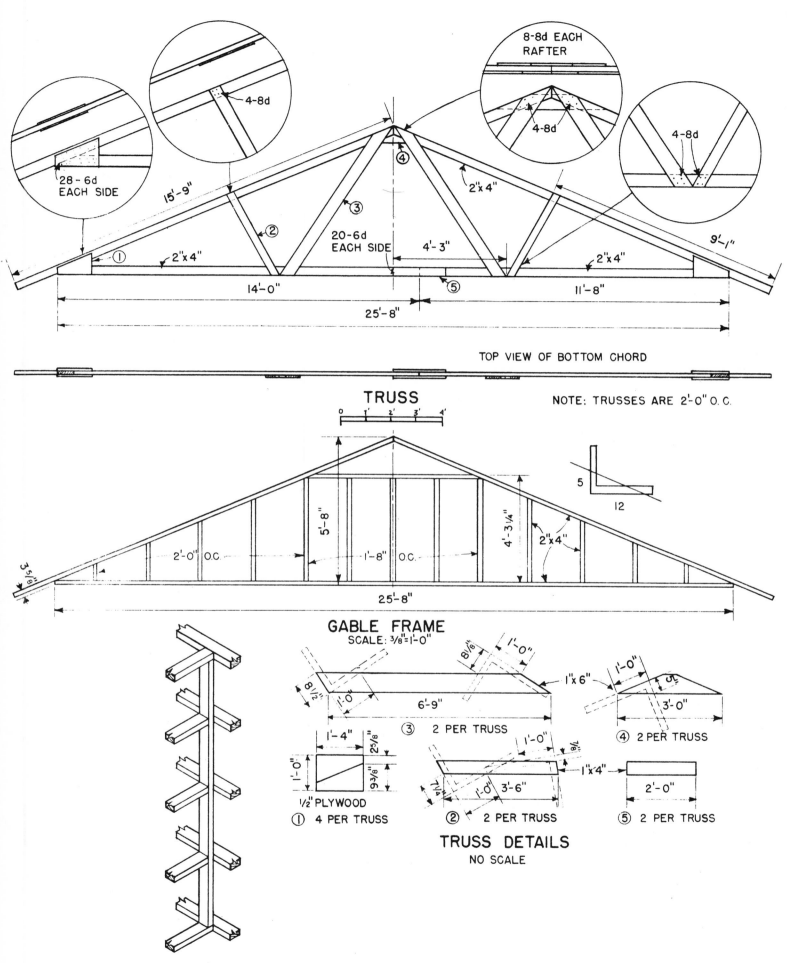

8-8d EACH RAFTER

4-8d

4-8d

4-8d

28-6d EACH SIDE

4-8d

15'-9"

2"x 4"

②

①

2"x 4"

20-6d EACH SIDE

③

④

4'-3"

⑤

2"x 4"

9'-1"

2"x 4"

14'-0"

11'-8"

25'-8"

TOP VIEW OF BOTTOM CHORD

TRUSS

0 1' 2' 3' 4'

NOTE: TRUSSES ARE 2'-0" O.C.

5'-8"

4'-3 1/4"

2"x 4"

2'-0" O.C.

1'-8" O.C.

3 5/8"

25'-8"

5

12

GABLE FRAME
SCALE: 3/8"=1'-0"

8/8"

1'-0"

8 1/2"

1'-0"

6'-9"

1"x 6"

③ 2 PER TRUSS

1'-0"

1'-0"

7/8"

3'-0"

④ 2 PER TRUSS

1'-4"

2 5/8"

1'-0"

9 3/8"

1/2" PLYWOOD

① 4 PER TRUSS

1'-0"

7/8"

7 1/4"

1'-0"

3'-6"

1"x 4"

② 2 PER TRUSS

2'-0"

⑤ 2 PER TRUSS

TRUSS DETAILS
NO SCALE

ISOMETRIC OF
CORNER IN PARTITION
FRAME
NO SCALE

16. TWO-BEDROOM TENANT HOUSE

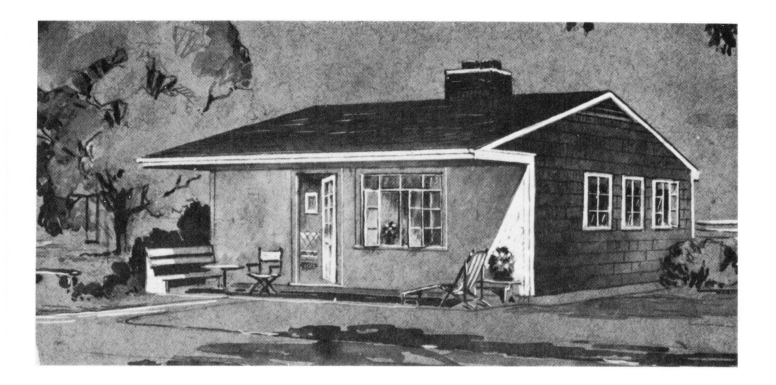

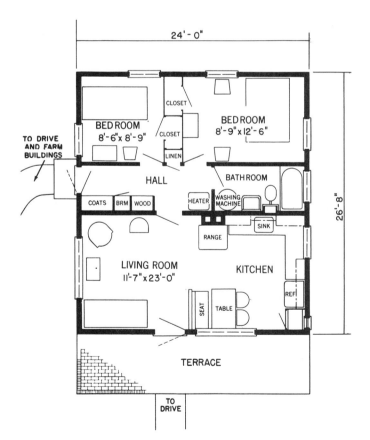

This basic structure is suitable for use as a tenant house or for the first home of a young couple.

For economy and good use of space, the living room, dining room, and kitchen are combined into one large room. Folding screens may be used to separate the kitchen area from the main living room.

A ventilated storage cabinet for food is provided next to the refrigerator.

A bunk bed could be used in the smaller of the two bedrooms. A deep, roll-rim sink in the bathroom serves as washbowl and laundry tray. There is space in the bathroom for a washing machine. In such a small house, the bathroom is a better place for doing the laundry than the cooking and living quarters.

A circulator heater or floor furnace can be installed in the back hall. The hall also contains clothes and utility closets.

The pipes for all plumbing fixtures are in one partition, which means that they can be installed with the greatest economy.

With the gable roof, the house can be expanded or the interior rearranged later at minimum expense. The roof is trussed, so there are no interior bearing partitions.

With the flat roof, the center partition of the house is a bearing partition, but other partitions can easily be moved. This style is usually a little cheaper to build than the gabled style.

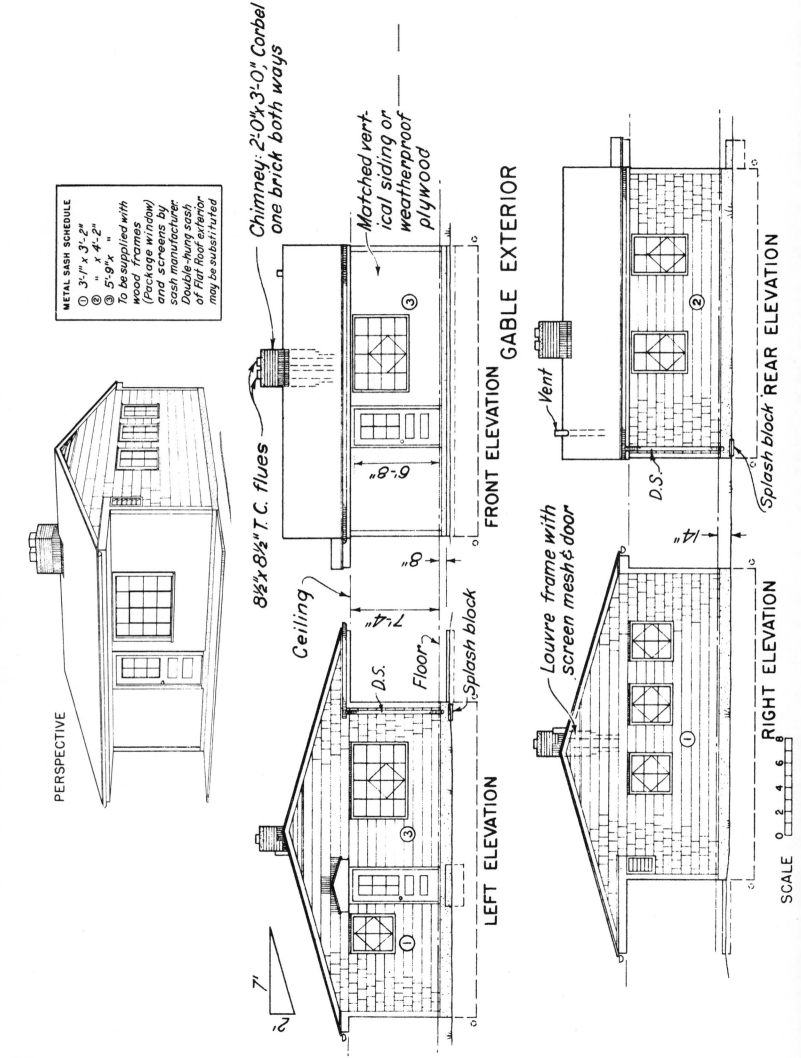

METAL SASH SCHEDULE

① 3'-1" x 3'-2"
② " x 4'-2"
③ 5'-9"x "

To be supplied with wood frames (Package window) and screens by sash manufacturer. Double-hung sash of Flat Roof exterior may be substituted

Chimney: 2'-0"x3'-0", Corbel one brick both ways

Matched vertical siding or weatherproof plywood

8½"x 8½" T.C. flues

Ceiling

Floor

D.S.

Splash block

6'-8"

8"

7'-4"

FRONT ELEVATION
GABLE EXTERIOR

LEFT ELEVATION

7'

2'

PERSPECTIVE

Vent

D.S.

Splash block REAR ELEVATION

14"

Louvre frame with screen mesh & door

RIGHT ELEVATION

SCALE 0 2 4 6 8

100

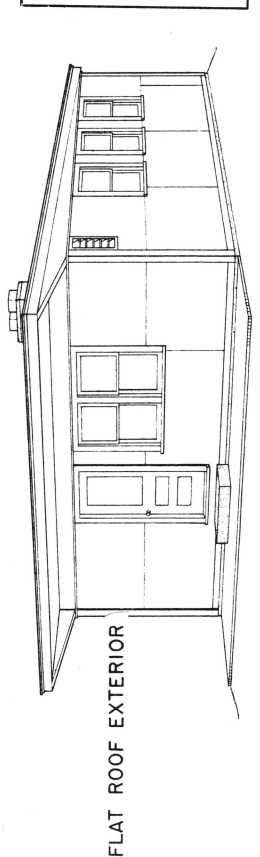

FLAT ROOF EXTERIOR

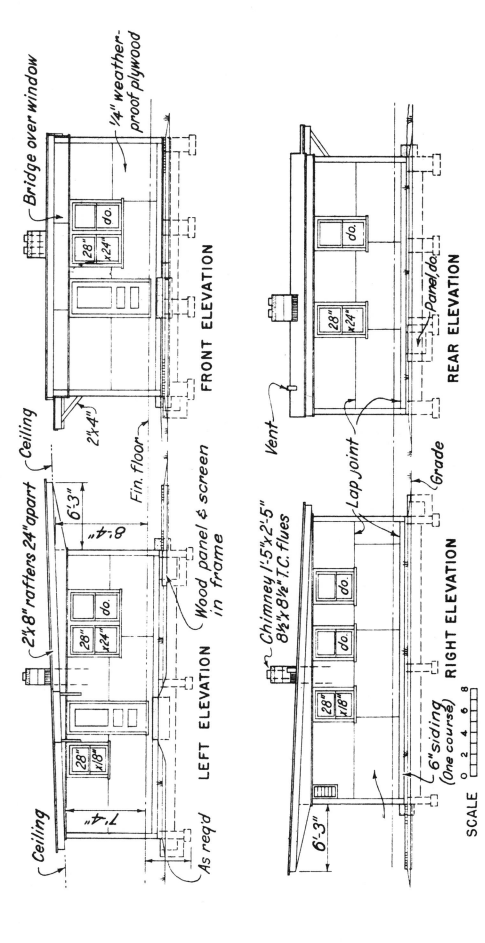

Bridge over window

¼" weather-proof plywood

28" x24" do.

FRONT ELEVATION

2"x4"

Fin. floor

2"x8" rafters 24"apart

Ceiling

6'-3"

8'-4"

28" x24" do.

Wood panel & screen in frame

LEFT ELEVATION

Ceiling

7'-4"

28" x/8"

As req'd

do.

REAR ELEVATION

Panel, do.

28" x24"

Vent

Grade

Lap joint

Chimney 1'-5"x 2'-5" 8½"x8½"T.C. flues

28" x/8" do. do.

RIGHT ELEVATION

6'-3"

6"siding (One course)

SCALE 0 2 4 6 8

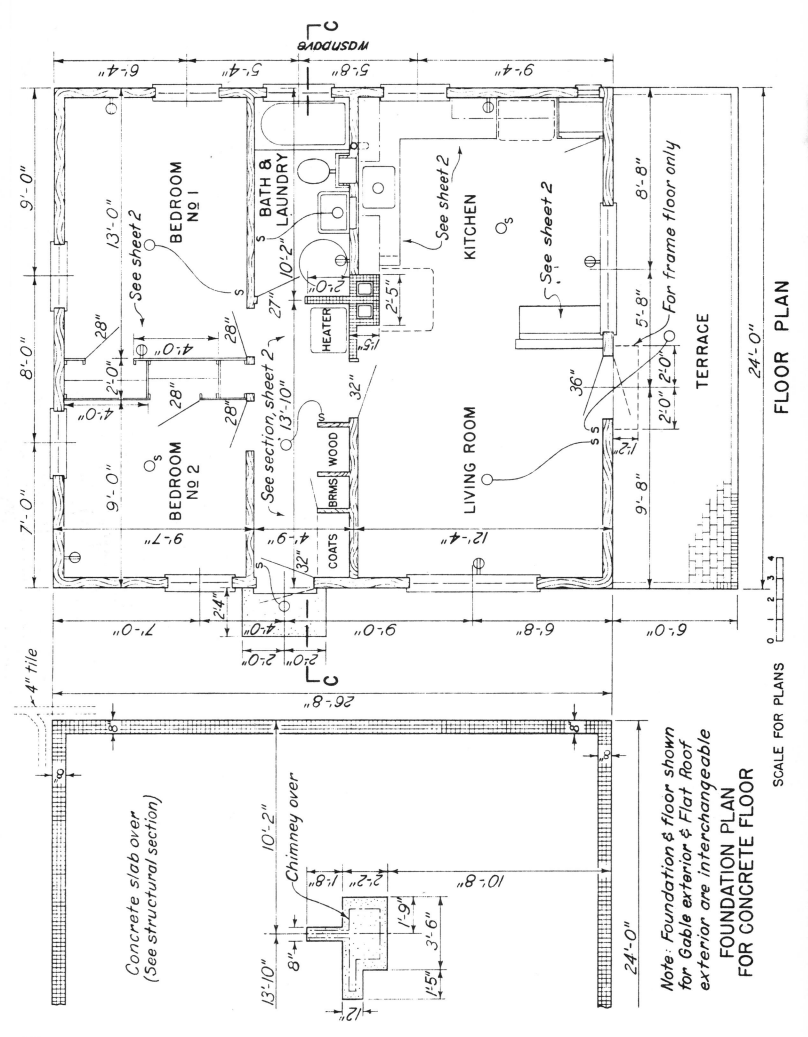

FLOOR PLAN

BEDROOM No 1

BATH & LAUNDRY

KITCHEN

See sheet 2

See sheet 2

See sheet 2

See sheet 2

See section, sheet 2

HEATER

WOOD

BRMS

COATS

BEDROOM No 2

LIVING ROOM

TERRACE

For frame floor only

washbowl

13'-0"

9'-0"

8'-0"

7'-0"

6'-4"

5'-4"

5'-8"

9'-4"

28"

28"

28"

28"

4'-0"

4'-0"

2'-0"

10'-2"

27"

2'-0"

2'-5"

1'-5"

32"

13'-10"

9'-7"

9'-0"

2'-4"

32"

12'-4"

4'-9"

4'-0"

2'-0"

2'-0"

9'-0"

6'-8"

6'-0"

24'-0"

8'-8"

5'-8"

36"

2'-0"

2'-0"

1'-2"

9'-8"

SCALE FOR PLANS

0 1 2 3 4

4" tile

Concrete slab over
(See structural section)

Chimney over

26'-8"

13'-10"

10'-2"

8"

8"

8"

8"

8"

1'-8"

2'-2"

10'-8"

1'-9"

3'-6"

1'-5"

12"

24'-0"

**FOUNDATION PLAN
FOR CONCRETE FLOOR**

Note: Foundation & floor shown
for Gable exterior & Flat Roof
exterior are interchangeable

102

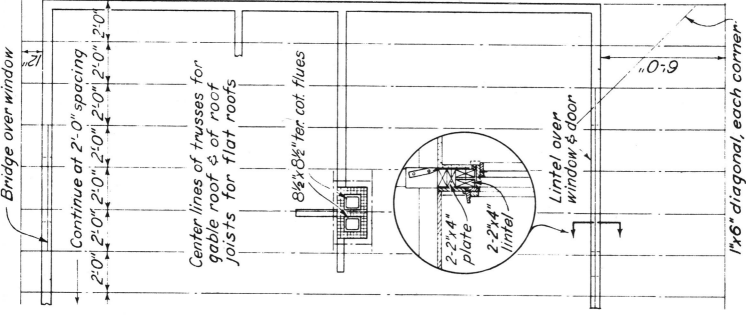

Bridge over window

Continue at 2'-0" spacing

2'-0" 2'-0" 2'-0" 2'-0" 2'-0"

12"

Center lines of trusses for gable roof & of roof joists for flat roofs

8½"x8½"ter. cot. flues

2-2"x4" plate

2-2"x4" lintel

Lintel over window & door

6'-0"

1"x6" diagonal, each corner

ROOF FRAMING PLAN

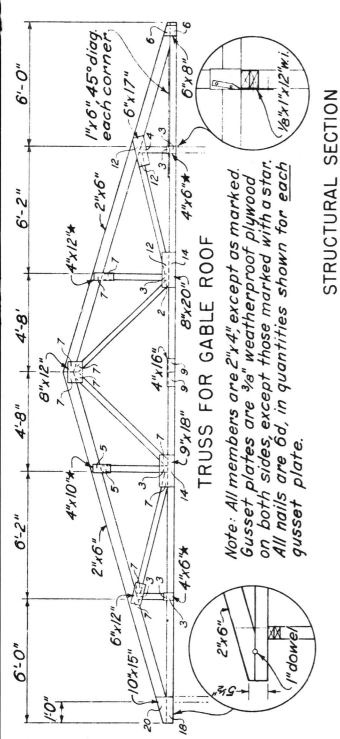

6'-0"

6'-2"

4'-8"

4'-8"

6'-2"

6'-0"

1'-0"

1"x6", 45° diag. each corner

6"x17"

6"x8"

⅛"x1"x12"w.i.

2"x6"

4"x6" ★

4"x12" ★

8"x20"

4"x16"

8"x12"

4"x10" ★

9"x18"

2"x6"

4"x6" ★

6"x12"

10"x15"

2"x6"

1"dowel

5½"

TRUSS FOR GABLE ROOF

Note: All members are 2"x4", except as marked. Gusset plates are ⅜" weatherproof plywood on both sides, except those marked with a star. All nails are 6d, in quantities shown for <u>each</u> gusset plate.

STRUCTURAL SECTION

SCALE 0 1 2

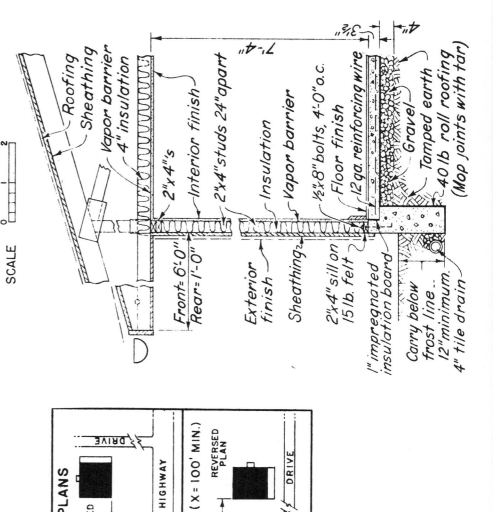

Roofing
Sheathing
Vapor barrier
4" insulation
Interior finish
2"x4"'s
2"x4" studs 24" apart
Insulation
Vapor barrier
½"x8" bolts, 4'-0" o.c.
Floor finish
12 ga. reinforcing wire
Gravel
Tamped earth
40 lb roll roofing
(Mop joints with tar)
1" impregnated insulation board
Carry below frost line... 12"minimum.
4" tile drain
Exterior finish
Sheathing
2"x4" sill on 15 lb. felt

Front = 6'-0"
Rear = 1'-0"

7'-4"

3½"

4"

SUGGESTED PLOT PLANS

NORTH

REVERSED PLAN
DRIVE
HIGHWAY
X

HIGHWAY
DRIVE
REVERSED PLAN

(X = 100' MIN.)

HIGHWAY
DRIVE
X
REVERSED PLAN

HIGHWAY
X
DRIVE

SECTION THROUGH HALL & BATH C-C

Flat roof ceiling

Interior finish

Shelf

13'-10"

Hooks

3'-8"

1'-6"

5'-6"

2'-0"

2'-0"

Matched boards or plywood

2"x4" buck

2'-8"

3'-4"

7'-0"

2'-8"

Heater

1'-0½"

1'-4½"

Hot water stor. tank

To range
From r'ge
From pump

Washing machine

Cold

14"x18"wd med. cab.

18½x24"sink

Hot

2'-0"

1'-8"

6"

12"

12"

12"

Tile wallboard

Dowel

Exposed Shelf

Diverter fitting

30x54"tub

1'-0"

2'-0"

Insulation
Vapor barrier

See kitchen elev's

Cleanout

Hatch

Flat roof ceiling

Slope ¼" per foot

Anchor girders to piers
with ⅛"x1"x18" w.i. straps.

20d nails, space 3" stagger."
4" curtain wall
8"x16" pier

2"x4" ledger

Joists 2"x4"

18"

SCALE 0 1 2

KITCHEN ELEVATIONS

B

(12"wide)
2'-0"

Screen mesh

Slide up door

7'-4"

Window shade

Window

2'-9"

3'-8"

3"

1'-0"

2"

1⅞"

1'-10"

Batten or plywood door

Lin. or tile wallb'd

3'-2"

¾"ply-wood top

2'-0"

1⅞"

1⅞"

2'-8½"

2'-2"

3½"

4"hole

Flat roof ceiling

1⅞"

A

Window shade

6" shelves

2'-9"

2'-8"

1⅞"

1⅞"

2'-8"

2'-4"

1⅞"

Linoleum or wallboard

Tank-range piping

Hot

Cold

3'-2"

2'-0"

2'-0"

2'-8½"

3½"

1⅞"

SCALE 0 1 2

104

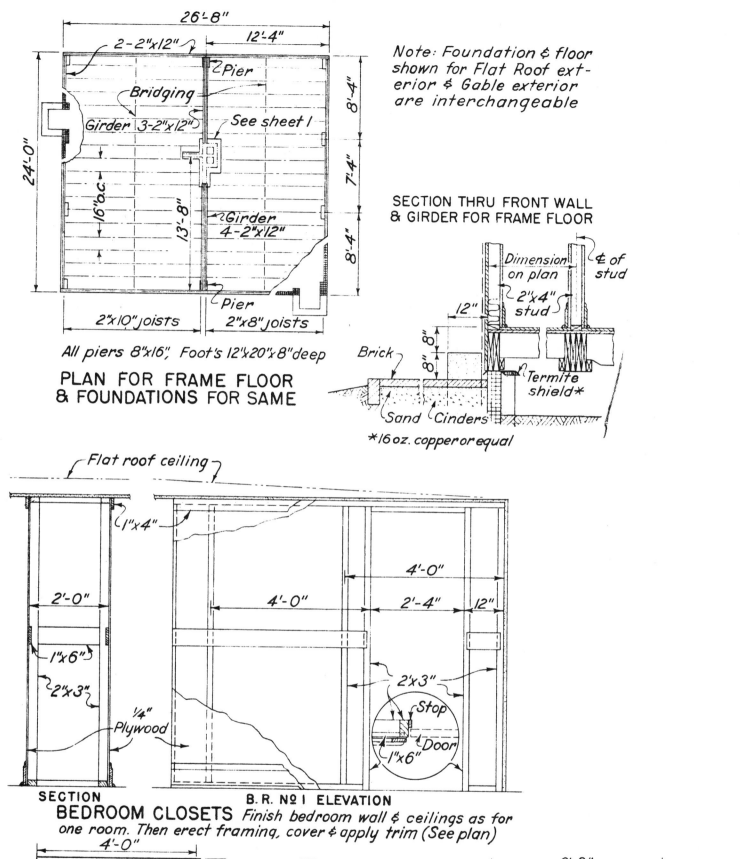

26'-8"

12'-4"

2 - 2"x12"

Pier

Bridging

See sheet 1

Girder 3-2"x12"

24'-0"

8'-4"

7'-4"

16"o.c.

13'-8"

Girder 4-2"x12"

8'-4"

Pier

2"x10" joists

2"x8" joists

All piers 8"x16", Foot's 12"x20"x8"deep

PLAN FOR FRAME FLOOR & FOUNDATIONS FOR SAME

Note: Foundation & floor shown for Flat Roof exterior & Gable exterior are interchangeable

SECTION THRU FRONT WALL & GIRDER FOR FRAME FLOOR

Dimension on plan

℄ of stud

2"x4" stud

12"

8" 8"

Brick

Termite shield*

Sand Cinders

*16 oz. copper or equal

Flat roof ceiling

1"x4"

2'-0"

4'-0"

4'-0"

2'-4"

12"

1"x6"

2'x3"

2"x3"

Stop

Door

1"x6"

¼" Plywood

SECTION

B.R. Nº1 ELEVATION

BEDROOM CLOSETS *Finish bedroom wall & ceilings as for one room. Then erect framing, cover & apply trim (See plan)*

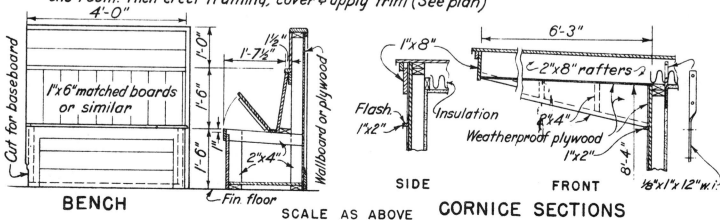

4'-0"

1'-0"

1'-6"

1'-6"

1½"

1'-7½"

1"

Cut for baseboard

1"x6"matched boards or similar

2"x4"

Fin. floor

Wallboard or plywood

BENCH

6'-3"

1"x8"

2"x8" rafters

Flash.

1"x2"

Insulation

2"x4"

Weatherproof plywood

1"x2"

8'-4"

⅛"x1"x12" w.i.

SIDE

FRONT

SCALE AS ABOVE

CORNICE SECTIONS